W0105768

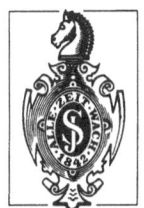

Exocrine Pancreatic Cancer

Edited by
H. Baumel and B. Deixonne

Foreword by H. Sarles

With 78 Figures, some in Color, and 36 Tables

Springer-Verlag Berlin Heidelberg New York
London Paris Tokyo

Professor Dr. Hughes Baumel
Dr. Bernard Deixonne

Centre hospitalier régional et universitaire de Nîmes
Chirurgie Digestive
Hôpital Caremeau, Rue du Prof. Robert-Debré
F-30006 Nîmes, France

The cover photographs showing microadenocarcinoma (*upper left:* see Fig. 2.10, p. 22), invasion of the major vessels by cancer (*upper right:* see Fig. 5.20, p. 81), and cancer of the pancreatic body: ultrasound *(bottom left)* and roentgenography *(bottom right).* See Fig. 5.3 a, b on p. 69.

ISBN-13: 978-3-642-71180-0   e-ISBN-13: 978-3-642-71178-7
DOI: 10.1007/978-3-642-71178-7

Library of Congress Cataloging in Publication Data.
Exocrine pancreatic cancer.
Includes bibliographies and index.
1. Pancreas - Cancer. I. Baumel, H. (Hughes) II. Deixonne, B. (Bernard)
[DNLM: 1. Pancreatic Neoplasms. WI 810 E956]
RC280.P25E95   1986   616.99'437   86-13831
ISBN 0-387-16530-4 (U.S.)

This work is subject to copyright. All rights are reserved, whether the whole or part of the material is concerned, specifically those of translation, reprinting, re-use of illustrations, broadcasting, reproduction by photocopying machine or similar means, and storage in data banks. Under § 54 of the German Copyright Law where copies are made for other than private use, a fee is payable to "Verwertungs-gesellschaft Wort", Munich.

© Springer-Verlag Berlin Heidelberg 1986.
Softcover reprint of the hardcover 1st edition 1986

The use of registered names, trademarks, etc. in this publication does not imply, even in the absence of a specific statement, that such names are exempt from the relevant protective laws and regulations and therefore free for general use.
Product Liability: The publisher can give no guarantee for information about drug dosage and application thereof contained in this book. In every individual case the respective user must check its accuracy by consulting other pharmaceutical literature.

2127/3145-543210

Foreword

For a long time, approximately since Oberlin and Guerin described the multifocal origin of pancreatic cancers and precancerous pancreatic lesions, no important study dealing with the entire subject of pancreatic cancer has been published in France and probably in the international literature. For some decades the knowledge acquired 40 years or more ago was not improved appreciably, though the frequency of the disease started to increase in occidental countries.

This has recently changed, and the progress of the medical sciences has spread to the pancreas. Although the surgical or medical prognosis of the most frequent form of pancreatic cancer, exocrine adenocarcinoma, remains very bad, recent studies have shown the multiplicity of its pathological forms, some being less severe so that curative surgery is possible. New experimental models, particularly in the hamster, and the use of carcinogenic drugs allow experimental studies on lesions similar to those in man. Oncologic immunology is still at its beginnings but shows promise for diagnosis and treatment. Though modern techniques of imaging – sonography, aspirative cytology, CT scan, endoscopic catheterism, arteriography, and maybe in the future nuclear magnetic resonance – have not yet significantly influenced prognosis, they have made the diagnosis easier and more precocious.

Yet in a disease that diffuses so rapidly to deep lymph nodes, it has not been proved whether early diagnosis can improve prognosis. Greater hope might result from the progress of epidemiology, which allows a better knowledge of the causative factors and will probably in the future help eradicate some risk factors, and from that in chemotherapy when some active new drugs will be discovered. Yet if epidemiology shows progress, chemotherapy and immunotherapy are just beginning and possibly still inefficient.

This book presents a good review on all the problems related to pancreatic cancer, both theoretical and practical. Based on a careful and extensive study of the literature, it is a document necessary to everyone, whether clinician, pathologist, or researcher, who intends to acquire a precise knowledge of pancreatic cancer. Besides a careful review of theoretical problems, the authors have produced a remarkable study of the practical problems that general practitioners, gastroenterologists, and surgeons have to face daily, and have proposed a simple and sensible strategy for diagnosis and treatment. This book, in the best clinical tradition, shows that the authors, besides having great knowledge of the disease, also have a very large amount of experience in treating patients; they are thus able to give a clear view of the difficult problems raised by the pancreatic cancer.

Marseille, June 1986

HENRI SARLES
Professor of Gastro-enterology

Preface

Known since antiquity, the pancreas was named by Rufus of Ephesus, who thought it to be an organ "totally of flesh", containing neither bones nor cartilage.

For a long time its anatomy was completely unknown. Vesalius, in the fifth volume of his work on human anatomy, did not recognize its excretory duct. It was not until 1642 that Wirsung, an anatomist in Padua, described the pancreatic duct; 100 years later Santorini described the minor pancreatic duct.

As far as the pathology is concerned, it was not much better. It seems quite surprising that the pancreatic origin of the most well-known metabolic disease, diabetes mellitus, was ignored for centuries; this was revealed only in 1881. As for pancreatic cancer, even though it was called a "very hard tumor" by Galen, it was not until the nineteenth century that Morgagni described five cases of carcinoma of the pancreas as a pathological entity.

Only at the end of the nineteenth century were the first attempts made in the treatment of pancreatic cancer. In 1882, Trendelenburg performed the first successful resection of a solid tumor of the body and tail of the pancreas. In 1887, Kappeler performed the first palliative bypass (cholecystojejunostomy) for a cancer of the head of the pancreas, with a survival time of 14.5 months. Merit is also due to Codovilla, who in 1898 successfully realized resections of the duodenal surroundings as well as a part of the head of the pancreas in a patient harboring a cancer, who died, however, 24 days later.

At the beginning of the twentieth century, several observations concerning bypass and resection were reported, but they remain isolated because of high mortality rates. In 1935, Whipple was the first to codify cephalic duodenopancreatectomy in two steps, and in 1940, with Nelson's help, he performed the same surgical intervention in one step, and this procedure has been named after him.

Up until the 1940s there were only a few surgeons who dared to perform such a resection. Advances in the general surgical environment facilitated the increase of resections and at the same time decreased surgical mortality. However, on a carcinological level, these resections were not completely satisfactory. Their disastrous results led a large number of surgeons in the 1960s to question the validity of resections relative to bypasses, since the survival rates were the same.

In 1958, Porter, considering the evolution of ideas in the field of pancreatic surgery, delineated three periods:

1. The *Pioneer Period* was initiated by Whipple at the Columbia Presbyterian Medical Center of New York in 1935 and lasted until 1947.

2. The *Radical Period*, from 1948 through 1952, saw more and more extensive resections and total pancreatectomies performed, with an increase in the number of cured cases.

3. The *Rational Period,* from 1953 through 1957, initiated the process of selection for the best resectable cases.

On a diagnostic level, development was not much faster. It is doubtless the anatomical localization of this organ, remote and silent, which caused these delays. It also explains the prolonged latency of carcinoma of the pancreas and is the main reason for its late diagnosis, and partly for its very special severity as well – it is the most serious of all carcinomas that have been studied to date. Actually, all evolutionary stages combined, the 5-year survival rate does not exceed 1%–2%, depending upon the series and the mean life prolongation remains inferior to 6 months. Moreover, the frequency of pancreatic cancer is increasing in western countries. What are the reasons for such a poor prognosis? Can we, taking into account our present means of diagnosis and therapy, find cause to feel optimistic about the future, to expect an improvement in the results?

If we consider the past 20 years (1965–1985) with developments in the techniques of both diagnosis and therapy, we see that we are capable of great progress. Indeed, during this period we have witnessed a real explosion in the number of tools at our disposal, in particular the techniques of imaging, gastrointestinal endoscopy, and cytology diagnosis. This allows Longmire to add to Portner's three periods a fourth – the *Diagnostic Period.* These advances permit an increase in the number of positive diagnoses and a reduction of the duration between the onset of symptoms and therapy, but they rarely allow early diagnosis. Our performance at a diagnostic level has not greatly improved; carcinomas revealed by the classical symptoms are usually in a later stage of development, whereas the discovery of small tumors occurs rarely and quite by chance.

Therefore, the results of therapy do not improve: even with more therapeutic possibilities, we cannot remarkably influence the evolution of bad cases, except to slightly increase the median survival. Our long-range plan, then, must be to improve therapy, and above all to diagnose cases for earlier treatment.

Earlier diagnosis must be based on more precise epidemiological knowledge, allowing a better recognition of high-risk groups. Physicians must learn to recognize the signs of lesser pancreatic lesions, and this implies the implementation of surveys among the general population and those at high risk. Providing that we arrive at a definitive diagnosis, we must then search for the best therapy. This must be based on a very methodical appraisal of the lesion, including a complete locoregional and general examination. This appraisal leads to the establishment of therapeutic indications, dependent upon the patient's general condition and the degree of tumor development. Thus, we must think in terms of therapy, with either a curative aim (surgical exeresis) or just a palliative one (surgery or other treatment); unfortunately, the latter is more common than the former.

Indeed, at present only about 25% of pancreatic carcinomas are resectable, and very few patients survive 5 years without recurrence. We have a long way to go!

We cannot hope for a striking change in therapy in the coming decade. We must therefore concentrate on furnishing a better diagnosis in order to give the therapist more curable patients.

These are very difficult objectives, perhaps even too hopeful, but we hope that this book will assist us in reaching them.

Nîmes, June 1986   H. BAUMEL

Table of Contents

Coauthors

FRANÇOISE D'ATHIS, M.D.
Professor of Anesthesiology, University of Montpellier,
Department of Anesthesiology, Hôpital G. Doumergue,
30000 Nîmes, France

HUGHES BAUMEL, M.D.
Professor of Surgery, University of Montpellier,
Department of Digestive Surgery, Hôpital Caremeau,
30000 Nîmes, France

JEAN MICHEL BRUEL, M.D.
Professor of Radiology, University of Montpellier,
Department of Medical Imaging, Hôpital Saint-Eloi,
34000 Montpellier, France

BERNARD DEIXONNE, M.D.
Department of Digestive Surgery, Hôpital Caremeau,
30000 Nîmes, France

ALAIN DUBOIS, M.D.
Department of Internal Medicine, Hôpital Caremeau,
30000 Nîmes, France

JEAN JACQUES ELEDJAM, M.D.
Department of Anesthesiology, Hôpital Caremeau,
30000 Nîmes, France

FRANÇOIS MICHEL LOPEZ, M.D.
Professor of Radiology, University of Montpellier,
Department of Medical Imaging, Hôpital Caremeau,
30000 Nîmes, France

PAUL LOPEZ, M.D.
Department of Radiology, Hôpital Lapeyronie,
34000 Montpellier, France

CHRISTIANE MARTY-DOUBLE, M. D.
Professor of Pathology, University of Montpellier,
Department of Pathology and Cytology, Hôpital G. Doumergue,
30000 Nîmes, France

THIERRY NARBONI, M. D.
Department of Medical Imaging, Hôpital G. Doumergue,
30000 Nîmes, France

CHRISTINE PIGNODEL, M. D.
Department of Pathology and Cytology, Hôpital Caremeau,
30000 Nîmes, France

CLAUDE RAFFANEL, M. D.
Department of Gastroenterology, Hôpital Caremeau,
30000 Nîmes, France

1 Epidemiology

A. Dubois

To day, the etiology of pancreatic cancer is still unknown. It is increasing in frequency in many parts of the world and its mortality is high. The advances in therapy do not greatly help the prognosis. The new methods of exploration (ultrasound, retrocholangiopancreatography, computer tomography) have not improved its detection at an earlier stage of the disease [47]. These points reinforce the interest in undertaking more profound epidemiological studies in order to define the high-risk population. The epidemiological studies concerning age, sex, geographical, and racial variations facilitate the characterization of the disease (descriptive epidemiology). However, they do not help to define the etiological factors (causal epidemiology). The epidemiological inquiries mainly concern adenocarcinoma of the exocrine pancreas, which is the most frequent histological type. However, due to the lack of surgical samples, histological confirmation is sometimes not possible.

1.1 Frequency

The frequency of pancreatic cancer is increasing worldwide [3, 4, 7]. Its death rate is nearly the same as its incidence (number of cases diagnosed per year) since the survival rate is low [13, 42].

In the United States 24000 new cases were diagnosed in 1981 [51]. The death rate, which was once 3/100000 inhabitants, reached up to 10/100000 in 1977 [45]. In the United States it is the fourth most common cause of cancer death for men and the fifth most common for women [51]. It is the second most common digestive malignancy, and ranks fourth overall, after carcinomas of the lung, colon, and breast [45]. The highest incidence appears in the industrialized countries [56] (Table 1.1).

In France, the risk has increased from one generation to another proportionally with an increase of the death rate by 48% for men and 27% for women between 1955 and 1969. In 1975, carcinoma of the pancreas represented the fourth cause of digestive cancer death after cancers of the colon (+rectum), stomach, and esophagus [3].

In 1975 alone, 4265 patients died of pancreatic cancer, representing 3% of all cancer deaths [4]. In 1960, the death rate was only 9.85 per 100000 men and only 7.65 per 100000 for women. Between 1970 and 1980, it increased by 98% for men and 61% for women. The north and east of France are the regions most at risk [12].

1.2 Descriptive Epidemiology

1.2.1 Incidence by Age and Sex

The curve of incidence as a function of age (Fig. 1.1) shows that risk increases with age, and that its incidence is highest after 55 years [17]. The death rate for pancreatic cancer increases in a linear fashion with age up to 60 years [3]. Among the black population of the United States the rate with respect to age-group is highest at 70 years and then decreases, whereas it continues to increase for every successive age-group in the white population [33]. The sex ratio (male/female) is 2/1 before the age of 50 and then subsequently decreases, but without ever reaching unity [58]. The sex ratio varies according to the region studied [34, 56] (Table 1.1), ranging from 2.9/1 for cancers of the body and tail of the pancreas to 1.8/1 for cancers of the head of the pancreas [45], and also according to race with extremes ranging from 0.75 for American Indians to 6.83 for Filipinos [34]. A study of the standard mortality undertaken in 34 countries between 1950 and 1978 proved the rate to be higher for men than for women [2].

1.2.2 Geographical, Racial, and Social Variations

Aoki and Ogawa [2] divided the 34 countries into three variable-risk groups: a high-risk group including the United States, England, the Scandinavian countries, and Israel; a low-risk group including Southern Europe and South-East Asia. France appears to pertain to a middle group [3]. The precise evaluation of the risk is difficult. It should be done according to regional cancer registrations which are more precise than simple death certificates. Such registers would be helpful to underline the important variations in risk from one region to another within the same country. Hence, the register of digestive cancers initiated in the Côte d'Or region of France on January 1, 1976 allows a census of all the new cases of pancreatic cancer and places this region of France in the high-risk group, as well as showing significant discrepancies between two distinct areas of the same region [17]. For many years, the risk seemed to be higher in urban areas than in rural ones. If this difference is still meaningful in Europe [17, 34], it is no longer the case in the United States [34, 40]. The incidence of pancreatic cancer is higher among the black population of the United States than among Caucasians [34]; the rates are 43% higher for black men and 48% higher for black women [59]. The reason for such a high incidence among Blacks is still unknown. The pancreatic cancer death rate is lower for male American Indians (69% of the rate for Caucasians) but higher for American Indian women (103% of the rate for Caucasians). However, this rate is still lower than that for black women [41].

Other high-risk populations are the Hawaiians and the Maoris of New Zealand [6]. These ethnic groups present a larger risk than that of the Caucasians living on

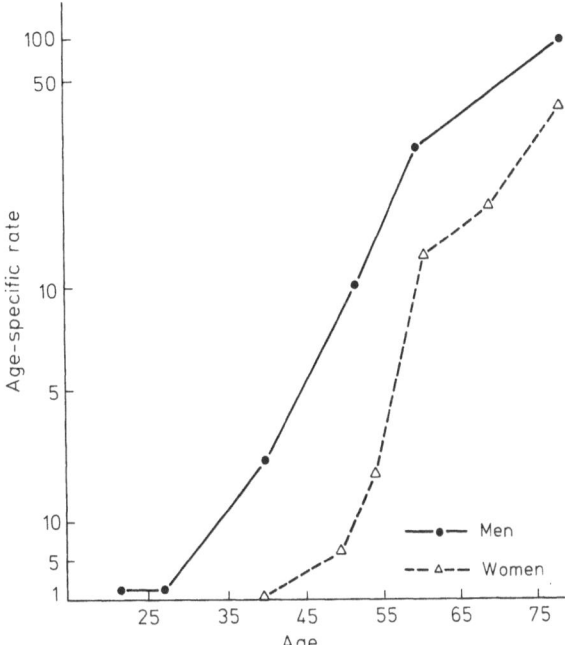

Fig.1.1. Incidence of pancreatic cancer according to age and sex (decimal logarithm of age-specific rate at 10-year intervals; from Faivre [17])

Table 1.1. Incidence of pancreatic cancer in certain parts of the world (standard rate per 100000 persons between 1968 and 1972; from Waterhouse, in Faivre [17])

Countries	Regions	Men	Women	Sex ratio
New Zealand	Maori	13.0	4.5	2.9
Switzerland	District of Geneva	11.4	5.4	2.1
Rhodesia	Bulawayo	10.9	3.6	3
Finland	–	9.8	3.6	2.7
France	Côte d'Or	8.7	3.1	2.8
United States	Connecticut	8.6	5.8	1.5
Great Britain	Oxford	7.8	5.0	1.6
Federal Republic of Germany	Hamburg	7.8	4.2	1.9
Japan	Myagi	7.3	4.5	1.6
Poland	Cracow	5.4	3.4	1.6
Colombia	Cali	3.7	3.4	1.1
Spain	Saragossa	3.2	1.5	2.1
India	Bombay	1.8	1.0	1.8

these two islands. The hypothesis proposing a genetic factor is intriguing because these races are also at high risk for diabetes [19].

A large number of studies seem to show that the incidence of pancreatic cancer is higher among the lower classes [15, 50]. Actually, it is very difficult to interpret these results, as a high consumption of alcohol and tobacco is frequently correlated to poverty [6].

1.3 Causal Epidemiology

1.3.1 Chronic Pancreatitis

Studying 70 cases of chronic pancreatitis (with or without lithiasis), Schultz and Finkler [48] did not find any cancer. The same authors, in a study based on 181 cases of pancreatic cancer, did not find any calcification in the 123 patients studied; only six patients had a past history of acute or chronic pancreatitis. Paulino-Netto et al. [44] find an analogy between the pancreatic calcification-pancreatic cancer association and the cholelithiasis-gallstone cancer association.

Johnson and Zintel [26] did not find any pancreatic calcification in 113 cases of pancreatic cancer. In the same report, the authors reviewed the medical literature of Great Britain from 1925 to 1962 and found 24 cases of pancreatic cancer among 653 cases of pancreatic calcification (3.7%), which is much higher than the usual findings in adult patients. More recently, Brooks [9] assessed the evidence of a positive relation between calcifying chronic pancreatitis and pancreatic cancer. These findings are also confirmed by Amman et al. [1]. A high incidence of carcinoma of the pancreas in patients with hereditary pancreatitis (calcifying pancreatitis) is an additional argument [4, 36]. In some families, some persons are affected by chronic pancreatitis and others by cancer of the pancreas [29]. Finally, even if the literature does not always provide congruent data, it seems that the presence of gallstones in the pancreatic ducts is a predisposing factor in the onset of cancer of the pancreas.

The role played by noncalcifying chronic pancreatitis in the development of pancreatic cancer is still dubious. It is frequently (10%–50% of cases) complicated by an upper pancreatitis secondary to the neoplastic obstruction [4]. To date, no causal relationship has been determined between chronic pancreatitis and pancreatic cancer. The coexistence of the two may possibly be chance.

1.3.2 Diabetes Mellitus

Many studies have shown that pancreatic cancer occurs more frequently in diabetic patients. It represents 5%–20% of all cancer occurring in diabetics, as against 4% in the nondiabetic population [28]. Since pancreatic cancer happens to give rise to diabetes during the course of the disease, an overestimation of the frequency of this carcinoma in diabetic patients is to be feared. Therefore, we will consider only cases where the onset of diabetes preceded that of cancer by 1 year. Studies show that the risk of pancreatic cancer in such cases was 2–6 times higher in the female diabetic patient [30]. There does not appear to be a positive correlation for men in the United States [8, 58]. Pancreatic cancer and diabetes occur frequently in two ethnic groups of Polynesian origin: the Maoris and the Hawaiians [6, 19].

At present, it is impossible to say whether all diabetic patients run the same risk of cancer or if this risk affects only a subpopulation [6]. Nevertheless, it seems clear that of all deaths among the diabetic population, only a few of them are due to cancer of the pancreas.

1.3.3 Dietary Habits

1.3.3.1 Diet

The role played by diet in the occurrence of pancreatic cancer has been suggested by studies of migrant populations. The increasing frequency of pancreatic cancer among Japanese people living in the United States as compared with those living in Japan could thus be partially explained by a change in their dietary habits [4].

In Japan, the risk of pancreatic cancer is positively related to the consumption of meat and negatively to the consumption of vegetables [23]. Segi et al. [49], on the basis of an international workshop, point out a clear positive correlation between the rate of pancreatic cancer rate and the consumption of fat. The role of the conversion of cholesterol to cholesterol epoxide was raised [58]. In another study [21], the incidence of carcinoma of the pancreas is positively correlated to the consumption of dietary fat, oil, sugar, and protein. Two recent studies in France lead to the same conclusions [5, 16].

Finally, the incidence of pancreatic cancer tends to increase in countries whose populations consume a "western" diet, rich in fat. This also explains the frequency of its relation to cancer of the colon, which is also greatly influenced by diet.

1.3.3.2 Coffee

The role of coffee in pancreatic cancer was suggested for the first time in 1970 by Stocks [52]. He found a positive correlation between the consumption of coffee and pancreatic cancer mortality in 19 countries between 1964 and 1965. This correlation was highly significant for men, but not for women. In a study carried out in Boston between 1974 and 1979, MacMahon et al. [38], assessed a strong association between the consumption of coffee and the pancreatic cancer rate for both sexes. According to these authors, one to two cups of coffee a day would double the risk of pancreatic cancer, and three or more would triple the risk. This study was subject to some strong criticisms with respect to the control group [37] and the methodology [18]. Since then, only one study has found a positive correlation between the two [43], whereas three others revealed no correlation [20, 25, 31]. Lin and Kessler [35] found no association either, but they suggested an association between the consumption of decaffeinated coffee and pancreatic cancer in women. A country-by-country analysis has produced no correlation between daily coffee consumption and pancreatic cancer in men [7] (Fig. 1.2).

1.3.3.3 Alcohol

The involvement of alcohol in the occurrence of pancreatic cancer is controversial. In a retrospective study of 83 pancreatic cancers, Burch and Ansari [11] noted chronic alcoholism in 75% of the cases. Recently, Lin and Kessler reported a correlation between wine consumption and pancreatic cancer [35]; unfortunately, the value of this study is limited by several methodological errors [39].

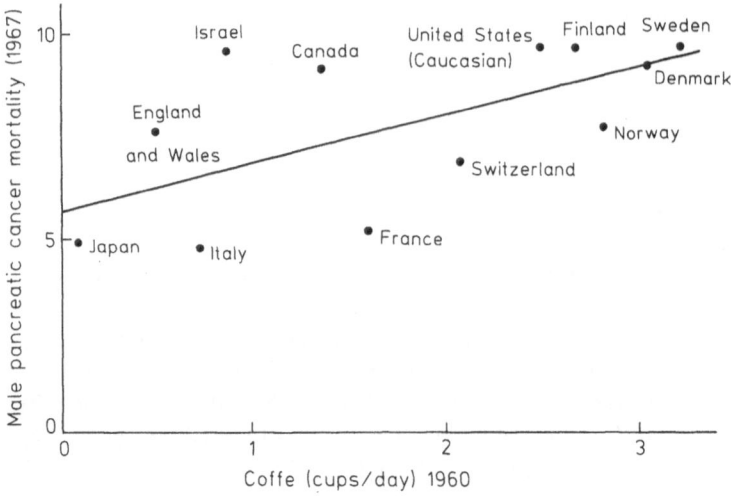

Fig. 1.2. Scattergram of male pancreatic cancer mortality 1966–1967 as against per capita coffee consumption in 1960 for 12 countries (*P*<0.05; from Benarde and Weiss [7])

According to some [8, 46, 55], this relationship is not meaningful. In France during the Second World War, the decrease in alcohol consumption did not influence the rate of pancreatic cancer, which continuously increased, unlike carcinomas of the esophagus and the larynx [54].

In a Norwegian prospective study, Heuch et al. found a strong relationship between alcohol consumption and pancreatic cancer, the relative risk being 5.4 times higher in drinkers than in nondrinkers [24].

In a recent French study, Durbec et al. [16], also showed that alcohol was a major factor in the etiology of pancreatic cancer. In a multifactorial analysis that included tobacco and alcohol, the latter seems to be the predominant factor. The incidence of pancreatic cancer seems to be higher in beer drinkers than in wine drinkers. (This difference might be explained by the larger quantity of nitrosamine in beer). Nevertheless, the exact role played by alcohol or by the various elements of alcoholic drinks is not precisely known.

1.3.3.4 Tobacco

Cigarette smoking seems to be a well-established factor in the exogenous risk of pancreatic cancer [6, 14, 22, 27, 39]. The risk of carcinoma of the pancreas is doubled by a daily consumption of 25 g of tobacco or of 40 cigarettes [Table 1.2]. This risk increases with the number of cigarettes smoked per day, but such a relationship has not been proven for pipe or cigar smokers [27, 38].

In comparison with the onset of cancers more closely linked to cigarette smoking, such as lung or bladder cancer [14, 22, 27] and hepatoma [HBs negative] [53], this association is not as strong. It is even less than the one recently assessed between cigarette smoking and chronic pancreatitis [39]. In order to explain the car-

Table 1.2. Relative risk of pancreatic cancer according to current level of cigarette consumption in three follow-up studies (from Mac Mahon [39])

Study	Nonsmokers	Cigarette smokers				
		Light	Moderate		Heavy	
Kahn [27]	1.0	1.1	1.4	1.8	2.2	2.7
Doll and Peto [14]	1.0	1.0	1.3		1.9	
Hammond [22]						
Men	1.0		2.4			
Women	1.0		1.8			

Table 1.3. Multifactorial etiological model for pancreatic cancer in man (from Lin and Kessler [35])

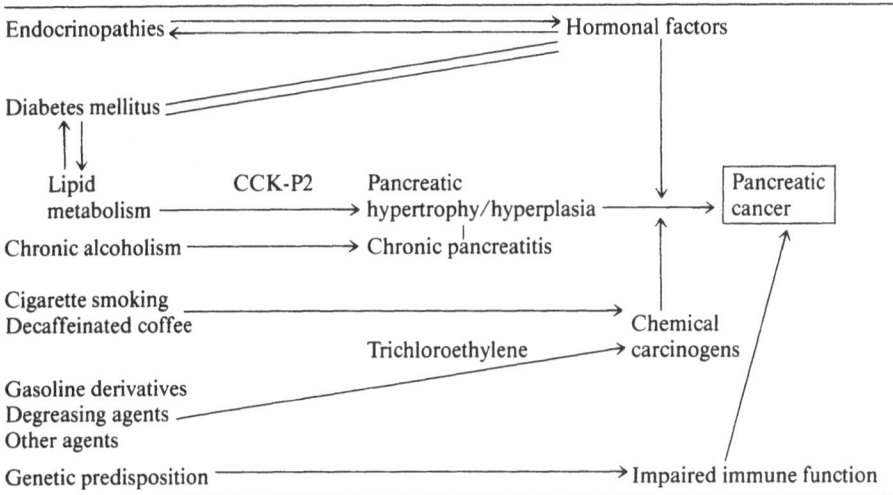

cinogenic role of tobacco in the pancreatic cancer process, Wynder [58] suggested that the carcinogenic elements (mainly nitrosamines) reached the pancreas via the blood vessels or the bile ducts by reflux towards the common bile duct or the duct of Wirsung.

1.3.4 Chemical and/or Industrial Agents

There is no proven relationship between the pancreatic cancer rate and the atmospheric pollution index [32] or diverse industries [8]. As of 1973, Wynder et al. [57] reported an abnormally high frequency of pancreatic cancer in workers and chemists exposed to naphthylamine and benzidine (benzidine alone does not seem to be a carcinogenic factor for the pancreas). A large number of professions have been involved in the onset of pancreatic cancer [6], but none of them has been formally implicated [10].

Hence, epidemiological studies point to a multifactorial etiology of pancreatic cancer [35] (Table 1.3). Some factors may be positively related to this cancer: male sex, cigarettes, dietary fat, diabetes in women. Other factors are not well delineated: alcohol, chronic pancreatitis, obesity, diabetes in men. For early detection, the high-risk population must be defined, as this is the only guarantee of an effective therapy.

References

1. Amman RW, Akovbiantz A, Largiader F, Schueler G (1984) Course and outcome of chronic pancreatitis. Longitudinal study of a mixed medical surgical series of 245 patients. Gastroenterology 86: 820–828
2. Aoki K, Ogawa H (1978) Cancer of the pancreas international mortality trends. World Health Stat Q 31: 2–27
3. Audigier JC, Euvrard P, Tuyns AJ, Lambert R (1976) Mortalité par cancer du pancréas en France. Arch Fr Mal App Dig 65: 107–114
4. Audigier JC, Lambert R (1979) Epidémiologie des cancers du pancréas. Ann Gastroenterol Hepatol 15: 159–162
5. Benhamou S, Clavel F, Revzani P, Doyon F (1982) Etude de la relation entre la mortalité par cancer du pancréas et certaines consommations alimentaires et de tabac en France. Biomedicine 36: 389–392
6. Berg JW, Connelly RR (1979) Updating the epidemiologic data on pancreatic cancer. Semin Oncol 6: 275–283
7. Benarde AM, Weiss W (1977) A cohort analysis of pancreatic cancer. Cancer 39: 1260–1263
8. Blot WJ, Fraumini JF, Stone BJ (1978) Geographic correlations of pancreas cancer in the United States. Cancer 42: 373–380
9. Brooks JR (1983) Surgery of the pancreas. Saunders, Philadelphia, pp 263–298
10. Buncher CR (1980) Epidemiology of pancreatic cancer. In: Moossa AA (ed) Tumors of the pancreas. Wilkins and Wilkins, Baltimore
11. Burch EG, Ansari A (1968) Chronic alcoholism and carcinoma of the pancreas. A correlative hypothesis. Arch Intern Med 122: 273–275
12. Czernichow P, Lerebours E, Azambourg JC, Hecketsweiler P, Colin R (1985) Mortalité par cancer du pancréas: épidémiologie temporo-spatiale française et internationale. Gastroentérol Clin Biol 9: 207 A
13. Cutler SJ, Myers MH, Green SB (1975) Trends in survival rates of patients with cancer. N Engl J Med 293: 122–124
14. Doll R, Peto R (1976) Mortality in relation to smoking: 20 years' observations on male British doctors. Br Med J 2: 1525–1536
15. Dorn HF, Culter SJ (1959) Morbidity from cancer in the United States. Public Health Service, Washington
16. Durbec JP, Chevillotte G, Bidart JM, Berthezene P, Sarles H (1983) Diet, alcohol, tobacco and risk of cancer of the pancreas. A case control study. Br J Cancer 47: 463–470
17. Faivre J, Gouget N, Michiels R, Dusserre P, Bastien H, Klepping C (1980) Incidence du cancer du pancréas dans le département de la Côte d'Or (1976–1978). Ann Gastroenterol Hepatol 16: 5–8
18. Feinstein AR, Horwitz RI, Spitzer WO, Battistas RN (1981) Coffee and pancreatic cancer: the problems of etiologic science and epidemiologic case control research. JAMA 246: 957–961
19. Fraumini JF (1975) Cancers of the pancreas and biliary tract: epidemiologic considerations. Cancer Res 35: 3437–3446
20. Goldstein HR (1982) No association found between coffee and cancer of the pancreas. N Engl J Med 306: 997
21. Gordis L (1980) Epidemiology of pancreatic cancer. In: Lilienfeld AM (ed) Reviews of cancer epidemiology, vol 1. Elsevier, New York, pp 84–117
22. Hammond ED (1966) Smoking in relation to the death rates of one million men and women. Natl Cancer Inst Monogr 19: 127–204

23. Hastings PR, Beazley RM, Cohn I (1982) Progress with pancreatic cancer. Prog Clin Cancer 8: 319-332
24. Heuch I, Kvale G, Jacobsen BK, Bjelke E (1983) Use of alcohol, tobacco and coffee and risk of pancreatic cancer. Br J Cancer 48: 637-643
25. Jick H, Dinan BJ (1981) Coffee and pancreatic cancer. Lancet 2: 92
26. Johnson JR, Zintel H (1963) Pancreatic calcification and cancer of the pancreas. Surg Gynecol Obstet 117: 585-588
27. Kahn HA (1966) The Dorn study of smoking and mortality among US veterans: report on eight and one-half years of observation. Natl Cancer Inst Monogr 19: 1-125
28. Karmody AJ, Kyle J (1969) The association between carcinoma of the pancreas and diabetes mellitus. Br J Surg 56: 362-364
29. Kattwinkel J, Lapey A, Di Sant'Agnese PA, Edwards WA (1973) Hereditary pancreatitis: three new kindreds and a critical review of the literature. Pediatrics 51: 55-69
30. Kessler II (1970) Cancer mortality among diabetics. J Natl Cancer Inst 44: 673-686
31. Kessler II (1981) Coffee and cancer of the pancreas. N Engl J Med 304: 1605
32. Krain L (1972) Cancer incidence. The crossing of the curves for stomach and pancreatic cancer. Digestion 6: 356-366
33. Levin DL, Connelly RR (1973) Cancer of the pancreas. Available epidemiologic information and its implications. Cancer 31: 1231-1236
34. Levin DL, Connelly RR, Devesa SS (1981) Demographic characteristics of cancer of the pancreas: mortality, incidence and survival. Cancer 47: 1456-1465
35. Lin RS, Kessler II (1981) A multifactorial model for pancreatic cancer in man - epidemiological evidence. JAMA 245: 147-152
36. Logan AJ, Schicke CP, Manning GB (1968) Familial pancreatitis. Am J Med 115: 112-117
37. Löwenfels AB (1982) Coffee and cancer of the pancreas. JAMA 247: 979-980
38. MacMahon B, Yen S, Trichopoulos D, Warren K, Nardi G (1981) Coffee and cancer of the pancreas. N Engl J Med 304: 630-633
39. MacMahon B (1982) Risk factors for cancer of th the pancreas. Cancer 50: 2676-2860
40. Maruchi N, Brian D, Ludwig J, Elveback CR, Kurland LT (1979) Cancer of the pancreas in Olmsted County, Minnesota 1935-1974. Mayo Clin Proc 54: 245-249
41. Mason TJ, McKay FW, Hoover R et al. (1976) Atlas of cancer mortality among US non whites: 1950-1969. US Department for Health, Education and Welfare, Washington
42. Moosa AR, Lewis MH, Macie CR (1979) Surgical treatment of pancreatic cancer. Mayo Clin Proc 54: 464-474
43. Nomura A, Stemmerman GM, Heilbrun LK (1981) Coffee and pancreatic cancer. Lancet 2: 415
44. Paulino-Netto A, Dreiling DA, Baranofsky ID (1960) The relation-ship between pancreatic calcification and cancer of the pancreas. Ann Surg 151: 530-537
45. Russel RI (1980) Clinical and diagnostic aspects of pancreatic cancer. Schweiz Med Wochenschr 110: 827-831
46. Sarles H (1973) An international survey on nutrition and pancreatitis. Digestion 9: 389-403
47. Savarino V, Mansi C, Bistolfi L, Zentilin P, Celle G (1983) Failure of new diagnostic aids in improving detection of pancreatic cancer at a resectable stage. Dig Dis Sci 28: 1078-1082
48. Schultz RE, Finkler NJ (1980) Pancreatic calficiation and pancreatic carcinoma: the relationship reconsidered. Mt Sinai J Med (NY) 47: 622-626
49. Segi M, Kurimara M, Matsuyama T (1969) Cancer mortality for selected sites in 24 countries (1964-1965). Department of Public Health, Tokohu University School of Medicine, Sendai
50. Seidman H (1970) Cancer death rates by site and sex for religious and socio-economic groups in New York City. Environ Res 3: 234-250
51. Silverberg E (1981) Cancer statistics. CA 31: 13-28
52. Stocks P (1970) Cancer mortality in relation to national consumption of cigarettes, solid fuel, tea and coffee. Br J Cancer 24: 215-225
53. Trichopoulos D, MacMahon B, Sparros L, Merikas G (1980) Smoking and hepatitis B negative primary hepato cellular carcinoma. J Natl Cancer Inst 65: 111-114
54. Tuyns AJ, Audigier JC (1976) Double wave cohort increase for oesophageal and laryngeal cancer in France in relation to reduced alcohol consumption during the second world war. Digestion 14: 197-208
55. Tuyns AJ, Pequignot G, Gignoux M, Valla A (1982) Cancers of the digestive tract alcohol and tobacco. Int J Cancer 30: 9-11

56. Waterhouse J, Muir C, Correa P, Powell J (1976) Cancer incidence in five continents, vol 3. IARC, Lyon (IARC scientific publication no 15)
57. Wynder EL, Mabuchi K, Maruchi N, Fortner JG (1973) Epidemiology of cancer of the pancreas. J Natl Cancer Inst 50: 645–667
58. Wynder EL (1975) An epidemiologic evaluation of the causes of cancer of the pancreas. Cancer Res 35: 2228–2233
59. Young JL, Asire AJ, Pollack ES (1978) SEER program cancer incidence and mortality in the United States 1973–76. Bethesda, Maryland, Department of Health, Education and Welfare

2 Pathological Anatomy

B. Deixonne, C. Marty-Double, and C. Pignodel

2.1 Macroscopic Study

This chapter is focused on the study of the gross morphology of cancer of the pancreas and on the distribution of its intraglandular localizations. A good knowledge of these localizations is very important, as they directly affect the therapeutic management.

2.1.1 Macroscopic Morphology

Carcinoma of the pancreas frequently presents a large volume (several centimeters in diameter; Fig. 2.1 a, b), particularly in the cephalic localization. It has a roughly spherical or ovoid shape, and on section it looks like an area of induration, ill bounded, with star-shaped or geographical grayish-white margins (Fig. 2.2). The fluid from curettage is turbid. Its special sclerous density has sometimes caused it to be called *pancreatic scirrhus,* and some calcifications may appear as well. The tumor tissue rarely appears homogeneous on gross examination: the brownish-red hemorrhagic foci and the yellowish necrotic plaques, even if excavated, have a rather polychrome appearance. In pancreatitis associated with cancer there are certain peculiar very scirrhous types in which the sclerosis dries up the organ, giving no fluid from curettage on dry slides.

In a few cases, carcinoma of the pancreas presents, from a macroscopic point of view, an *encephaloid* shape: a grayish, flabby, and friable mass which disintegrates under the knife at dissection. The encephaloid shape represents a particularly dense tumor necrosis, often hemorrhagic.

The *extratumoral pancreas* is sometimes normal. Most of the time, however, it is modified, particularly in the cephalic types, by lesions of the upper pancreas called *epineoplastic pancreatitis.* This condition will be described in more detail in a following paragraph.

Scirrhus and encephaloid tumors are the typical macroscopic features of carcinoma of the pancreas. Other aspects, more rarely seen, are also possible; they are related to special pathological-histological forms and will be discussed later.

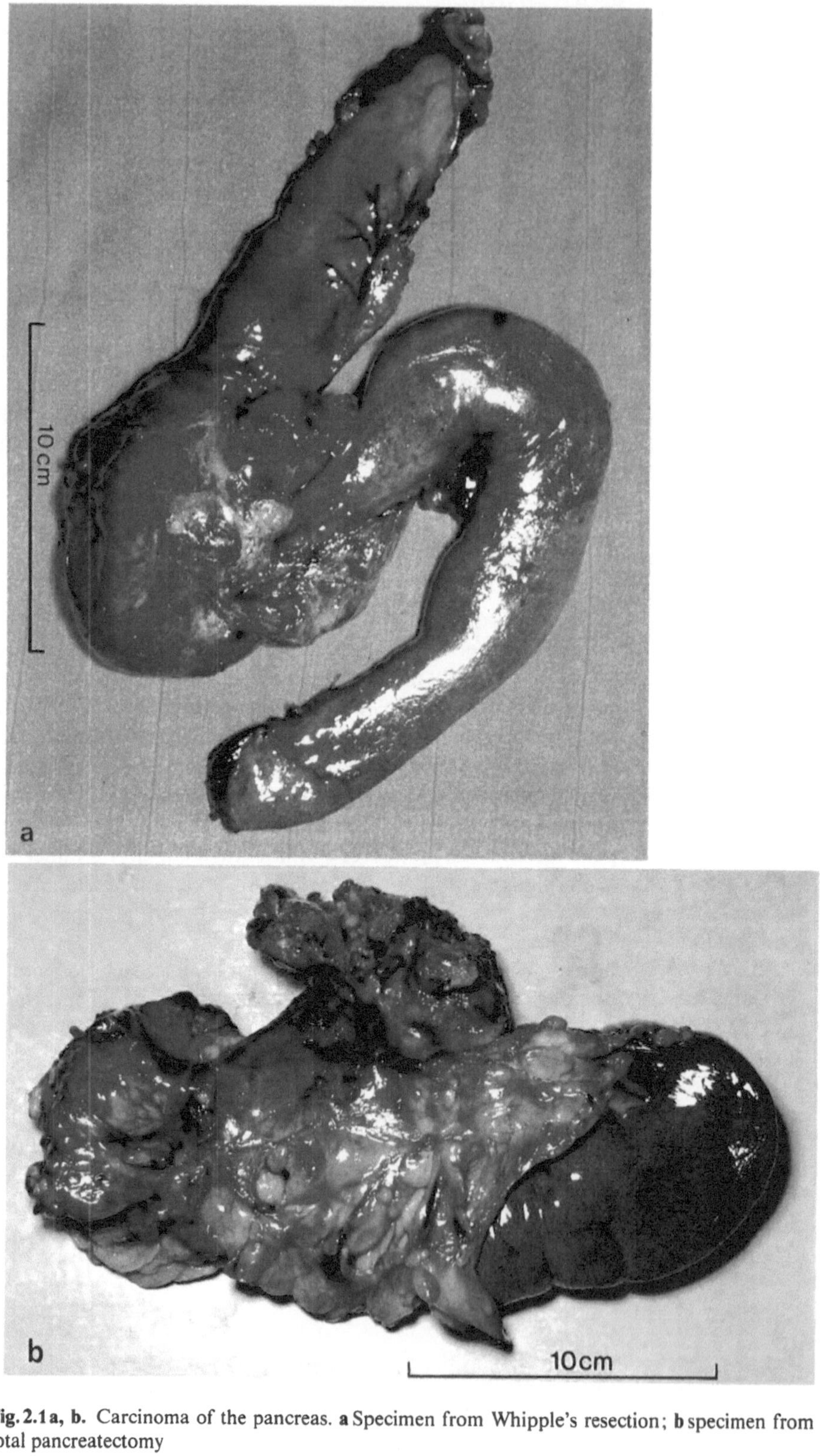

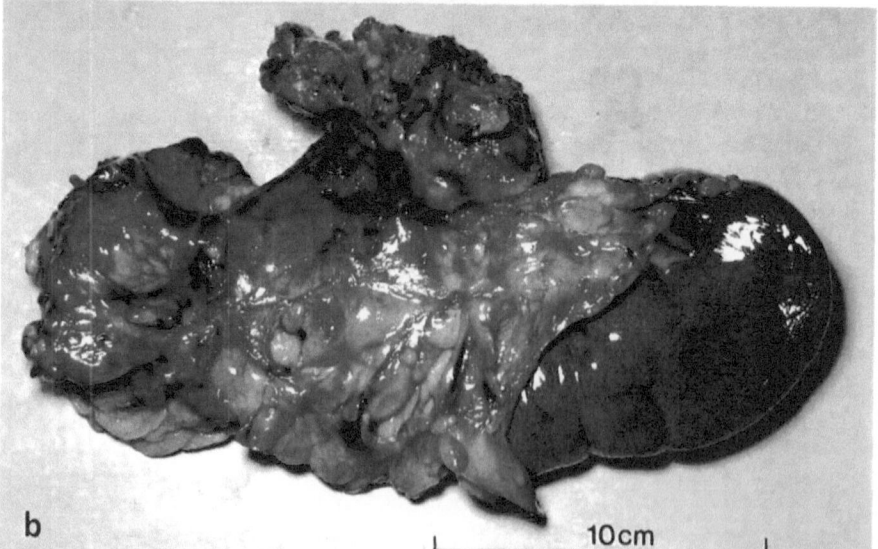

Fig. 2.1 a, b. Carcinoma of the pancreas. **a** Specimen from Whipple's resection; **b** specimen from total pancreatectomy

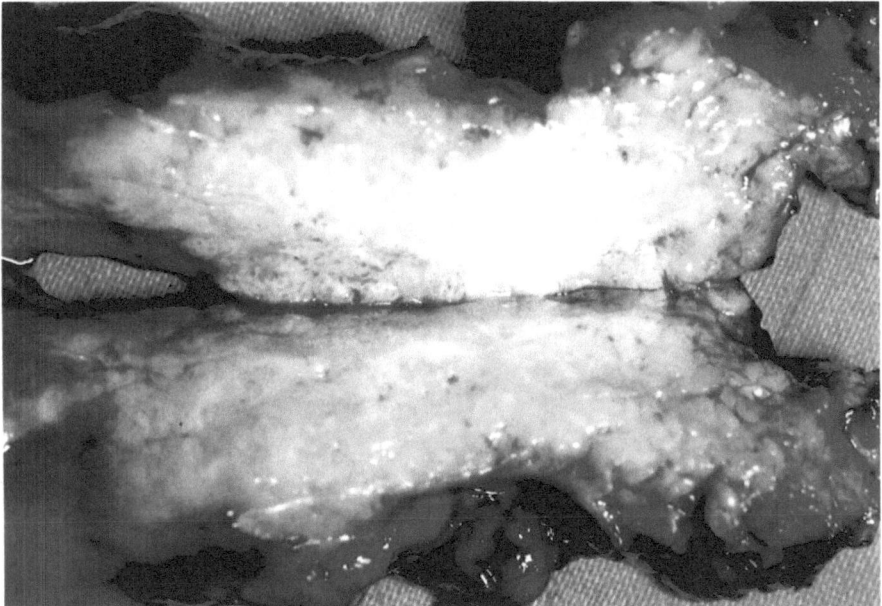

Fig. 2.2. Carcinoma of the pancreas at section. Tumor tissue is poorly delimited, with grayish-white margins

2.1.2 Intraglandular Localization

Classical anatomy divides the pancreas into three parts – the head, the body, and the tail. However, we think this distinction is artificial and prefer the following nomenclature: a right and left pancreas divided by an isthmus, located in front of the portomesenteric vascular axis. This point will be further developed along with the anatomosurgical bases of resection in the chapter on therapy. At present, referring to other authors and to a statistical series based on classical anatomical methods, we will continue to use this early nomenclature to localize exocrine pancreatic cancer.

Recently, Van Kemmel [71] induced a sector-based three-part classification which was not exactly congruent with the classical anatomical pattern of head, body, and tail of the pancreas (Table 2.1). Of a total of 45 patients showing a multiple sector-based disease, he found 19 bisector-based localizations and 26 trisector-based ones. The identification was mainly macroscopic.

In a series of 380 exocrine pancreatic cancers, Cubilla [18] observed 61% to be in the head, 13% in the body, and 5% in the tail of the pancreas. In the remaining 21% the tumor was found in various sites. Similar percentages of localization are to be found in other studies, reflecting some clinical reality. The localization in the head of the pancreas is by far the most frequent and thus easily explains why duodenopancreatectomy, or Whipple's operation, was for so long the operation of choice in that type of cancer. However, through careful examination of pancreatic sections from resected specimens which had been said to be macroscopically healthy or nor-

Table 2.1. Van Kemmel's sector-based classification [71]

Part A: cephalic, included in the duodenal region
Part B: median isthmocorporeal and retrovenous, in relation with the superior arteriovenous mesenteric axis
Part C: body and tail, in relation with the spleen

Table 2.2. Frequency of multicentric localization of exocrine pancreatic cancer, according to the literature

Reference	Reported frequency (%)
Herter [30]	2.4
Hermreck [29]	6.5
Shapiro [63]	7
Solassol [64]	10
Ihse [35]	16
Pliam [56]	19
Cubilla [18]	21
Piorkowski [53]	23
Fortner [23]	27
Van Heerden [70]	31
Tryka [69]	38

mal, anatomopathologists discovered that they had been invaded by the tumor process in about 30% of the cases. In 1954, Ross [60] described a discontinuous tumor 13 cm in length, extending from the head toward the tail of the pancreas, in a patient who had by chance undergone a total resection of the gland. Since then, a plethora of cases have shown multiple sector-based or multicentered exocrine pancreatic cancers, and such cases in these studies range from a few to 38% (Table 2.2).

After having established that 38% of pancreatic head cancers spread far beyond the palpable tumor of the head itself, Tryka and Brooks [69], proceeded to describe three different types of intraglandular extensions (Fig. 2.3). In type I the tumor reaches the main bile duct. In type II it passes through the isthmus and reaches the body of the pancreas. Type III consists of multiple foci forms with invasive or non-invasive islets interspersed throughout the healthy pancreas. Tumor cells can also be seen in the lumen of the pancreas ducts, but the gland itself is not invaded, except with tumor in the head of the pancreas. For example, Gaston [25] discovered some tumor cells 13 cm above the primary tumor of the head, and Matsui et al. [47] also found tumor cells in the upper duct of Wirsung in four of the five invasions by contiguity reported. In agreement with these findings, it has been mooted that there was a causal relationship between the discovery of tumor cells in the caudal duct of Wirsung and the recurrence of tumors after Whipple's procedure. Whether or not this was the case, it seems difficult to determine that the link is meaningful.

The question now arises to why multiple-foci forms appear in roughly a quarter of the cases. Sommers et al. [65] put forward the hypothesis of a malignant transformation arising from a duct hyperplasia. They found an associated duct hyperplasia in 41% of 141 resected specimens from adenocarcinoma. In four cases observed they found a simple hyperplasia, an in-situ cancer, and an invasive carcinoma ap-

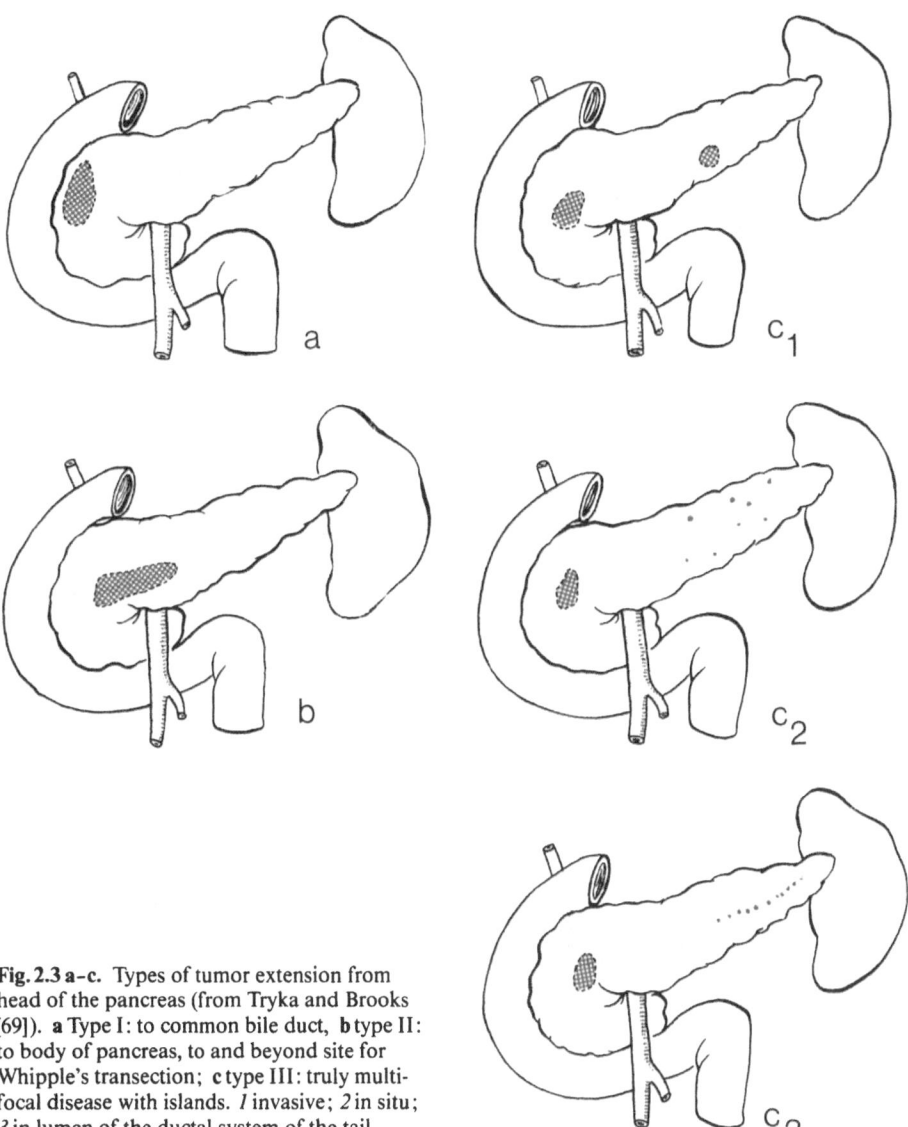

Fig. 2.3 a–c. Types of tumor extension from head of the pancreas (from Tryka and Brooks [69]). **a** Type I: to common bile duct, **b** type II: to body of pancreas, to and beyond site for Whipple's transection; **c** type III: truly multifocal disease with islands. *1* invasive; *2* in situ; *3* in lumen of the ductal system of the tail

pearing simultaneously, suggesting a transition from hyperplasia to the invasive form. This relation was confirmed by the findings of Kozuka et al. [39], who defined three types of hyperplasia and showed that they appear more frequently in cases of exocrine pancreatic cancer than in noninvaded pancreas (Table 2.3). When invasive, these multifoci forms are easily discernible macroscopically, but when noninvasive, they totally elude discovery during surgery.

An additional component of intraglandular tumor localization is the exact volume of the tumor. This is difficult to determine with precision due to its association

Table 2.3. Comparison of incidence of hyperplasia in pancreas with infiltrating carcinomas and in those without (from Kozuka et al. [39])

	Pancreas with infiltrating carcinoma (%)		Pancreas without infiltrating carcinoma (%)	
Total number	24	(100)	713	(100)
Atypical hyperplasia	7	(29.2)	5	(0.7)
Papillary hyperplasia	9	(37.5)	74	(10.4)
Nonpapillary hyperplasia	19	(79.2)	182	(25.5)
No hyperplasia	3	(12.5)	452	(63.5)

with pancreatitis. In its primitive form, as well as in the multiple-foci pattern, it is revealed only by means of a microscopic examination of the resected specimens. On the basis of 23 total pancreatectomies, Pliam and Remine [56] reported an extensive distal pancreatitis (making the boundary between tumor and inflamed tissue virtually impossible to identify) in 67% of the cases. According to Cubilla [16], the operative macroscopic size estimate should be 1 cm longer than that of the histological measurement.

Given the difficulties linked both to a precise estimate of the volume of the tumor and to the location of other carcinogenic islets in some multiple-foci forms, there is a very important bias towards total resection of the gland. This will be discussed elsewhere.

2.2 Microscopic Study

Since publication of Oberling and Guerin's *Le Cancer du Pancréas* in 1931 (Doin, Paris), the knowledge of pathologic anatomy of pancreatic cancer has not been basically modified: It has, however, been enriched by differentiation of some histological types, by the progress of medical imagery allowing cytodiagnosis, and by modern microscopic techniques (such as ultrastructure and immunohistochemistry) facilitating the comprehension of anatomoclinical forms already described so well by Oberling and Guerin.

2.2.1 Histological Types

The exocrine pancreas consists of acinar and excretory ducts arranged in lobules, which are themselves divided by conjunctive fibrous walls. Each of these constitutive features can become cancerous with variable frequency (Table 2.4): carcinoma of the ducts, whose site of origin is the excretory system, is by far the most frequent; acinar cell carcinomas, only recently diagnosed, are more rarely found. Primary

Table 2.4. Histological types of pancreatic cancer

Type	Percent of cases
I - Duct Carcinomas	
Duct adenocarcinoma	75-80
Giant cell adenocarcinoma	
– pleomorphic type	4
– epulis-type (osteoclastoma)	1
Adenosquamous carcinoma	4
Microadenocarcinoma	3
Mucinous (colloid) adenocarcinoma	2
Mucinous cystadenocarcinoma	1
II - Acinar cell carcinoma	
Acinar cell adenocarcinoma	1-2
Solid and cystic acinar cell tumor	2
Acinar cell cystadenocarcinoma	1 case
III - Cancer of uncertain histogenesis	
Pancreatoblastoma	1
Cystic papillary carcinoma	1
Small cell anaplastic carcinoma	1.5
Mixed carcinoma	1
IV - Sarcoma	0.5

pancreatic sarcoma remains an exceptional finding, historically recorded. We will introduce into this classification a last category regarding cancers of uncertain histogenesis, sarcomas or carcinomas, ductal or acinous, exocrine or endocrine [14, 37].

2.2.1.1 Duct Carcinomas

Duct cell adenocarcinoma is the major pancreas duct cancer, appearing in 75%-80% of all cases. Its topography concerns essentially the head of the pancreas.

On an architectural level, this kind of carcinoma creates quite uneven glandular cavities, differing in size and possibly voluminous, and more or less elaborated (pseudoglandular in appearance). On a cytological level, the tumor cells usually have a cylindrical morphology, along with clear cytoplasm, occasionally cubic with a reduced cytoplasm, and, less frequently, presenting a completely goblet cell appearance. Mucin secretion is irregular, but rarely absent. Mucus is present in the apex of tumor cells more or less abundantly and is also found in the glandular lumen (Figs. 2.4-2.6). Electron microscopy corroborates the presence of mucigenous granules in most duct adenocarcinomas. The significant desmoplastic stroma reaction surpasses the tumor and extends to the extratumoral pancreas, creating either atrophy or duct ectasia as well as dystrophic alterations of contacting acini. Additional hemorrhagic or necrotic foci may occur, including foci of fat necrosis. Exocrine pancreatic adenocarcinoma is subject to morphological variations, with papillary features in 10% of patients and pseudocystic features in 6%.

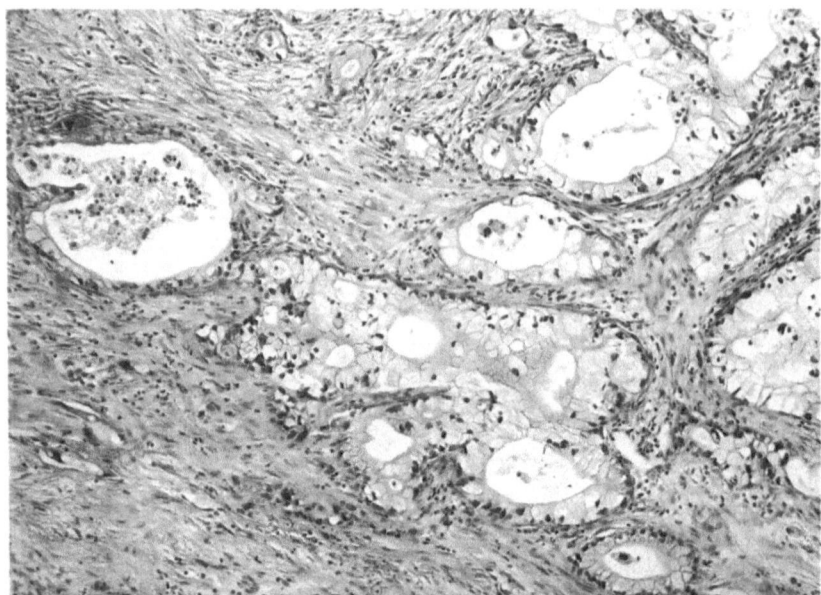

Fig. 2.4. Differentiated duct adenocarcinoma. × 52

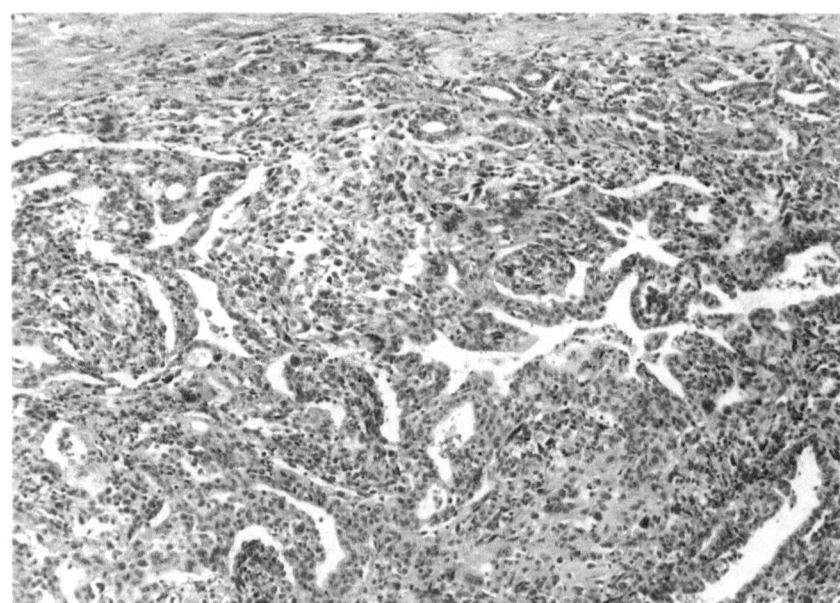

Fig. 2.5. Undifferentiated duct adenocarcinoma. × 52

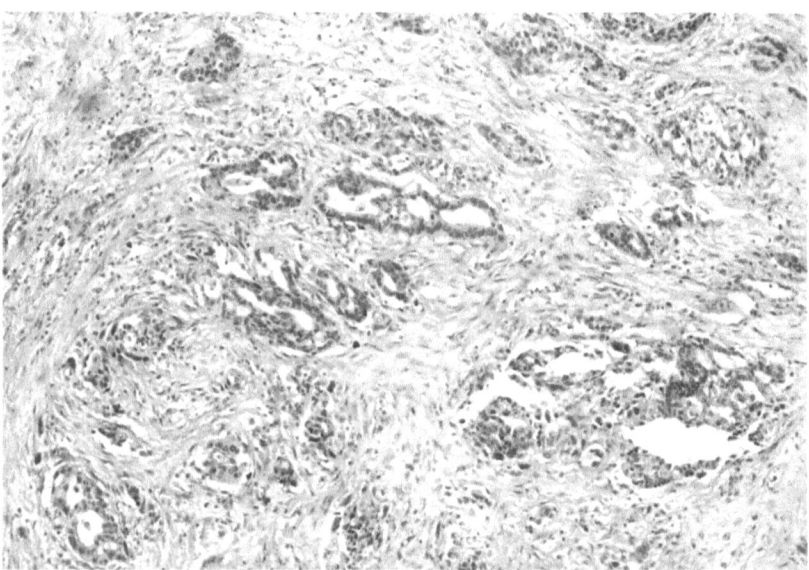

Fig. 2.6. Poorly differentiated duct adenocarcinoma. × 52

Giant cell adenocarcinoma is rarely observed. However, this is a classical and very well-known tumor: on observing a distant metastasis of giant-cell type, the pathologist always suggests the pancreas as the possible site of origin. This tumor presents two different aspects. *The pleomorphic form* (4% of cases) has preferentially a cephalic topography, but localizations in the tail and the body of the pancreas are sometimes found as well. Macroscopically, the excavated tumor is voluminous, presenting a pseudocystic aspect with necrotic-hemorrhagic material inside. Regarding its histological features, the glandular cavities and the pseudoglandular structures indicate the ductal nature of this carcinoma, but their characterization is compromised by the fact that it is drowned in a proliferation of giant cells (Fig. 2.7). The giant cells, truly monstruous, are overwhelmingly obvious on observation. They are huge and multinucleated, often vacuolized, having a large prominent nucleolus as well as an intensely, colored chromatin, aggregated in big lumps, and finally an abundant dense and intensively basophilic cytoplasm. Some fusiform cells are also to be found, typically mononucleated and occasionally with fibrillary cytoplasm; the malignant features are obvious and these cells may participate in the development of the pseudoglandular structures. A last cellular type is represented by small, round elements of regular morphology, with a pale cytoplasm, arranged in clumps or clusters, and rich in mitoses. The special coloration portrays a mucin secretion in the pseudoglandular structures, more rarely found in giant cell cytoplasm. *The giant cell adenocarcinoma, epulis type, or osteoclastoma,* even more rare (1%), appears to be a more differentiated form [14] and results in a less severe prognosis [37]. The giant cells are predominant, they range from monstrous giant cells (as in the pleomorphic carcinoma described above) to the osteoclastic type of plasmode (non-atypic, with no malignant appearance). Joining this proliferation is a fusiform popula-

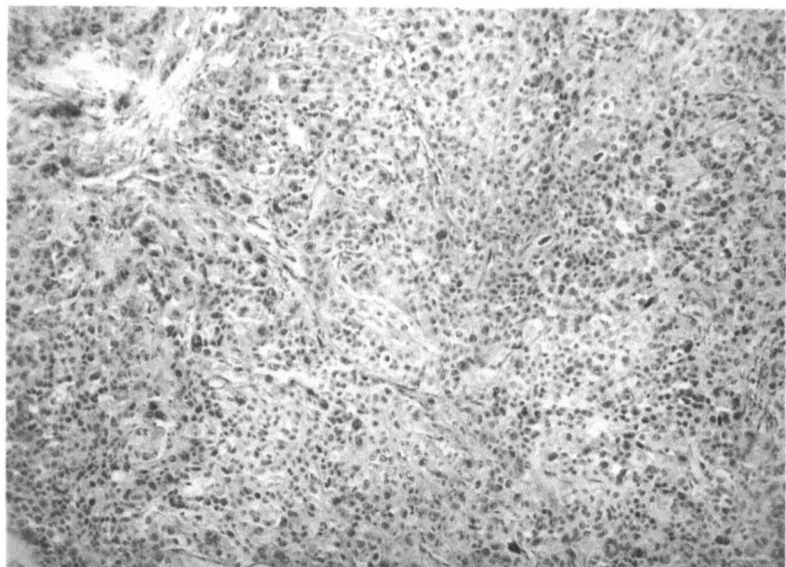

Fig. 2.7. Giant cell pleomorphic carcinoma. × 52

tion, either fibroblastic in appearance with no malignant features or properly neoplastic (Fig. 2.8). A great number of osteoid foci can be seen in the stroma. Finally, in some observations, foci of the ductal type of adenocarcinoma are seen. Electron microscopy shows real desmosomes in osteoclasts and proves the epithelial nature.

Adenosquamous carcinoma is rare in the pancreas but very well-known in other organs (uterus, bronchi, stomach) and is also called epidermoid adenocarcinoma. It is an established fact that it represents about 4% of malignant tumors of the pancreas. The role played by anterior abdominal irradiation has been elsewhere discussed [68].

The carcinoma corresponds to a linked proliferation of an adenocarcinomatous contingent, more or less well differentiated, and of a malpighian contingent, generally well differentiated, including intracytoplasmic bridges and keratin pearls (Fig. 2.9). These two components are proportionally variable, and sometimes it is necessary to perform many resections in order to find both. In most cases, staining by mucicarmine gives positive results in adenocarcinomatous cells.

Microadenocarcinoma: The prefix 'micro' relates to the size of proliferating glands, not to the size of the carcinoma, which is more than 10 cm in diameter. This kind of tumor consists of sheets or tumoral lobules hollowed by small glandular cavities. The small proliferating cells have regular round or ovoid nuclei and a rather pale and scanty cytoplasm. The gross global appearance matches a carcinoid, and, in fact special staining shows the mucinous feature of the tumoral elements (Figs. 2.10, 2.11). Moreover, both Grimelius' stain and differential techniques aimed at showing

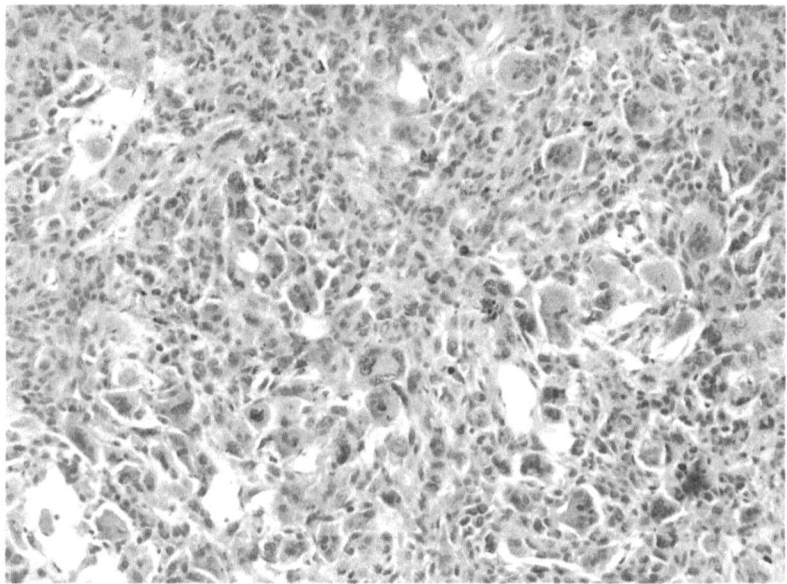

Fig. 2.8. Giant cell epulis-type carcinoma. × 52

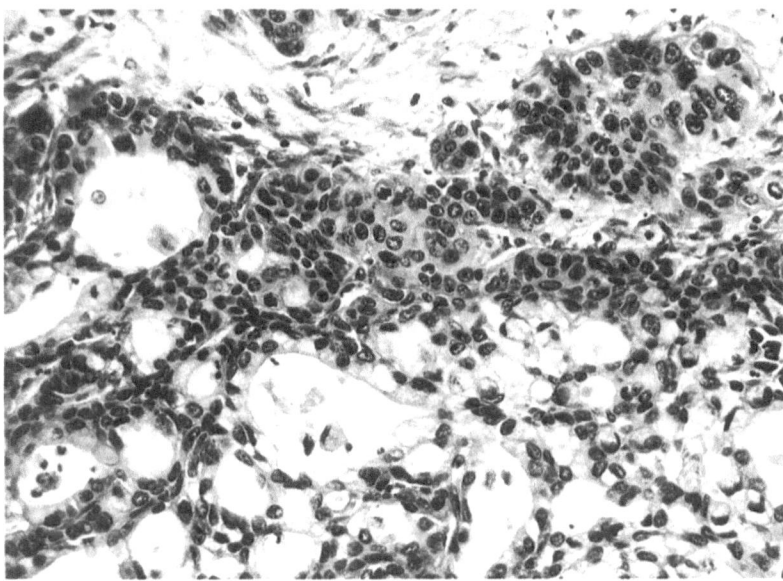

Fig. 2.9. Adenosquamous carcinoma. × 130

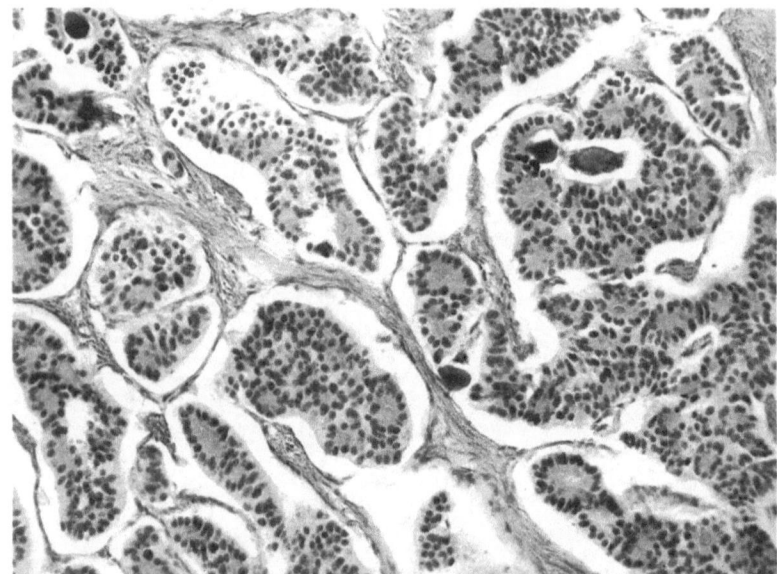

Fig. 2.10. Microadenocarcinoma. × 52

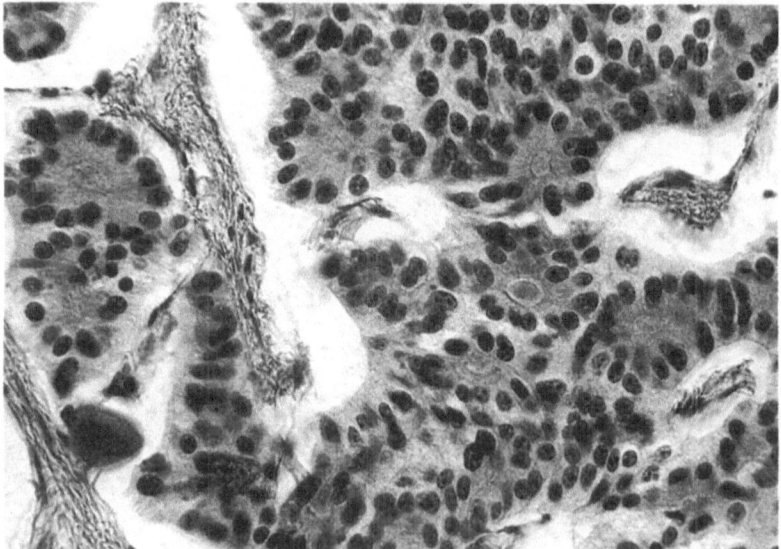

Fig. 2.11. Microadenocarcinoma. × 130

endocrine pancreatic cells are negative. Strong evidence for the ductal origin of this neoplasm is that neurosecretory granules are not observed with electron microscopy. In a critical study on the classification of Cubilla and Fitzgerald [14] Klöppel [37] questioned the microadenocarcinoma as an antomoclinical entity: in his view it is only an undifferentiated form of duct adenocarcinoma.

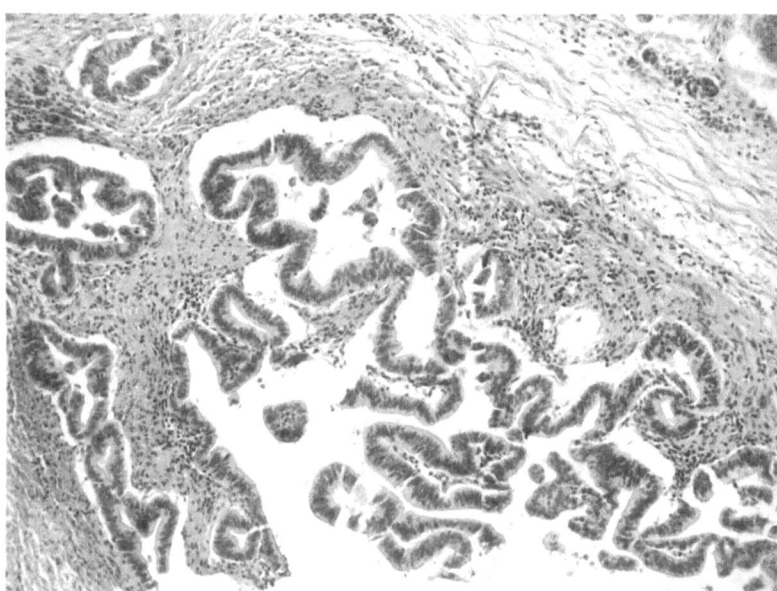

Fig. 2.12. Cystadenocarcinoma: the cyst wall. × 52

Mucinous adenocarcinoma, also referred to as colloid or gelatinous adenocarcinoma, is rarely found (2% of cases). It occurs most often in patients with a long history of pancreatic disease.

The tumor, located mainly in the head of the pancreas, is voluminous, smooth, and resistant to pressure. On a microscopic level, it appears as either vast cystic cavities, rich in mucus and bordered by a high cylindric epithelium, or lakes of mucus, among which a more or less voluminous aggregate of floating cells may outline some glandular structures. The mucinoid lakes may be very poor in cells (peculiarly of the signet-ring type) or even completely cell free.

Cystadenocarcinoma has recently [8] been isolated from the benign cystadenomas. It occurs in about 1% of all pancreatic cancers. It has a mucinous and macrocystic appearance and clearly differs from the serous and microcystic cystadenomas, which never degenerate. Cystadenocarcinomas are located mainly in the body and the tail of the pancreas and can reach up to 30 cm in diameter. Macroscopically, one can see a cystic mass, uniform or plurilobed, containing mucus intermingled with red blood clots and necrotic fragments. The cavities are covered by high cylindrical epithelium, sending out papillary invaginations into the lumen of the cysts (Fig. 2.12). Cytological and architectural signs of malignancy are sometimes not very apparent, and multiple sections are often necessary to arrive at a diagnosis. Yet, according to Alexandre [1], any mucinous carcinoma free of them must be considered potentially malignant and must be treated as such. The preoperative differential diagnosis with a false cyst is often difficult to establish and pre- and peroperative histological evaluation is of great value, permitting successful oncological surgery. The 5-year survival, is around 68%, far higher than for any other kind of pancreatic cancer [32].

2.2.1.2 Acinar Cell Carcinomas

The variation in frequency of acinar cell carcinomas is high: 15% of all pancreatic cancers according to Leach [42], 10% according to Webb [73], 2% for Becker [2], only 1% for Cubilla and Fitzgerald [14], and 11% according to Horie et al. [33].

Their clinical presentation as numerous subcutaneous nodules and adiponecrosis is classical but rarely observed. Horie et al. have described a significant elevation of the serous rate of carcinoembryonic antigen in acinous carcinomas, as contrasted with other pancreatic cancers. This was demonstrated through the positive immunoreactivity of acinocarcinomatous cells to peroxidase-labeled anti-CEA. In the head, the body, or the tail of the pancreas, the tumor mass is largely modified by the necrosis. The malignant voluminous and polygonal cells have a round nucleus and abundant granular cytoplasm. They form compact clusters, among which acini with a slight central lumen, bordered by polarized cells (basal nucleus, apical cytoplasmic granulations) can be observed. The tumor cytoplasm is occasionally PAS positive, and immunoperoxidase techniques reveal amylase-positive and α_1-antitrypsin-positive granules in the malignant cells. Tubular formations resembling pancreatic ducts are frequently observed during proliferation. Ultrastructural studies have seldom been undertaken for this type of cancer, but they confirm the acinous nature of the tumor by revealing actual intracytoplasmic zymogen granules.

The **solid and cystic acinar cell tumor** isolated by Klöppel in 1981 [36] must be related histologically to the acinar cell carcinoma. Young women predominated in the observations (average age 28.5 years). The large, well delimited tumor has a preferentially cephalic topography. It associates some solid pseudopapillary sheets with fibrous stroma to pseudocystic necrotic foci; granulomas of a more or less giant cell type are present, frequently surrounding cholesterol crystals. The tumor cells are monomorphic and present a granular cytoplasm, sometimes vacuolated and containing PAS-positive secretions, as well as being α_1-antitrypsin, amylase, and lipase positive to immunoperoxidase. Finally, electron microscopy reveals the presence of zymogen granules. In the rare studies reported, the evolution has always been considered positive.

No correlation could be established with the **acinar cell cystadenocarcinoma** described by Cantrell et al. in 1981 [11], since on the basis of only one case reported, the evolution was the same as that of other exocrine pancreatic cancers. As are cystic cavities, it is separated by conjunctive splits and bordered by a planed epithelium, either cubic or cylindrical. Immunohistochemistry discloses the presence of trypsin in tumor cells, and electron microscopy presents evidence of zymogen granules.

2.2.1.3 Cancers of Uncertain Histogenesis

Pancreatoblastoma is unique and appears in the very young child. Small cells with clear or amphophilic cytoplasm develop in a dense mass. A few images of homologue differentiation can be seen: glandular lumen including mucin, or more voluminous cells with granular cytoplasm (and zymogen granules shown by electron microscopy). An heterologous differentiation is also possible among the blastomatous sheets: concentric arrangement of epidermoid cells, well-differentiated chondroid or osteoid substances, and even true bone plates. This tumor presents a pessimistic prognosis, due to rapid metastasis. In a recent study, Nagaraj and Polk [50] have revised this classical pessimistic prognosis when the margins of the tumor are circumscribed, and propose that radical surgery would be beneficial. There is little information available on the histogenesis of this rare tumor. The blastomatous appearance of these proliferating cells and the possibility of both homologous and heterologous differentiation have given it the name "pancreatoblastoma", by analogy with other blastomas of the region. Nevertheless, the authenticity of a pancreatic blastoma is still to be embryologically demonstrated.

Papillary cystic carcinoma: The predominant pattern is that of sheets of small cells, with cavities containing red blood cells, sometimes bordered by papillary structures whose cells adopt a perithelial arrangement around the blood vessels (a reminder of the choroid plexus). This strange tumor has already been described by Frantz [24] and has also been studied by Hamoudi et al. [27] and Oertel [51]. To date, about 60 cases have been reported; the evolution is generally benign, and metastatic dissemination was noted in only two cases.

Anaplastic small cell carcinoma is still relevant to Cubilla and Fitzgerald's classification [14] and to the more recent one of Klöppel et al. [37]. It is consistently endocrine in nature. Its common association with ectopic hormonal secretion, ACTH [13, 31], parathormone [31], calcitonin [46], and the observation with electron microscopy [46] of neurosecretory granules gives some support to this theory. It is morphologically superimposable with the anaplastic small cell carcinoma of the lung, having more or less necrosed dense sheets of small oat cells, cytonuclearly atypical (Fig. 2.13).

Mixed carcinoma: Ductal, insular, ductal-acinar, or even ductal-acinoinsular types have been reported. One must keep in mind that in most cases they happen to be the continuation of normal pancreatic structures among the tumor proliferation. There have been some striking observations [14, 21] of associated tumor proliferation of two or more of these components, one of them being more prominent.

Given the uncertain histogenesis of the oncocyte, the only case of primary pancreatic **oncocytoma** so far must belong to this classification. Huntrakoon [34] reported a case in which the architecture and tumor cytology were consistent with those of the classical oncocytomas of the salivary glands or the kidney. The malignancy of the proliferation was assessed by the invasion of the perineural sheathes, by the extension to the splenic parenchyma, and finally by lymph node metastases.

2.2.1.4 Sarcomas

Some primary pancreatic sarcomas have been reported: among them malignant fibrous histiocytoma, leiomyosarcoma, malignant hemangiopericytoma, osteogenic sarcoma [21], rhabdomyosarcoma [21], and pancreatic determinations of malignant lymphomas [52].

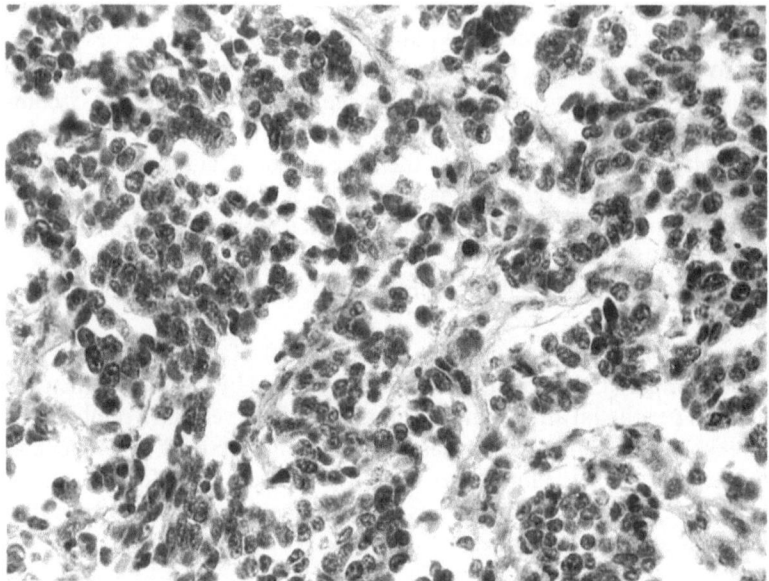

Fig. 2.13. Small cell anaplastic carcinoma. × 130

2.2.2 Epineoplastic Pancreatitis

Under this nomenclature two conditions can be distinguished: one is a pancreatitis involved with cancer, having a stroma reaction value; the other is a pancreatitis that is only distantly related to cancer, contributing to a gross alteration of the pancreas, the most significant form being the obstruction of the upper pancreas. Both of these lesions may appear in the same gland. In such a case, it is impossible, when presented with a surgical specimen of pancreatic cancer associated with pancreatitis, to decide which of the lesions is primary, and it is an open question whether a pancreatitis-cancer relation is possible. We will then proceed in this chapter to describe pancreatic lesions whose origin appears to be secondary to the developing cancer. The precancerous lesions will be discussed under duct hyperplasia-carcinoma relations.

2.2.2.1 Pancreatitis Associated with Cancer

The development of cancerous tissue in the pancreas, as in any organ, breeds a stroma reaction; this latter may be perceived as an inflammatory reaction of the connective tissue, developing in correlation with parenchymatous destruction. It is essentially a fibroblastic inflammatory reaction, with collagenous strands of variable thickness, more or less well vascularized. This sclerosis tends to be extensive, and the compression due to tumor tissue and the secretion of proteolytic enzymes by cancer cells explain the destruction of the noninvaded parenchyma. The necrosis of

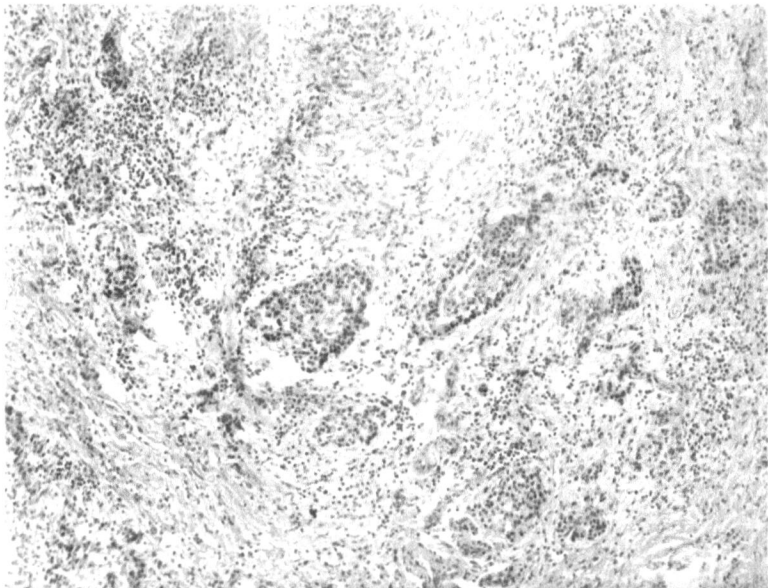

Fig. 2.14. Epineoplastic pancreatitis. × 52

the lobules frees the lipases, inducing a necrosis of the adipose tissue; these necrotic foci are themselves subject to a secondary fibrosis. The fibrosis circumscribes the lobules and invades and holds the acini and ducts; the latter then present degenerative alterations of varying degree: ductal dedifferentiation of the acini, pseudocystic dilatation, and metaplastic alterations of the ducts and ductules. This deep disruption in the architecture of the pancreatic parenchyma is closely related to the neoplastic development, especially in the region surrounding the invasion. There are a large number of consequences: first, the volume of the tumor increases through the lesions, which are not necessarily cancerous; second, quantification of the exact volume of the tumor is difficult. These difficulties are not necessarily resolved by microscopic examination, especially if there is indication for a biopsy. It is often difficult, even with paraffin embedding, to distinguish reasonably a dystrophic duct compressed by the fibrosis from a cancerous ductule that is relatively orthoplasic and infiltrating the connective tissue. The reason is that these two structures may be contiguous in the same microscopic field (Fig. 2.14).

2.2.2.2 Pancreatitis Distantly Related to Cancer

This type appears in most cases as pancreatitis of the head and body of the pancreas; rarely, it occurs as pancreatic atrophy with a parenchyma reduced to a grayish moniliform thread melting into the adipose pancreatic tissue. Generally, this pancreatitis induces an irregular hypertrophy of the gland, loss of the lobular surface, and unequal induration, but occasionally it presents flocculent embossment.

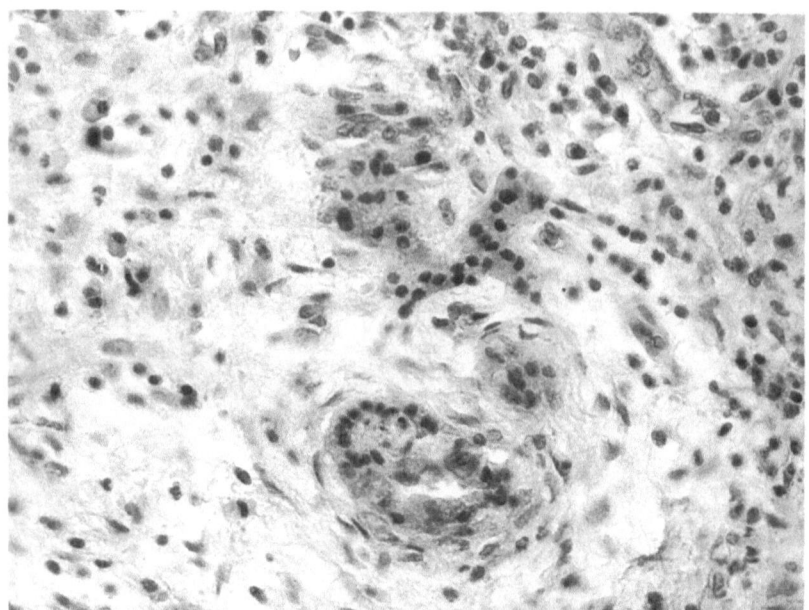

Fig. 2.15. Epineoplastic pancreatitis: dystrophic ductules. × 130

On section, the irregular dispersion of the grayish-white foci of sclerosis can be seen alternating with cystic cavities of various size and with foci of fat necrosis. The latter may also sometimes be seen on the peripancreatic peritoneum, where calcium deposits are possible. Microscopic findings are those of classical chronic pancreatitis. The main feature being the irregular disposition of the lesion sites: the processes of the foci become confluent, but quasi-normal lobules remain. The acini undergo regressive dystrophic alterations resulting either in atrophy by fibrous compression, or more frequently in dilatation by ductal dedifferentiation. In this case, a large number of dedifferentiated acini may converge, giving birth to microcysts, with polycyclic contours. Ducts - whatever their diameter - are altered. They are visually dilated but in an irregular way and they present a tortuous track with retentional cystic dilatation of unequal volume (up to 1 or 2 cm in diameter). Their lumen either is empty or includes mucous concretions, sometimes calcified. Their wall is flattened, endotheliform or in epidermoid metaplasia (sometimes filled with horny lamellae), or mucoid (with goblet cells). The interstitial tissue supports a permanent periductal fibrosis, peri- and intralobular. It is a collagenous fibrosis more or less rich in fibroblasts, more or less well vascularized, and generally poor in inflammatory elements. This fibrosis is frequently interspersed with foci of fat necrosis. As in all chronic pancreatitis, the islets of Langerhans are remarkably preserved even in the most profoundly modified lobules. This upper pancreatitis complicates surgical evaluation since it suggests a total cancer, taking in the whole pancreas. A histological differential diagnosis between the lesions of dystrophic pancreatitis and real invasive cancer is often difficult to establish, especially with a specimen biopsy, but preoperative cytodiagnosis is less prone to error (Figs. 2.15, 2.16).

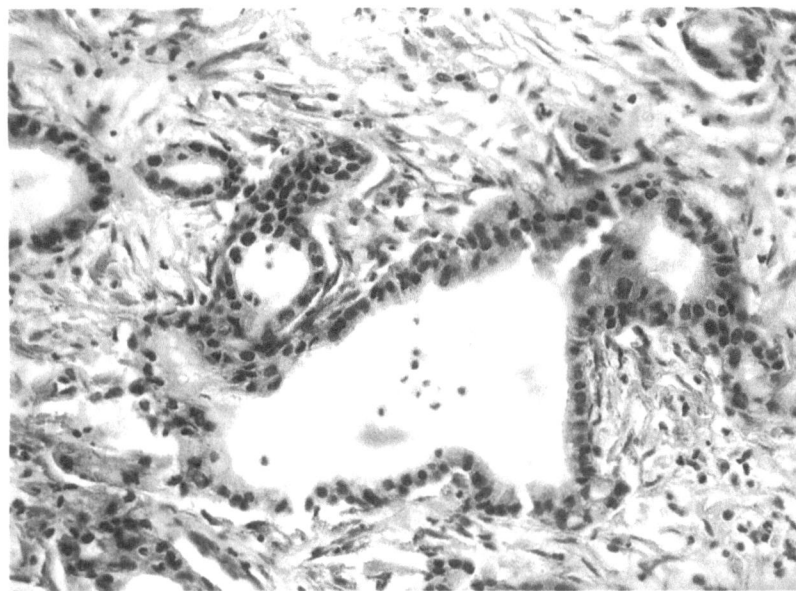

Fig. 2.16. Differentiated duct cell carcinoma with a striking resemblance to dystrophic chronic pancreatitis. × 130

2.2.3 Pancreatic Cytology

Although this method of diagnosis has been known for a long time now, cytology has only recently been used in the detection of carcinoma of the pancreas. It was in the 1970s that some Scandinavian authors, notably Christoffersen and Poll [12] and Forsgren and Orel [22], reported some interesting results on cytodiagnosis applied to pancreatic pathology. Since then, little by little, the method has been developed, particularly in France [6, 7]. One of the techniques used in cytological examination is to study a sample of the pancreatic juice taken by endoscopy. Initially, secretion samples were obtained by duodenal aspiration [44, 58]; now they are taken during selective catheterization of the duct of Wirsung [20, 38], injected with secretine. The results obtained are sometimes cytologically deceptive, with a large number of false negatives (20%–50%, according to Tatsuta [67]); however, a cytological examination is logical when catheterization is performed, and we cannot neglect this method of diagnosis even if cytology is less reliable in this case than any of the other techniques of withdrawal.

Already used as a method of detection for other deep cancers, thin-needle cytoaspiration is currently the method of choice in pancreatic cytology. This examination may be pre- or peroperatively performed.

Preoperative cytoaspiration is performed to confirm a doubtful diagnosis, and is guided by another morphological method of exploration (ultrasound echography, tomodensitometry). The investigation is usually done transcutaneously, less frequently by means of endoscopy.

Peroperative cytoaspiration is easily performed by the direct anteroposterior route or by transduodenal aspiration. In both cases, the reading will be immediate, taking from 10 to 20 min, allowing to determine the quality of samples and to make a quick diagnosis which will guide the surgeon [4, 5, 20, 41].

2.2.3.1 Cytological Techniques

The actual aspiration techniques will be described in a later chapter. However, a few points should be stressed here. One must avoid spreading this material as the cells are fragile; slight spreading may be carried out avoiding any destruction of the preparation. According to the staining technique chosen, the slides are either fixed at once or air dried. If sufficient tissue specimens are obtained, they are placed in a fixative and then embedded in paraffin. Many methods of staining are possible: May-Grunwald-Giemsa staining on unfixed slides or Papanicolaou or Harris-Shorr staining on fixed slides. Simple staining with hematoxylin and eosin may be used also, with consistent results.

2.2.3.2 Results

From an analytical point of view, the following features are studied: the background of the preparation, which can be hemorrhagic, more or less inflamed, or even necrotic; the density of the cells, which contributes to orientation; the mode of cellular aggregation; and the cytological features, with or without cytonuclear atypia.

If the puncture is done in a normal region, the acinar cells are easily recognized: frequently isolated or with bare nuclei, they may be grouped in rosettes. They have a regular nucleus and scant cytoplasm. Some ductal cells are also found, grouped in unicellular bundles, coherent, and without any irregular nuclei. The background is clear, including only some bare nuclei and a few polynuclear cells. In the course of chronic pancreatitis, some bundles of unicellular duct cells appear, as well as stressed anisokaryosis. The background is inflamed, with altered polynuclear and sometimes squamous cells issued from cystic foci. When fibrosis is marked, the distribution of cells is poor.

Regarding pancreatic cancer, we describe here the most frequent manifestation of exocrine duct adenocarcinoma. Generally, there is strong cell density, but there may be fewer cells in the fibrous areas. The neoplastic cells are enlarged with a high nuclear-cytoplasmic ratio. The nuclei are usually clear and strongly nucleolated, but they may be hyperchromatic with nonuniform chromatin (Fig. 2.17) arranged in large lumps. Their margins are irregular and angular, with anisokaryosis. The cytoplasm, not easily discernible, may be abundant in the differentiated forms when the cytonuclear atypia is less marked. It is important to note the intergrouping of the cells: the neoplastic cells are generally settled in thick tridimensional layers of little coherency, and highly suggestive of malignancy (Fig. 2.18). It is also important to screen all slides in detail. The frequency of epineoplastic pancreatitis is known, and emphasis must be placed on the search for neoplastic cells associated with normal

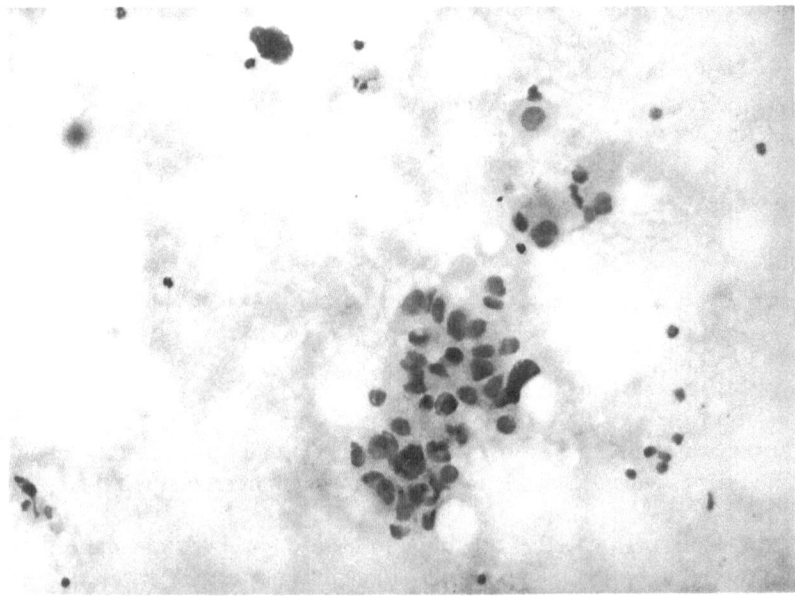

Fig. 2.17. Pancreatic cytology. Small group of malignant cells from a patient with an adenocarcinoma. × 130

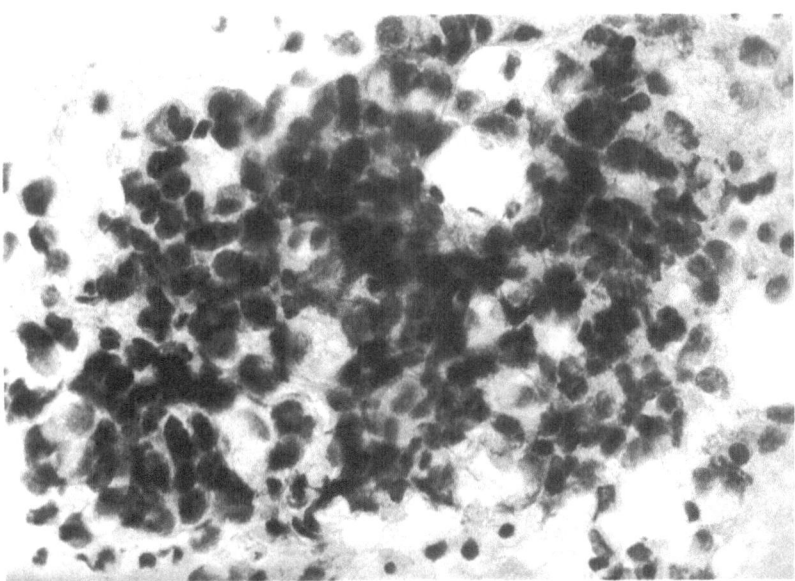

Fig. 2.18. Pancreatic cytology. An irregular clump of cells in duct cell adenocarcinoma, the nuclei show marked pleomorphism and the cytoplasm is scant. × 130

or dystrophic epithelial cells. Finally, the borderline cases must be stressed, as the diagnosis here is difficult, particularly if there are some papillary structures: they appear as small tridimensional but coherent epithelial pearls, sometimes showing cytonuclear atypia. One should then suspect a ductopapillary or atypical hyperplasia, the importance of which is known in the onset of carcinoma of the pancreas [39, 40]. Consequently, the discovery of such structures should lead to follow-up investigations.

2.2.3.4 Advantages of and Limits to Cytology

Cytology has several advantages over biopsy:

Simplicity: A definite diagnosis can be made without surgical intervention. Transcutaneous cytopuncture [6] seems to be the most common method used nowadays.

Innocuousness: The needles are thin and lead to fewer complications than are seen subsequent to biopsy (hemorrhage, pancreatitis or necrosis, fistulas).

Reliability: Cytology is more reliable than biopsy, since cytopuncture allows the study of a larger area of the pancreas by the multiplication of deeper punctures in diverse directions, bypassing peritumor pancreatitis when it exists. An exact diagnosis is established in 75%–85% of cases (Bret, from a series of 116 punctures [7]), even in 90% of cases, according to Diebold [19].

False-positive results are rare. Assessment of malignancy depends on the quality of the cytological samples and on the cytologist's experience. In case of uncertainty, the examination is said to be inconclusive, and it is likely that the lack of false positive results leads to an increase in false-negative or inconsistent results. Some false-negative results are not due to cytology, particularly in primary cancers, as owing to its small size the tumor is difficult to reach. The results are dependent upon the method of withdrawal. Tatsuta et al. [67] stress the superiority of percutaneous cytopuncture over endoscopy for obtaining pancreatic secretions (20%–50% of the latter are false negatives). Cytopuncture provides a larger sample, and the better preservation of the cells improves the efficiency of the cytological evaluation by diminishing the number of dubious cases. Another puncture can be made pre- or postoperatively if the first one happens to be blank. Concerning the true negatives, it may be difficult to establish an accurate diagnosis of the lesions since it is sometimes possible to conclude only that there is a lack of malignant cells. The cell alterations found in chronic pancreatitis are rather worrying and they must be known to the cytologist. In case of an absolutely benign and normal cytological distribution, and especially if doubt remains from the clinical examination, the diagnosis is uncertain. However, only positive results have an absolute value; the negative ones can never be interpreted to determine the most efficient way to use this method. In a series of 19 patients affected with pancreatic cancer, Tatsuta et al. [67] complemented the cytological examination with a dosage of CEA in the sample taken at puncture; this gave positive results in 100% of cases.

Finally, the cytological examination is dependent on the sample-taking techniques. It may sometimes be difficult to ascertain nonmalignancy, particularly in the case of chronic pancreatitis. It is important to be able to differentiate between it and borderline cases of duct hyperplasia. Whatever the method, cytology obviously relies on the other complementary ways of exploration, morphological or surgical. It is not a truly screening method; pancreatic cytodiagnosis can be based only on clinical features or morphological abnormalities. But cytology diminishes the exploration necessary for complete examination in case of pancreatitis, and it provides prompt answers for a quicker diagnosis.

2.2.4 Duct Hyperplasia-Cancer Relationship

The relationship between pancreatitis and pancreatic cancer has been dealt with in Chap. 1, with reference to clinical and epidemiological procedures. In this chapter we will try to conclude whether a precancerous state can be defined in the pancreas, based on morphological studies (specimens from biopsy or autopsy). There are two methods: examination of the extratumoral pancreas for pancreatic cancer from resected specimens and systematic examination of the pancreas by nonselective autopsy.

2.2.4.1 Resected Specimens

A large number of studies have been done of resected specimens, but the results are generally rather deceiving, for, as we have already said in a previous chapter, it is quite impossible to determine from the specimens where lesions of pancreatitis and cancer are juxtaposed or even intermingled, which process occurs prior to the other, keeping in mind that the cancer itself can contribute to the pancreatitis. As was reported by Becker [2], there are controversial histological factors in the possible relationship between pancreatitis and cancer.

Arguments Against a Relationship. Epidermoid metaplasia of the ductules during pancreatitis is an almost constant lesion, but adenosquamous cancers are exceptional (2%–4% only). However, Harstock and Fischer [28] reported a plurifocal in-situ malpighian epithelioma in the tail of the pancreas.

Plurifocal pancreatic cancers are also rare (7%, according to Becker [2]). The lesions of chronic pancreatitis are said to be diffuse, but if it were true that chronic pancreatitis preceded cancer, we should find more plurifocal cancers. Finally, lesions of pancreatitis are rarely confirmed before the invasion of the cancer process. Some lucky observations are nevertheless cited, such as that of Watanobe et al. [72], where a calcified pancreatitis of the head and the body of the pancreas was radiologically proven to have appeared 2 years prior to the carcinoma of the tail of the pancreas. Watanobe emphasizes the role as an irritant played by the intraductal calculi in the origin of this carcinoma.

Arguments for a Relationship. A test of an old inflammatory process can be deceptive, considering the duct and the acinar modifications. However, if we look at the indirect, nonpancreatic features on a parenchymatous level, the research may provide some interesting results. Thus, the intimal fibrosis of the vessels and the hyperplasia of Brunner's duodenal glands would be markers of age of the inflammatory lesions. According to Becker [2], they appear in 17% of resected specimens from pancreatectomy in the case of pancreatic cancer. Another, even more indirect bias is based upon the main histological feature of pancreatic cancer. Acinar cell cancer is rare (2%–11% of cases, according to statistics). On the other hand, pancreatic cancer is a ductal carcinoma (in more than 80% of cases), i.e., a cancer born from structures capable of multiplication and therefore of regeneration. As in other types of general oncology (cervix, uteri, bronchi, gallbladder), after a prolonged irritation followed by regeneration, the pancreas may lose its power of self-regulation, and thus change into a cancerous proliferation.

2.2.4.2 Nonselected Specimens

We refer essentially to Kozuka's results [39, 40], based on 1174 pancreas taken at autopsy, recently reconfirmed by Stamm [66] with 112 autopsy sections. These authors define duct hyperplasia as a lesion of ducts whose cells are enlarged (two-fold) and abundant in neutral mucin and sialomucin, as opposed to the normal duct epithelium, which is abundant in sulfomucin.

It is not real hyperplasia, but rather cell hypertrophy associated with histochemical metaplasia or crinin imbalance. Duct hyperplasia develops in three stages. The first is *simple hyperplasia,* which is nonpapillary and involves ducts of any diameter. It is frequently found in the ducts of medium-sized lumen presenting as adenomatous tubular hyperplasia. It is observed in 18.1% of patients older than 19 years. The second is *papillary hyperplasia,* related to medium-sized or large ducts and often associated with simple hyperplasia, having transitional features between these two types of hyperplasia. It can be seen in 6.6% of patients older than 34 years, accompanied by a certain degree of fibrosis. *Atypical hyperplasia* constitutes the third stage. It was observed in only 13 cases in Kozuka's series and in two cases of Stamm. It is a pseudostratification of the duct walls with cytonuclear atypia, such as anisokaryosis or mitosis, and without basement membrane destruction. Transitional features of the two previous stages are frequently seen. In seven of the 13 cases reported by Kozuka atypical hyperplasia was associated with a duct cancer. This lesion is observed in patients ranging from 42 to 72 years of age. Taking age into consideration (these lesions appear in 50% of cases in patients older than 80; one-third of pancreatic cancers appear in the seventh decade), then topography (atypical hyperplasia is observed mainly in the head of the pancreas), and finally frequency relative to the general population (simple hyperplasia: 18.1%; papillary: 6.6%; atypical: 1.1%; pancreatic cancer: 1.87%), Kozuka thinks the following sequence is possible: simple hyperplasia →papillary hyperplasia →atypical hyperplasia →cancer.

In a more recent work [40] Kozuka confirms these previous results, as well as the precancerous features of atypical hyperplasia. Provided with additional morphological reports (1388 autopsies), the author tried to find the cause of duct hyperplasia. The lesion does not come only with senescence. It is also seen in pancreas that are impaired by a necrosing pancreatitis, often minimal (small foci of fat necrosis). The lesional process would thus be as follows: small necrosing lesions with fat necrosis, then granuloma of resorption followed by fibrosis, then regenerative duct hyperplasia, potentially atypical.

2.2.4.3 Definition of a Precancerous Pancreatic State

This definition seems possible: duct hyperplasia, preceded by simple hyperplasia, then papillary hyperplasia with slight alteration of the mucin secretion at the beginning and removal or reduction of the acid sulfomucin, benefitting the neutral mucin as well as the acid sialomucin.

Advances in medical imaging and in cytodiagnosis by means of transcutaneous puncture will soon allow the detection of lesions that are not yet invasive in a high-risk population (necrosing pancreatitis, at least) and the discovery of a curative treatment.

2.3 Extraglandular Extension

Knowledge of the extraglandular extension of pancreatic duct cancer is at least as important as knowledge of its intraglandular topographical distribution. For, as in any other cancer, it adds to the seriousness and takes on a peculiar relief owing to its location and to the anatomical relations of the gland. Extraglandular extension arises from contiguity with the adjacent organs and with the veinous and lymphatic vessels.

2.3.1 Spreading by Contiguity

Spreading by contiguity initially includes extension to the common bile duct that we have already mentioned, matching type I of Tryka and Brooks [69]. An ascending parietal infiltration – macroscopically difficult to evaluate – toward the intraductal vegetations requires resection of the upper part of the main bile duct. Moreover, the spreading can include the prepancreatic peritoneum and adjacent organs, and the duodenum in case of invasion of the head of the pancreas. Extension may also involve the stomach, and the transverse colon through the mesocolon. This spreading to neighboring organs, particularly to the stomach and transverse colon, indicates an advanced tumor of large volume, but if isolated, primary invasion does not compromise the resectability of large tumors.

Extension of the tumor to the retroisthmic vascular axis has a different importance. A carcinoma presenting posterior development by means of direct contiguity, and by the right and left retropancreatic lamina will invade the venous and arterial axis formed by the superior mesenteric artery at the convergence of the retropancreatic process. It is essential to know whether the adventitia of the artery has been invaded. In case of invasion, only a total Fortner type-II resection of the gland may be considered as surgical intervention. At present without, and sometimes in spite of, preoperative angiography, the exact degree of extension of the tumor can be determined only by means of cautious dissection.

Nowadays, intraoperative ultrasonography gives the surgeon precise information regarding the relationship between the tumor and the superior mesenteric artery. However, the distinction between a simple repression and an invasion is easier to see in the main veins, which consist of the splenic vein, the splenomesaraic trunk, and the mesentero-portal axis. Looking at their localizations, calibers, and walls, the distinction is easier to make. Indeed, in giving the surgeon very precise information on the extension to the retroisthmic vascular axis, ultrasonography is a valuable aid to diagnosis.

2.3.2 Spreading via the Venous Network

The neoplastic embolism passes directly through the vein to reach the liver, where it can metastasize. However, it can also cross the hepatic filter to the pulmonary filter, which can in turn be crossed, resulting in metastases throughout the system including in our experience, the brain.

Considering the findings of Lisa et al. [45], we note that they emphasized the frequency of secondary pulmonary localizations, especially when the primary tumor is located in the left pancreas (Table 2.5). At this point, anatomical knowledge of the venous collaterals is not as important as it is in the exploration of some endocrine tumors. What does appear to be important, when no metastases are found, is whether or not the exeresis should include the mesenterico portal venous axis.

Table 2.5. Visceral metastases in carcinoma of the pancreas (from Lisa et al [45])

Site of tumor	No. of cases	Liver	Lung	Intes-tine	Adre-nal	Stomach	Kidney	Spleen	Biliary tract
Head	47	29	13	14	8	5	7	4	7
Tail	19	8	10	2	6	3	3	1	0
Body	10	8	2	1	2	2	1	1	3
Body and tail	13	11	10	6	5	2	2	3	1
Head, body, and tail	9	5	4	2	0	3	0	1	0
Head and body	5	3	3	1	4	0	0	0	0

2.3.3 Spreading via Lymphatic Effluents

This takes a particular form, given the location of the pancreas in relation to the ret-ropancreatic process. The posterior collecting vessels reach the peri-aorticocaval nodes after only a few centimeters.

Credit goes to Pissas [54] for having described the lymphatic drainage of the pancreas and its lymphatic channels (Fig. 2.19). His description of these lymphatics as draining into five main regions is somewhat at odds with that of Rouviere [61]. But Pissas also noted that when dealing with the pancreas it was difficult to speak of systemic and independent regions, owing to the large number of intraparenchyma-tous anastomoses appearing between the anterior and posterior face, as well as be-tween the right and left pancreas. From the anatomical studies of resected speci-mens, it appears that there are two preferential lymphatic flows, a right and a left, divided by the isthmus. The lymphatic drainage into the anterior face of the gland passes (except for the superior margin of the left pancreas) through two nodal branches prior to reaching the central collecting vessels. In contrast, the posterior drainage needs only one branch before reaching the retroperitoneal node. We will not consider Winslow's pancreas, which has no nodal branches between the gland and the central collecting vessels (Table 2.6).

Thus, we are presented with a complex concept of lymphatic drainage that is difficult to describe, with preferential regions and currents. Knowledge of the main

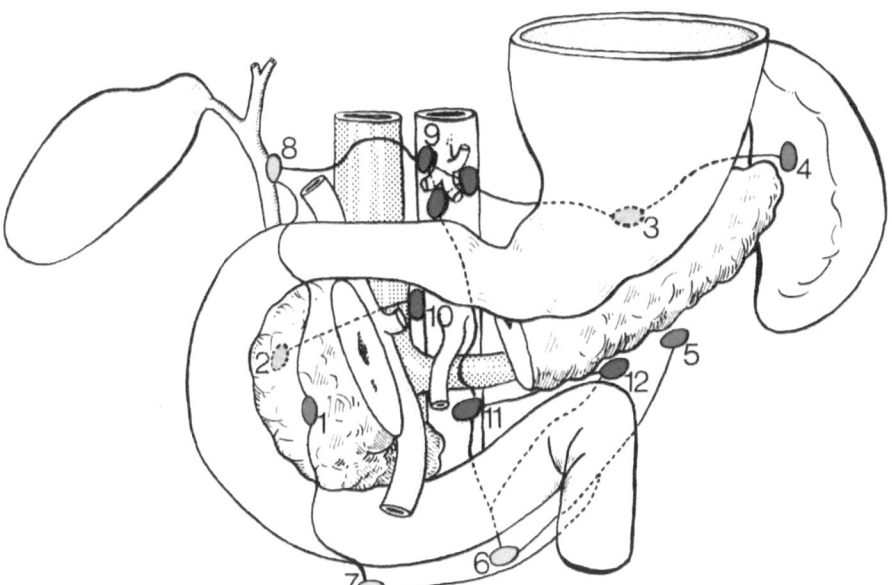

Fig. 2.19. Lymphatic drainage of the pancreas and its major relays. First relay nodes *(blue): 1* anteri-or pancreaticoduodenal; *2* posterior pancreaticoduodenal; *3* superior body; *4* splenic; *5* inferior body. Second relay nodes *(yellow): 6* jejunal; *7* midcolic; *8* hepatic chain. Third relay nodes *(red):* *9* celiac; *10* interaorticocaval; *11* left subnephric; *12* left paranephric

Table 2.6. Lymphatic drainage of the pancreas (from Pissas [54])

Right pancreas	*Anterior* face	I relay:	anterior pancreatico-duodenal nodes
		II relay:	common bile duct, midcolic or posterior pancreatico-duodenal nodes
		III relay:	celiac or left paranephric nodes
	Posterior face	I relay:	posterior pancreatico-duodenal nodes
		III relay:	interaorticocaval nodes
Left pancreas	*Anterosuperior* face	I relay:	superior body and splenic nodes
		III relay:	celiac and left paranephric nodes
	Anteroinferior face	I relay:	inferior body nodes
		II relay:	midcolic and/or jejunal nodes
		III relay:	sub- and left paranephric nodes
	Posterior face	I relay:	splenic, superior, or inferior body nodes
		III relay:	sub- and left paranephric nodes
Uncus		III relay:	interaorticocaval and/or left subnephric nodes

nodal ductules is essential for satisfactory surgery. We stress again the fact that the posterior lymphatic flow uses the right and left retropancreatic process to reach the peri-aorticocaval nodes. Another important point is the short distance and the few or absent nodal ductules, which explain the quick and systematic invasion in the case of carcinoma of the pancreas.

Accurate knowledge of the intraglandular topography of the exocrine pancreatic cancer and of its extraglandular extension leads us now to consider its classification with respect to its developmental stages.

2.4 Classification of the Stages of Development

Classification appears to be necessary when comparing the effects of different therapies on tumors at the same stage of development. To avoid guesses and errors, this staging must be precise, but at the same time, neither too long nor too tedious, so as not to discourage users. It must also include the diagnosis, any therapeutic advances, and the progress in the evolution of the disease.

Many classifications are used to define the evolutionary stages of exocrine pancreatic cancer. We will put aside that of Leadbetter et al. [43] used in the state of Vermont (USA) for tumor registration. This classification differentiates between three developmental stages without distinguishing the nodal groups or the invasion of the adjacent tissues. On the other hand, Sato et al. [62] accord great prognostic importance to this latter invasion. These classifications are, except by their authors, less frequently used now, and the most well-known and clinically used references are the TNM, Hermreck's and Cubilla's classifications.

Table 2.7. Staging of cancer of the pancreas according to Cancer of the Pancreas Task Force [10]

T 1:	No direct extension of the primary tumor beyond the pancreas
T 2:	Limited direct extension (to duodenum, bile ducts, or stomach) possibly still permitting tumor resection
T 3:	Further direct extension, incompatible with surgical resection
T X:	Direct extension not assessed or not recorded
N 0:	Regional nodes not involved
N 1:	Regional nodes involved
N X:	Regional involvement not assessed or not recorded
M 0:	No distant metastases
M 1:	Distant metastatic involvement
M X:	Distant metastatic involvement not assessed or not recorded

Stage I: T 1, T 2, N 0, M 0
No (or unknown) direct extension, or limited direct extension of tumor to adjacent viscera, with no (or unknown) regional node extension and absence of distant metastases. Limited direct extension was defined as involvement of organs adjacent to the pancreas (duodenum, common bile duct, or stomach) that could be removed in bloc with the pancreas if a curative resection was attempted.

Stage II: T 3, N 0, M 0
Further direct extension of tumor into adjacent viscera, with no (or unknown) lymph node involvement and no distant metastases, and which preclude surgical resection

Stage III: T 1-3, N 1, M 0
Regional node metastases without clinical evidence of distant metastases

Stage IV: T 1-3, N 0-1, M 1
Distant metastatic disease in liver or other sites present

2.4.1 TNM Classification

By far the best known by oncologists, the TNM classification was settled on at the International Congress on Pancreatic Cancer in New Orleans in 1980 [10] (Table 2.7). However, we have some criticisms. The first concerns the differentiation of T; the only one between T2 and T3 concerns a possible extension of T2 where a resection is still feasible and not in T3. This assessment is very subjective, for even without taking into account any adjacent invaded organs, it depends only on the surgeon's experience and skills. The reports of a surgical series undertaken by Fortner et al. [23] and Moossa et al. [48] include enlarged pancreatectomies in some patients who elsewhere had undergone simple exploratory laparotomy, for their tumors had been judged to be unresectable by surgeons less qualified or simply less trained in this practice.

Second, in the extensive nodal network there is no gradation between N0 and N1, and it seems to follow the all-or-nothing-rule. We disapprove of and challenge the term "regional lymph nodes" because of its lack of accuracy. Finally, the four-stage classification combining T, N, and M is only approximate. In particular, the forms in stage II (T3, N0, M0) would not benefit from curative surgery, whereas some forms of stage III (T2, N1, M0) would benefit from a regional curative pancreatectomy when the retroperitioneal nodes are free from metastases.

Table 2.8. Staging of pancreatic cancer (from Hermreck et al. [29])

Stage I	Local disease
Stage II	Invasion into surrounding tissues (duodenum, portal vein, mesenteric vessels, and the like)
Stage III	Regional lymph nodes
Stage IV	Generalized carcinoma (liver metastases, peritoneal implants, etc.)

2.4.2 Hermreck's Classification

In 1974, taking into account the studies of Broders, Hermreck et al. suggested a four-stage classification of pancreatic adenocarcinoma [29] (Table 2.8). It has often been used, but in the past few years it has lost importance.

The major disadvantage is at the level of gradation of the disease. For instance, Hermreck considers stage-III invasion of the duodenum equal in value with stage-III invasion of the superior mesenteric artery. We do not agree, as we feel that an invasion of the adjacent digestive system (common bile duct, duodenum, stomach, transverse colon) permits of curative resection; the extension is comparable to some forms of colorectal carcinomas at curative stage D. In contrast, it is probable that an invasion of the portal vein or of the superior mesenteric artery would lead to distant metastases, frequently subclinical at operation. Moreover, stage II should be less severe than stage III, where invasion of the regional lymph nodes is possible, this being criticism similar to that of the TNM classification.

2.4.3 Cubilla's Classification

This classification is said to be the most current, thanks to its simplicity, as it consists of only three different stages of development [17]. It is named after Cubilla, a pathologist who worked at the Memorial Sloan Kettering Cancer Center of New York, and who redescribed the peripancreatic node groups and the frequency of their invasion during the process of pancreatic duct cancer [17]. His findings are striking, based on a systematic examination of all the nodes found in the resected specimens that surgeons had given him. Thus, he has been able to describe five main collecting vessels and five node groups, i.e., superior, inferior, anterior, posterior, and splenic, each of the groups being divided into subgroups (Table 2.9). From the records he kept on the invasion of the node groups, Cubilla then classified exocrine pancreatic cancers according to three stages (Table 2.10).

This classification however, gives little information on the invasion of the adjacent organs. In 1978, Cubilla et al. stated in the Journal of Surgical Oncology [16]: "In some cases, involvement of contiguous organs such as the duodenum occurred, and these were classified as stage II." Should we also regard the invasion of the mesenteric and portal vessels as stage II? As for the other classifications, there is a lack of precision regarding stage-II invasion of the regional nodes. Cubilla et al. talk

Table 2.9. Distribution of lymph nodes (from Cubilla [17])

1. Superior:	gastric superior head superior body
2. Inferior:	inferior head inferior body midcolic
3. Anterior:	pyloric anterior pancreatico-duodenal mesenteric
4. Posterior:	posterior pancreatico-duodenal common bile duct
5. Splenic:	tail of pancreas and splenic

Table 2.10. Staging of pancreatic cancer (from Cubilla [18])

Stage I:	confined to the gland
Stage II:	regional lymph nodes involved
Stage III:	distant metastases present

of group-IV lymph nodes, that is to say, those from the posterior group: "They empty into the posterior pancreatic-duodenal lymph nodes, as well as into the common bile duct lymph nodes, right latero-aortic lymph nodes, and into some nodes at the origin of the superior mesenteric artery" [17]. Hence, the distinction between the juxtapancreatic node groups and the retroperitoneal group is not clearly established. In fact, Cubilla et al. did not research the lymph drainage of the pancreas on an anatomosurgical level, but described the main peripancreatic lymph groups and the frequency of their involvement, regarding the tumor distribution. The merit of this work is to indicate which of the node groups are to be resected during Whipple's operation of the head of the pancreas – a regional, total, or subtotal pancreatectomy. Moreover, they demonstrated that more node groups than those regularly resected during Whipple's operation could be involved in cases of cancer of the head of the pancreas. They thus gave a formal pathological bias toward total or regional pancreatectomy.

2.4.4 A New Proposal

At present, we are more familiar with intrapancreatic tumor invasion as we have just mentioned, in particular with the various aspects and the frequency of the multiple-foci forms, as well as with lymph flow and node relay. In other words, we can now explore the pancreas prior to and during surgery. Tumor assessment and extensive examinations are easier. We can get a rapid cytodiagnosis and biopsies of the gland and of the distant metastases. We will not detail the diagnostic techniques, but we would like to say that nowadays, in a center for digestive surgery managed by experienced surgeons, we should be able to classify developmental stages of exocrine pancreatic cancers in a more complete and exact manner that is, however, neither tedious nor difficult.

Taking into account recent findings, we envisage this classification as divided into the following four stages:

Stage I: the tumor is localized to the gland
Stage II: invasion of the juxtapancreatic nodes or the first relay nodes
Stage III: extension into the second relay nodes and/or to the adjacent tissues
            a) duodenum, stomach, colon
            b) superior mesenteric artery, portal vein, and the afferents
Stage IV: involvement of the third relay nodes and/or distant metastases

More specifically, in stage I the tumor is strictly limited to the gland. The peripancreatic peritoneum is not invaded, but the common bile duct may be. Regarding stage II, the term "juxtapancreatic/first relay nodes" refers to the anterior and posterior duodenum pancreatic nodes, the splenic chain, the nodes of the gastrohepatic omentum and the inferior pancreatic chain. At stage III the adjacent tissues are involved, and the cancer spreads to the peripancreatic peritoneum, the duodenum, the stomach, and the transverse colon, which form the subgroup "a", and to the arteriovenous axis, subgroup "b", as outlined above. We differentiate these two directions of spreading because even if it is macroscopically possible to do enlarged curative resections in the first case, it seems difficult to do so when there is invasion of the vessels. Vascular resection is still possible, but can we then continue to speak of curative resection? Stage III includes the nodes of the transverse mesocolon root and the mesenteric and hepatic pedicula, all of which are what we have called nodes of second relay.

Finally, stage IV includes distant metastases and the nodes of third relay, i.e. the node groups localized in the main retroperitoneal lymph ducts, particularly the laterocaval, lateroaortic, interaorticocaval, and left sub- and paranephric nodes and the celiac bundle.

In conclusion, taking into account lymphatic drainage with its various node relays, we attempt in this classification to rank the developmental severity of the disease. We also attempt to differentiate between extension to neighboring gastrointestinal structures and those to vascular axes, as we feel that each type has a distinct prognostic value. Doubtless, the staging in four parts is far from perfect, but considering that since Fortner, regional pancreatectomies have been performed in specialized centers and are considered routine operations, we believe is provides an objective understanding of the therapeutic results.

References

1. Alexandre JH, Billebaud TH, Molkhou JM, Soubielle C, Laget JL (1984) Cystodeno-carcinome pancréatique. A propos d'un cas et revue de la littérature. J Chir (Paris) 121 (2): 77–80
2. Becker V (1978) Carcinoma of the pancreas and chronic pancreatitis. A possible relationship. Acta Hepatogastroenterol (Stuttg) 25: 257–259

3. Bienhayme J, Gross P (1975) Tumeurs malignes du pancréas chez l'enfant. Présentation de deux cas. Ann Chir Infant 17: 131
4. Boutelier P, Callard P, Champault G (1981) La cytoponction per-opératoire dans les tumeurs solides du pancréas. Chirurgie 107: 568
5. Boutelier P, Callard P, Champault G (1984) La cytoponction per-opératoire dans les tumeurs solides du pancréas. Forum. In: Actualités chirurgicales. 85° Congrès Français de Chirurgie. II. Chirurgie abdominale et digestive (2ème partie). Masson, Paris, pp 84-85
6. Bret P, Labadie M, Moulin B, Descos P, Palliard P, Lambert R (1981) Place de la cytoponction guidée par voie transcutanée en pathologie digestive. Gastroenterol Clin Biol 5: 151 A
7. Bret PM (1984) La ponction percutanée du pancréas à l'aiguille fine. In: Actualités chirurgicales. 85° Congrès Français de Chirurgie. II. Chirurgie abdominale et digestive (2ème partie). Masson, Paris, pp 86-93
8. Campagno J, Oertel J (1978) Mucinous cystic neoplasms of the pancreas with overt and latent malignancy. Am J Clin Pathol 69: 573-580
9. Camprodon R, Quintanilla E (1984) Successful long term results with resection of pancreatic carcinoma in children: prognosis for an uncommon neoplasm. Surgery 95 (4): 420-426
10. Cancer of the Pancreas Task Force (1981) Staging of cancer of the pancreas. Cancer 47: 1631-1637
11. Cantrell BB, Cubilla AL, Erlandson RA, Fortner J, Fitzgerald PJ (1981) Acinar cell cystodenocarcinoma of human pancreas. Cancer 47: 410-416
12. Christoffersen P, Poll P (1970) Peroperative pancreas aspiration biopsies. Acta Pathol Microbiol Scand [Suppl] (1973) 212: 28
13. Corrin B, Gilby E, Jones N, Patrick J (1973) Oat cell carcinoma of the pancreas with ectopic ACTH secretion. Cancer 31: 1523-1527
14. Cubilla AL, Fitzgerald PJ (1975) Morphological patterns of non-endocrine human carcinoma. Cancer Res 35: 2246
15. Cubilla AL, Fitzgerald J (1979) Cancer of the pancreas. A suggested morphologic classification. Semin Oncol (1978) 6 (3): 285-297
16. Cubilla AL, Fitzgerald PJ, Fortner JG (1978) Pancreas cancer - duct cell adenocarcinoma: survival in relation to site, size, stage and type. J Surg Oncol 10: 465-482
17. Cubilla AL, Fortner J, Fitzgerald PJ (1978) Lymph node involvement in carcinoma of the head of the pancreas area. Cancer 41: 880-887
18. Cubilla AL, Fitzgerald PJ (1979) Classification of pancreatic cancer (non endocrine). Mayo Clin Proc 54: 449-458
19. Diebold MD, Pluot M, Caulett, Payen L, Patey M (1984) De l'intérêt de l'examen cytologique extemporané au cours des affections pancréatiques. Arch Anat Cytol Pathol 32 (1): 58
20. Endo Y, Morii T, Tamura H, Okuda S (1974) Cytodiagnosis of pancreatic malignant tumors by aspiration, under direct vision, using a duodenal fiberscope. Gastroenterology 67: 944-951
21. Fitzgerald PJ (1981) Pancreatic cancer (non-endocrine) at a Cancer Hospital (1949-1978). Pancreatic cancer. UICC Rep 57: 13-29
22. Forsgren L, Orel S (1973) Aspiration cytology in carcinoma of the pancreas. Surgery 73: 38
23. Fortner JG, Kim DK, Cubilla AL, Turnbull A, Pahnke LD, Shils ME (1977) Regional pancreatectomy. Ann Surg 186: 42-50
24. Frantz VK (1959) Tumors of the pancreas. Armed Forces Institute of Pathology, sect 7, fasc 27 and 28: 27-73
25. Gaston EA (1948) Total pancreatectomy. N Engl J Med 238: 345-354
26. Grosfeld JL, Clatworthy HW, Hamoudi AB (1970) Pancreatic malignancy in children. Arch Surg 101: 370
27. Hamoudi AB, Misugi K, Grosfeld JL, Reiner CB (1970) Papillary epithelial neoplasm of pancreas in a child. Report of a case with eledion microscopy. Cancer 26: 1126-1134
28. Haarstock RJ, Fisher ER (1961) In situ carcinoma of pancreas. Arch Surg 82 (5): 674-678
29. Hermreck AS, Thomas CY, Friesen SR (1974) Importance of pathologic staging in the surgical management of adenocarcinoma of the exocrine pancreas. Am J Surg 127: 653-657
30. Herter FP, Cooperman AM, Ahlborn JN, Antinori C (1982) Surgical experience with pancreatic and periampullary cancer. Ann Surg 195: 274-281
31. Hobbs RD, Stewart AF, Ravin RD, Carter D (1984) Hypercalcemia in small cell carcinoma of the pancreas. Cancer 53 (7): 1552-1554

32. Hodgkinson DJ, Remine WH, Weiland LH (1978) A clinicopathologic study of 21 cases of pancreatic cystadenocarcinoma. Ann Surg 188: 679-684
33. Horie Y, Gonyuda M, Yukihiro K (1984) Plasma carcinoembryonic antigen and acinar cell carcinoma of the pancreas. Cancer 53 (5): 1137-1142
34. Huntrakoon M (1983) Oncocytic carcinoma of the pancreas. Cancer 51 (2): 332-336
35. Ihse I, Lilja P, Arnesjo B, Bengmark S (1977) Total pancreatectomy for cancer. An appraisal of 65 cases. Ann Surg 186: 675-680
36. Kloppel G, Morohoshi T, John HD (1981) Solid and cystic acinar cell tumor of the pancreas. Virchows Arch 392: 171-183
37. Kloppel G, Held G, Morohoshi T, Seifert G (1982) Klassifikation exokriner Pankreas-Tumoren. Pathologie 3: 319-328
38. Kozu T (1972) Duodenoscopic collection of intraductal pure pancreatic juice and its application to the cytodiagnosis. In: Endoscopy of the small intestine with retrograde pancreato-cholangiography. International Workshop at Erlangen. Thieme, Stuttgart
39. Kozuka S, Sassa R, Taki T, Masamoto K (1979) Relation of pancreatic duct hyperplasia to carcinoma. Cancer 43: 1418-1430
40. Kozuka S (1980) Pathogenesis of duct hyperplasia in the pancreas. Digestion 20: 234-247
41. Labadie M, Descos L, Berger F (1980) La fonction cytologique du pancréas. Etude préliminaire. Arch Anat Cytol Pathol 28 (3): 175-179
42. Leach WB (1950) Carcinoma of the pancreas. A clinical and pathological analysis of 39 autopsied cases. Am J Pathol 26: 333-347
43. Leadbetter A, Foster RS, Haines CR (1975) Carcinoma of the pancreas - Results from the Vermont Tumor Registry. Am J Surg 129: 356-360
44. Lemon H, Byrnes W (1949) Cancer of the biliary tract and pancreas. Diagnosis from cytology of duodenal aspirations. JAMA 141: 252-257
45. Lisa JR, Trinidad S, Rosenblatt MB (1964) Pulmonary manifestations of carcinoma of the pancreas. Cancer 17: 395-401
46. Marty-Double C, Balmes P, Pignodel C, Raffnel C, Prat P, Deixonne B (1981) Carcinome pancréatique à stroma amyloïde avec sécrétion de calcitonine. Etude ultra-structurale. Ann Pathol 1 (1): 99-101
47. Matsui Y, Aoki Y, Ishikawa O, Iwigana T, Wada A, Tateishi R, Kosaki G (1979) Ductal carcinoma of the pancreas: rationales for total pancreatectomy. Arch Surg 114: 722-726
48. Moossa AR, Lewis MH, Mackie CR (1979) Surgical treatment of pancreatic cancer. Mayo Clin Proc 54: 468-474
49. Morohoshi T, Held G, Kloppel G (1983) Exocrine pancreatic tumours and their histological classification. A study based on 167 autopsy and 97 surgical cases. Histopathology 7 (5): 645-661
50. Nagaraj H, Polk HC (1984) Pancreatic carcinoma in children. Surgery 95 (4): 505
51. Oertel JE (1975) Personal communication cited by Cubilla and Fitzgerald (1979)
52. Oguma S, Nippo K, Ketsueki T, Gakka-Sasshi S (1983) Plasmacytoma of the head of the pancreas. 5 cases. J Clin Pathol 36: 147-152
53. Piorkowski RJ et al. (1982) Pancreatic and periampullary carcinoma. Am J Surg 143: 189-193
54. Pissas A (1982) Essai d'anatomie clinique et chirurgicale sur la circulation lymphatique du pancreas. Medical dissertation, University of Bobigny
55. Pissas A (1983) Préliminary study of the lymphatic drainage of pancreas. Folia Angiol 10-12
56. Pliam MB, Remine WH (1975) Further evaluation of total pancreatectomy. Arch Surg 110: 506-512
57. Pour PM, Sayed S, Sayed G (1982) Hyperplastic, preneoplastic and neoplastic lesions found in 83 human pancreas. Am J Clin Pathol 77: 137-145
58. Raskin H, Wenger J (1958) The diagnosis of cancer of pancreas, biliary tract, and duodenum by combined cytologic and secretory methods. Exfoliative cytology and description of rapid method of duodenal intubation. Gastroenterology 34: 996-1008
59. Rosai J (1968) Carcinoma of pancreas simulating giant cell tumor of bone. Cancer 22: 333-344
60. Ross DE (1954) Cancer of the pancreas, a plea for total pancreatectomy. Am J Surg 87: 20-33
61. Rouviere H (1948) Anatomie humaine descriptive et topographique, vol 1/2. Masson, Paris
62. Sato T, Saitoh Y, Noto N, Matsuno S (1978) Factors influencing the late results of operations for carcinoma of the pancreas. Am J Surg 136: 582-586

63. Shapiro TM (1975) Adenocarcinoma of the pancreas. A statistical analysis of biliary by pass US. Whipple resection in good risk patients. Ann Surg 182: 715-721
64. Solassol C, Joyeux H, Yakoun M, Blanc F, Bories P (1984) La pancréatectomie régionale dans le traitement de l'adénocarcinome du pancréas. Gastroenterol Clin Biol 8: 17-21
65. Sommers SC, Murphy SA, Warren S (1954) Pancreatic duct hyperplasia and cancer. Gastroenterology 27: 629-640
66. Stamm BH (1984) Incidence and diagnostic significance of minor pathologic changes in the adult pancreas at autopsy. Hum Pathol 15 (7): 677-683
67. Tatsuta M, Yamamoto R, Yamamura H, Okuda S, Tamura H (1983) A cytologic examination and CEA Ca measurement in aspirated pancreatic material collected by percutaneous fine-needle aspiration biopsy. Cancer 52: 693-698
68. Trepeta RW (1981) Giant cell tumor (osteoclastoma) of the pancreas. A tumor of epithelial origin. Cancer 48: 2022-2028
69. Tryka AF, Brooks JR (1979) Histopathology in the evaluation of total pancreatectomy for ductal carcinoma. Ann Surg 190: 373-381
70. Van Heerden JA, Remine WH, Weiland LJ, McIlrath DC, Ilstrup DM (1981) Total pancreatectomy for ductal adenocarcinoma of the pancreas. Am J Surg 142: 308-311
71. Van Kemmel M, Rwamasirab OE, Lagache G (1983) 152 cancers du pancreas; classification sectorielle et options thérapeutiques. Chirurgie 109: 260-267
72. Watanobe K, Inamura S, Uehara T (1982) A case of pancreatic carcinoma presenting ascite as an initial sign (with special reference to possible precancerosites of chronic calcifying pancreatitis). Acta Hepato-Gastroenterol (Stuttg) 29: 216-219
73. Webb JN (1977) Acinar cell neoplasms of the exocrine pancreas. J Clin Pathol 30: 103-112

3 Clinical Features

A. Dubois

The diagnosis of pancreatic cancer is difficult, as it concerns an organ whose clinical and radiological exploration is awkward and because the deficiencies of its exocrine or endocrine functions are rare or difficult to determine. So far, a carcinoma of the pancreas is revealed only by late clinical and/or radiological associated symptoms, due to invasion of the contiguous organs. None of these signs are specific [6, 7, 8]. The evolution is accompanied by intense and rapid denutrition. All these facts explain the difficulty of diagnosis in the early stage of the disease, and this delay explains why curative surgery is usually impossible.

3.1 Classical Types

3.1.1 Painful

Pain is the most frequent symptom of pancreatic cancer, whatever its localization [6, 8] (Table 3.1). In more than half the cases, it is the first symptom to appear [7] and it can have a prolonged evolution [8, 32]. Classical studies report the seat of pain to vary according to the localization of the malignancy: right upper quadrant for cancer of the head, left upper quadrant for cancer of the tail, and upper abdominal for cancer of the body of the pancreas. Actually, there are no strict anatomoclinical parallelisms (Table 3.2). In a series of 255 patients presenting pancreatic cancer, Gambill [16] recorded the location of the pain as upper abdominal 23%, midepigastric 46%, right upper quadrant 18%, left upper quadrant 13%, lower abdominal 20%. Pain is very characteristic of carcinoma of the body and tail of the pancreas. Frequently associated with a systemic alteration of general health, it closely resembles the pancreatico-solar syndrome that Chauffard described in 1908 [9]. The pain is transfixing in 60% of cases, but it may sometimes develop in aberrant radiations. Facilitated by decubitus, such pain causes insomnia and rapidly becomes severe, agonizing; its intense paroxysmal evolution reminds one of tabetic attacks. It can sometimes be soothed by genupectoral posture or ventral decubitus. It may be located strictly in the back, confusing the diagnosis because the abdominal examination is normal. Unfortunately, such pain is a bad sign, indicating an invasion of the celiac region. Exploratory laparotomy generally uncovers a widespread and unresectable cancer.

Table 3.1. Frequency of main symptoms in pancreatic cancer according to the localization of the tumor (from Braganza and Howatt [6])

	Cancer of the head		Cancer of the body and of the tail	
	No	(%)	No	(%)
Total no. of cases	67		21	
Weight loss	56	(83)	15	(71)
Pain	47	(70)	19	(90)
Jaundice	57	(85)	5	(22.5)
Asthenia	26	(36)	7	(33)
Anorexia	29	(44)	11	(52)
Nausea	14	(21)	2	(9.5)
Vomiting	21	(32)	4	(19)
Constipation	9	(14)	5	(23.5)
Diarrhea	25	(38)	7	(33)
Mental symptoms	4	(6)	3	(14)
Thrombophlebitis	5	(8)	2	(9.5)

Table 3.2. Duration of ten most frequent symptoms, from onset of symptom to diagnosis: percentage based on 924 cases with presence of symptoms known (from Cancer of the Pancreas Task Force [8])

Symptom	Short duration <2 months (%)	Long duration >2 months (%)	Unknown duration (%)
Pain	31	38	9
Weight loss	20	47	9
Anorexia	25	26	6
Jaundice	33	8	4
Nausea	24	15	5
Light stool	26	10	5
Dark urine	28	7	4
Vomiting	21	9	4
Constipation	10	12	10
Abdominal distention	11	5	7

Any transfixing upper abdominal pain indicates a pancreatopathy.

A preoperative diagnosis of pancreatic cancer may be invalidated by an exploratory laparotomy, which sometimes reveals chronic pancreatitis, as exemplified by the case of a 63-year-old man who had been suffering postprandial epigastralgia for months. Then the pain changed, lying in the left upper quadrant and radiating in the back, but keeping its paroxystic postprandial character. There was a past history of alcohol and tobacco consumption. There was a weight loss of 3 kg within 3 months, and anorexia was noticeable; however, there was no diarrhea or fever. At clinical examination, cutaneous signs of alcoholic intoxication were seen. The liver was firm and 13 cm long on the midclavicular line. On a biological level, the sedimentation rate was 85; there was macrocytosis of $102\,\mu^3$, leukocytosis of $10000/mm^3$, with 82% of the white blood cells being polynuclear neutrophils, hyperamylasemia at 100 IU/liter (Nl 7–37), and hypocalcemia at 2.16 mmol/liter (Nl 2.20–2.40). Abdominal ultrasound showed a heterogeneous hypoechogenic region in the body of the pancreas, 3 cm in diameter, with a slightly globular tail. Retrograde pancreatography showed a stenosis of Wirsung's duct associated with a loss of the efferent ductules and upper dilatation. Laparotomy invalidated the diagnosis of pancreatic cancer by showing an enlarged pancreas with an inflammatory reaction and some steatonecrosis recalling pancreatitis. A resection of the body and the tail of the pancreas with splenectomy and cholecystectomy was performed. All of the diverse biopsy specimens were modified by significant lesions of fibrous chronic pancreatitis. At contact, the pancreatic acinar cells were being modified by very important degenerative alterations. In many sites, the chronic pancreatitis foci were increased by some necrotic pseudocysts. No tumor lesion could be found and the subsequent evolution proved to be favorable.

3.1.2 Jaundiced

Jaundice associated with pancreatic cancer appears progressively, is frequently preceded by pruritus, and is always accompanied by dark urine and pale, off-white stools in which the characteristic fat is not always found. In the beginning, general good health is retained and weakness is absent, in contrast to jaundice associated with viral hepatitis.

The jaundice is obstructive, with severe hepatomegaly. The discovery of an enlarged but painlessly distended gallbladder is of great semiological value (Courvoisier–Terrier law). The gallbladder is palpable in only one-third of patients harboring a cephalic tumor [6, 17] (Table 3.3). Hepatomegaly is found with cancer of the head of the pancreas in more than 70% of cases; usually, it implies the presence of cholestasis. Tumors of the body and tail of the pancreas appear in two-thirds of cases and are generally congruent with metastases [6, 17].

Table 3.3. Physical findings in pancreatic cancer (from Braganza and Howatt, in Sarles and Howatt [7])

	Cancer of the head		Cancer of the body and tail	
	No.	(%)	No.	(%)
Number of cases	67		21	
Hepatomegaly —with jaundice	52	(77)	4	(19)
Hepatomegaly —all cases	59	(88)	14	(66)
Gallbladder palpable —with jaundice	19	(29)	3	(14)
Gallbladder palpable —all cases	21	(31)	4	(19)
Pancreatic mass	7	(10)	6	(29)
Ascites	5	(8)	2	(9.5)
Splenomegaly	6	(9)	0	–

At an advanced stage the pancreatic biliary syndrome of Bard and Pic [3] appears; it associates jaundice, pruritus, massive loss of weight, enlarged cholostatic liver, and enlarged gallbladder with the rare deep epigastric tumor.

Discovery of an enlarged gallbladder on palpation of a jaundiced patient is almost always an indication of pancreatic cancer.

Actually, clinical examination is usually normal during the preliminary stage. The important thing when examining a jaundiced patient is to assess, by means of ultrasound, the dilatation of the biliary ducts and to determine clearly the localization and nature of the obstacle.

Jaundice associated with pancreatic cancer may be accompanied by symptoms of cholangitis linked with pain, febrile attacks, intermittent jaundice, and hyperleukocytosis. A diagnosis of cholelithiasis can also be made; the succession with in 48 h of pain, fever, and jaundice retains its significance. Diagnosis is frequently assessed by means of computerized tomography.

Only laparotomy permits confirmation of the diagnosis or the discovery of papillary cancer, common bile duct cancer, or even chronic pancreatitis. This differential diagnosis is difficult because pancreatitis can occasionally hide a small cancer.

The significance of this jaundice is far from univocal: it is a late symptom of extensive invasion of the head, or adenopathy, or liver metastases, and an early symptom that reveals primary cancer developing close to the papilla or in contact with the common bile duct in the retropancreatic region.

3.1.3 Cachectic

Loss of more than 10% of the ideal weight [27] is frequently significant, but has not yet been fully explained. Anorexia and maldigestion due to insufficient exocrine function and diabetes mellitus are contributing factors. Weight loss may appear alone but is frequently accompanied by pain or "little symptoms" such as hiccupping or dyspeptic troubles.

Any important or progressive loss of weight must prompt one to look for a gastrointestinal neoplasm, above all for a pancreatic cancer.

Case Report. A 55-year-old man was admitted to hospital because of a weight loss of 10 kg in 1 year (representing a loss of 15%) and of nonradiating left basis thoracalgia, maximal during the night. Six months before, diabetes mellitus had been diagnosed and treated by a low-carbohydrate diet. Clinical examination showed a left lumbar systolic murmur. An abdominal CT scan showed evidence of a heterogeneity in the body of the pancreas. Abdominal ultrasound confirmed this, but also showed stricture of the superior mesenteric vein and a stenosis of the splenic artery. Exploratory laparotomy revealed segmental portal hypertension, a pancreatic tumor mass in the body and tail, adherent to the posterior plane, some retroperitoneal adenopathy, and liver metastases. Exeresis was impossible. Histological examination confirmed an adenocarcinoma. Death occurred 60 days after surgery.

3.1.4 Tumor

The frequency of tumor varies, according to different authors, between 8% and 35% of cases [4, 21] (Table 3.3). Usually it appears as a deep and firm neoplasm that can transmit aortic throbbings, mimicking pseudoaneurysm. A CT scan of the abdomen and the retroperitoneum can change the previous diagnosis of an abdominal mass.

An epigastric mass leads one to consider an enlargement of the left quadrant lobe of the liver, carcinoma of the stomach, transverse colon, or body of the pancreas, or a retroperitoneal tumor. A mass in the left upper quadrant indicates a colic tumor, splenomegaly, enlarged kidney, or carcinoma of the tail of the pancreas.

The semiotic features of the mass (anterior margin crenated of a splenomegaly, lumbar contact, and abdominal bloating of an enlarged kidney, with the stony consistency of a neoplastic mass) and the associated symptoms allow one to approach a diagnosis. Auscultation of the abdominal mass in search of a systolic murmur must be done systematically. It is too often true that exploratory laparotomy reveals an unresectable tumor.

3.2 False Types

If the varied grouping of pain, jaundice, and weight loss indicates the classical symptoms of cancers of the head, body, and tail of the pancreas described 50 years ago, some pancreatic cancers may be revealed by an unique and sometimes deceptive symptom.

3.2.1 Rheumatological

Posterior pain may mimic that of a vertebral ailment because it appears at night with insomnia, is increased on coughing, and radiates in a hemi-lap belt. This pain is troubling by its persistence, tenacity, and above all the concomitant alterations in outward signs; it becomes more intense and sometimes evolves into paroxysms.

Clinical examination is astonishingly normal in view of the intensity of the pain. X-rays of the rachis may show no modifications on two successive examinations. The diagnosis is more difficult as the classical symptoms may be lacking. This is illustrated by the following case: A 48-year-old man was admitted to hospital due to a change in his general state of health (8 kg weight loss within months – 12% loss of weight) and to dorsal pains that had persisted for the past 18 months. The original posterior site of the pain had recently changed to become epigastric, with postprandial attacks increased by dorsal decubitus. Clinical evaluation was normal. No discosomatic lesions were revealed by X-rays of the rachis. Ultrasonography and a CT scan of the abdomen showed evidence of an ascitic lamina, a dilatation of the splenoportal trunk, and some retroperitoneal adenopathy. Exploratory laparotomy revealed chylous ascites, dilatation of the epiploic vessels and of the round ligament, diffuse peritoneal carcinosis, liver metastases, and a hard, fixed, tumor mass linked to the pancreas, the mesentery, and the transverse colon. The histological examination showed that it was an adenocarcinoma presenting, in places, ductular architecture. Death occurred 1 month after surgery.

Any persistent dorsal pain with normal lumbar X-rays of the rachis and with normal upper gastric tract endoscopy indicates, as a first priority, the search for a neoplastic invasion of the celiac region.

3.2.2 Gastrointestinal

3.2.2.1 Gastrointestinal Troubles

Dyspeptic troubles may create some digestive harassment associated, to some extent, with epigastric heaviness, postprandial flatulence, some regurgitation, and hiccupping. All of these symptoms may go along with or even precede by months some more suggestive symptoms. Attention must be paid to the digestive system, but gastrointestinal troubles rarely require exploration of the pancreas.

3.2.2.2 Ulceration   .

A typical ulceration syndrome may indicate pancreatic cancer [25]. Upper gastroendoscopy can easily rule out a gastroduodenal lesion. The actual difficulty exists when a gastric or duodenal ulcer is associated with pancreatic cancer. Diagnosis is falsely comforting and is further misled by the finding of the ulcer, which is temporarily relieved by efficient anti-ulcer therapy. Faced with a lesion in the duodenal region, it is essential to rule out pancreatic cancer before diagnosing an autonomic lesion [33].

3.2.2.3 Disorders of Elimination

In the early stage of pancreatic cancer transit disorders are sometimes the only symptoms. Their frequency is diversely reported [1, 28]. Constipation is important only in case of a recent manifestation. Diarrhea is rare, and steathorrea is inconstant. Malabsorption occurs only in patients in whom the output of pancreatic enzymes is reduced by 90% [11].

Case Report. A 64-year-old woman was admitted to the hospital for diarrhea which had been occurring for 6 months. It consisted in four or five loose and fetid stools per day and was associated with the recent onset of diabetes, anorexia, and a loss of 17 kg in 10 months. Clinical examination was normal. No mass was palpable, nor was there any abdominal murmur. The thyroid gland was not palpable either. The weight of the stools ranged from 600 g to 800 g per 24 h. No steatorrhea and, biologically, no symptoms of malabsorption were to be found. Hyperamylasemia and amylasuria were both found at times. Barium enema and gastroscopy were normal. Transit through the small intestine, except for an acceleration, was normal, as was a histological examination of the structure. Hypervascularization of the region of the body and tail of the pancreas and clotting of the splenic artery were proven by angiography of the celiac trunk. CT scan, abdominal ultrasound, and retrograde roentgenography indicated a mass localized in the body of the pancreas. This was confirmed during laparotomy with the finding of an unresectable tumor of the isthmus and body of the pancreas, including the mesenteric vessels. Histological findings showed an adenocarcinoma.

3.2.2.4 Duodenal Stenosis

Duodenal stenosis is exceptional. It occurs late after palliative therapy and may indicate a carcinoma of the head, the isthmus of the pancreas [5, 14, 24, 36].

Case Report. A 58-year-old man was admitted to the hospital because of a loss of 10 kg within 2 months, asthenia, anorexia, and epigastric pain alleviated by postprandial vomiting. An eccentric and irregular stenosis, 3 cm long, on the upper part of the second duodenum was brought to attention by an esophagogastroduodenal transit. The abdominal ultrasound indicated a carcinoma of the head of the pancreas. This diagnosis was confirmed by surgery which revealed a tumor localized in the head of the pancreas associated with a major duodenal stenosis. Peroperative ultrasonography visualized a stenosis of the portal vein; histology proved this to be an adenocarcinoma. The operation consisted of a subtotal duodenopancreatectomy with restoration of the continuity by means of choledochojejunal and gastrojejunal anastomoses with a Roux-Y loop and a hepatic metastasectomy.

3.2.2.5 Gastrointestinal Hemorrhage

Gastrointestinal hemorrhages are rare. Their mechanism is not simple. They can happen secondary to an invasion of the gastroduodenal mucous membrane or secondary to a compression or a thrombosis of the peripancreatic venous network with portal hypertension. Hemorrhage frequently indicates carcinoma of the body and the tail of the pancreas [18, 30, 37].

3.2.2.6 Ascites

Ascites is rarely of significance for diagnosis. It exists in 10%–20% of cases [6, 16] (Table 3.3). Generally, it appears very late in the course of the disease and indicates venous compression or peritoneal carcinosis [29]. The blocking of the retroperitoneal lymphatics may entail chylous ascites.

3.2.3 Psychic

Psychic types of pancreatic cancer have been reported by Yaskin [40] and Kohn [22]. Anxiety and depression appear in half of the cases but their pathogenesis is still obscure. Fras et al. [15] noticed mental symptoms in 76% of patients presenting a pancreatic cancer, as against 17% of patients suffering from a carcinoma of the colon.

3.2.4 Febrile

A lasting fever can be the only symptom of pancreatic cancer. It appears in 25% of cases and might be associated with a biological inflammatory syndrome.

When faced with an unexplained fever, it is the rule to look for a deep cancer, especially a pancreatic cancer.

3.2.5 Endocrine

The outbreak of *hyperglycemia* in a previously healthy patient, or the sudden aggravation of a diabetes that until then was well balanced, even though it is nonspecific, makes one suspect pancreatic cancer. A recent onset of diabetes mellitus occurs in 25% of all cases [17].

Renin secretion by the pancreatic tumor is exceptional [31]. It brings out hypertension which leads the patient to seek medical advice. The symptomatology is sometimes secondary to hypokalemia (poyluria, thirst, and muscle cramps).

Hypoglycemia is exceptional. It may reveal a tumor of the exocrine pancreas by a duct obstruction involving the head of the pancreas [26].

The apparition of diabetes mellitus after 40 years of age without any particular predisposition (obesity, heredity) or an unexplained aggravation of the same may be signs of pancreatic cancer.

3.2.6 Blood-Vascular

Phlebitis can be an indication of pancreatic cancer [12, 35]. Classically, it is superficial, with little inflammation, frequently taking on the appearance of the "wire of iron" described by Favre [13]. It is likely to recur or migrate to unusual areas (cervical region, thoracic or abdominal wall). It is sometimes associated with portal thrombosis and is then accompanied by gastrointestinal hemorrhage and splenomegaly.

A *systolic murmur* from the upper abdomen or left upper quadrant may be the only symptom of pancreatic cancer. Such an observation is not pathognomonic, but it does aid a definitive diagnosis [2, 39] and is an indication for superior mesenteric angiography. Because it gives evidence of stenosis of the splenic artery, systolic murmur is frequently synonymous with unresectability [2, 20].

> When pancreatic cancer is suspected, auscultation of the abdomen must be done systematically.

Case Report. A 55-year-old man was admitted to the hospital after losing 10 kg within 1 year. For months he had suffered left posterior basithoracic pain, nonradiating, moderate, and maximal at night. Diabetes mellitus had recently appeared. At clinical examination the only sign found was an aspirative systolic murmur, distant, and perceived in the left lumbar cavity. The electrocardiogram and thoracic X-rays were normal. Abdominal ultrasound and a CT scan showed a heterogeneity of the head and body of the pancreas, with compression of the superior mesenteric and splenic arteries. At surgery, a heterogeneous pancreatic mass of the head and body of the pancreas was found. There was adhesion to the posterior venous plane which compressed the superior mesenteric artery, as well as segmental portal hypertension, approximately ten liver metastases, 3–10 cm in diameter, and adenopathy at the level of the celiac trunk and of the mesenteric root. No radical surgery was possible. At cytology, some malignant cells proved the presence of adenocarcinoma in the region of the tail of the pancreas. The patient died 3 months after laparotomy.

This report underlines the lack of anatomoclinical parallelism as far as pancreatic cancer is concerned. Poor clinical symptoms are unfortunately related frequently to large and unresectable lesions.

3.3 Metastatic Types

Metastases can be revealing and are often accessible by means of needle aspiration or biopsy. They develop mainly at the level of the liver (invasion via the portal vein or the lymph vessels of the hepatic pedicle) and are too often responsible for isolated hepatomegaly. Invasion then reaches the mediastinial, supraclavicular, and cervical nodes. There are two particular forms: pleural effusion with elevated amylase activity, and steatonecrosis.

3.3.1 Pleural Effusion

Pleural effusion with elevated amylase activity is less frequent in pancreatic cancer than in pancreatitis [34]. Effusion is abundant, inexhaustible, and recurring. In order to be significant, the pleural amylase levels must be 5 to 10 times higher than those of serum amylase.

3.3.2 Steatonecrosis

Steatonecrosis, both cutaneous and systemic, can be encountered with carcinoma of the pancreas [19, 23, 38]. A relationship between the former lesion and nondegenerative febrile nodular panniculitis (Weber-Christian syndrome) has been hypothesized [10, 23]. The association of this syndrome with pancreatic cancer is rare and, when present, complicates diagnosis [10].

References

1. Ansari A, Burch GE (1968) A correlative study of proven carcinoma of the pancreas in 83 patients. Am J Gastroenterol 30: 456-475
2. Balmes JL, Alquier Y, Bert JM, Carriere J (1969) Le syndrome artériel des cancers du pancréas. Arch Fr Mal App Dig 58: 605-606
3. Bard L, Pic A (1888) Contribution à l'étude clinique et anatomo-pathologique du cancer primitif du pancréas. Rev Méd 8: 267-273
4. Berk JE (1941) Diagnosis of carcinoma of the pancreas. Arch Intern Med 68: 525-529
5. Blum M, Frank P, Legal Y (1965) Cancer de la tête du pancréas à expression duodénale. Arch Fr Mal App Dig 54: 1099
6. Braganza JM, Howat HT (1972) Cancer of the pancreas. Clin Gastroenterol 1: 219-237
7. Braganza JM, Howat HT (1980) Tumeurs du pancréas exocrine. In: Sarles H, Howat HT (eds) Le pancréas exocrine. Paris, pp 463-495
8. Cancer of the Pancreas Task Force (1981) Staging of cancer of the pancreas. Cancer 47: 1631-1637
9. Chauffard MA (1908) Le cancer du corps du pancréas. Bull Acad Med 60: 242-255
10. Delaware J, Capron JP, Chivrac D, Dupas JL, Gontier MF, Lorriaux A (1977) Syndrome de Weber-Christian et cancer du pancréas. Etude d'un cas et revue de la littérature. Gastroenterol Clin Biol 10: 789-798
11. Dimagno EP, Malagelada JR, Go VLW, Moertel CG (1977) Fate of orally ingested enzymes in pancreatic insufficiency: comparison of two dosage schedules. N Engl J Med 296: 1318-1322
12. Edwards EA (1949) Migrating thrombophlebitis associated with carcinoma. N Engl J Med 240: 1031-1035
13. Favre M (1953) La phlébite "fil de fer". Presse Med 61: 579-582
14. Fraisse M, Paysan G (1957) Sténose de l'angle duodéno-jéjunal par cancer de la tête du pancréas. Arch Fr Mal App Dig 46: 1040-1041
15. Fras I, Litin EM, Bartholemew LG (1968) Mental symptoms as an aid in the early diagnosis of carcinoma of the pancreas. Gastroenterology 55: 191-198
16. Gambill EE (1970) Pancreatic and ampullary carcinoma: diagnosis and prognosis in relation to symptoms, physical findings and elapse of time as observed in 255 patients. South Med J 63: 1119-1122
17. Gullik HD (1959) Carcinoma of the pancreas: a review and critical study of 100 cases. Medicine (Baltimore) 38: 47-84

18. Hurwitt ES, Altman JF, Gerst GR, Webber BM (1954) Gastro-intestinal bleeding due to splenic vein obstruction by pancreatic tumors. Arch Surg 68: 7
19. Jackson SH, Savidge RS, Stein L, Varley M (1952) Carcinoma of the pancreas associated with fat necrosis. Lancet 268: 962-967
20. Joyeux R, Mirouze J, Colin R, Dossa J, Lapeyrie H (1969) A propos du syndrome artériel du cancer du pancréas. Arch Fr Mal App Dig 58: 399-400
21. Justin Besancon L, Pequignot M, Etienne JP, Delavierre P, Thiroloix J (1966) Les aspects du cancer pancréatique en médecine générale. Sem Hop Paris 42: 417-421
22. Kohn LA (1952) The behavior of patients with cancer of the pancreas. Cancer 5: 328-335
23. Lievre JA, May V, Benichou C, Camus JP, Marlais J, Lievre JA (1964) Stéato-nécrose disséminée, ostéolyse stéato-nécrotique et cancer du pancréas. Discussion du syndrome de Weber-Christian. Bull Mem Soc Med Hop Paris 115: 755-771
24. Lindenauer SM, Reuter SR, Joseph RR (1968) Carcinoma of the head of the pancreas presenting as duodenal obstruction without jaundice: an uncommon manifestation with a note on visceral angiography as an aid in diagnosis. Am J Surg 115: 705-708
25. Lortat-Jacob JL (1966) Ulcères gastro-duodénaux et cancer du pancréas. Lyon Chir 62: 438-441
26. McBee JW, Lanza FL, Erickson EE (1966) Hypoglycaemia due to obstruction of pancreatic excretory ducts by carcinoma. Arch Pathol 81: 287-291
27. Malagelada JR (1979) Pancreatic cancer. An overview of epidemiology, clinical presentation and diagnosis. Mayo Clin Proc 54: 459-467
28. Moldow RE, Connelly RR (1968) Epidemiology of pancreatic cancer in Connecticut. Gastroenterology 55: 677-686
29. Parrish RA, Humphries AL, Moretz WM (1968) Massive pancreatic ascites. Arch Surg 96: 887-891
30. Peycelon R, Delore X, Jegou Y, Porta JP, Miouron JM (1965) Cancer du pancréas à forme occlusive et hémorragique. Lyon Chir 61: 404-406
31. Ruddy MC, Atlas SA, Salerno FG (1982) Hypertension associated with a renin-secreting adenocarcinoma of the pancreas. N Engl J Med 307: 993-997
32. Sahel J (1983) Progrès dans le diagnostic des cancers du pancréas. Actualités digestives médico-chirurgicales. Masson, Paris, pp 117-127
33. Schops R (1969) Niche du troisième duodénum et cancer du pancréas. Sem Hop Paris 43: 1189-1190
34. Siguier F, Godeau P, Herreman G, Kalifat R, Delluc G (1967) Epanchement pleural à activité amylasique élevée et cancer pancréatique. Bull Soc Med Hop Paris 118: 1287-1298
35. Sproul EE (1938) Carcinoma and venous thrombosis: the frequency of association of carcinoma in body or tail of the pancreas with multiple venous thrombosis. Am J Cancer 34: 566-585
36. Thomas M, Gillet M, Adloff M (1969) Cancer du pancréas révélé par une sténose duodénale aigüe isolée. A propos de 3 observations. Lyon Chir 65: 352-357
37. Vachon A, Romier H (1957) Les hémorragies gastro-intestinales au cours des affections pancréatiques. Sem Hop Paris 11: 641-649
38. Veyssier P, Siguier F (1970) Cyto-stéato nécrose sous-cutanée et cancer du pancréas. Ann Med Interne (Paris) 121: 975-977
39. Warter J, Storck D, Kieny R (1970) Valeur séméiologique de l'auscultation des artères de l'abdomen. Presse Med 78: 421-424
40. Yaskin JC (1931) Nervous symptoms as early manifestations of carcinoma of the pancreas. JAMA 96: 1664-1668

4 Biological Examinations

A. Dubois

Biological examinations have only a relative value in the detection of carcinoma of the pancreas, as they do not completely compensate for the weakness of clinical examinations. Considering the repercussions of the tumor process on the biliary pancreatic functions (cholestasis, diabetes mellitus, pancreatic insufficiency of the exocrine functions), disturbances of the biological parameters are frequently of indirect significance. The hope placed on the assays of certain tumor markers in blood and pancreatic juice, has been disappointing in almost all cases, due to the lack of specificity among the substances studied, regardless of their frequent presence in cancer of the exocrine pancreas.

4.1 Standard Biology

A specific biological systematic test for detection of pancreatic cancer does not exist [7] (Tab. 4.1). Iron deficiency **anemia** may appear secondary to the ulceration of periampullar proliferation or to malignant invasion of gastro-duodenal mucosa. **Hypersplenism** secondary to obstruction of the splenic vein by the pancreatic tumor and the deficiency due to metastatic medullar invasion are exeptional [5].

Table 4.1. Results of laboratory tests done in 10% or more of 924 patients (from Cancer of the Pancreas Task Force [7])

Laboratory test	Test done (%)	Test result (% of cases having test done)		
		Depressed	Normal	Elevated
WBC count	88	7	60	32
Hemoglobin	85	48	49	3
Hematocrit	83	43	54	3
Serum bilirubin	77		40	60
Serum alkaline phosphatase	75	3	25	72
Serum SGOT	66	1	33	66
Prothrombin time	50	13	57	30
Platelet count	48	10	78	12
LDH	47	4	50	46
Serum amylase	44	15	64	21
Serum SGPT	23		36	64

Carcinoma of the head of the pancreas is often expressed by a **cholestatic syndrome** combined with hyperbilirubinemia, as well as by an increase in alkaline phosphatases, gammaglutamic transferase and 5'nucleotidase. There is no correlation between hyperbilirubinemia and the increase in alkaline phosphatases [4]. **Cytolysis** appears in two thirds of all patients [8]; sometimes, initially, it may appear at the onset of the disease, thus, leading to a false diagnosis.

An **inflammation** is frequently found in the febrile types. An insulin-dependent **diabetes** exists in 34% of all patients before surgical intervention [31]. An oral glucose-tolerance test is pathological in 47% of cases [42].

Elevated **amylase** and **lipase** activities are less frequent [27].

Gullick's study reports the detection of **blood in stools** with 54% of patients [22]; the frequency was comparable regardless of the tumor's localization.

Frequency of **steatorrhoea** is variable, however, it does never exceed 25% in the reported series. It seems to be more frequent with head tumors than with body and tail tumors [4].

4.2 Pancreatic Function Tests

Sensitivity of functional tests is variable. Most of them show advanced pancreatic insufficiency only, with clinical evidence of malabsorption. More sensitive ones, require a duodenal intubation and stimulation of pancreatic secretion. The obstruction of the main pancreatic duct leads to diminution of volume of the secretions collected in the duodenum after secretin stimulation [6, 13]. Reduction rate of debit depends on the localization of the tumor. In the secretin test, Dreiling [15] reported reduced volumes in 95% of patients with cancer of the head, in 59% of patients with cancer of the body, whereas only 3% with cancer of the tail. Similar rates were found by other authors with the cholecystokinin test [11, 12].

Progressive deterioration of pancreatic functions affects initially, with preference, the enzymatic secretion stimulated by pancreozymin rather than bicarbonates secretion after secretin [6, 11].

In fact, whatever the method of stimulation of exocrine pancreatic secretion, duodenal intubation shows a decrease of the pancreatic secretory capacity in 90% of patients whose cancer is localized in the head, and in 80% of the patients whose cancer is localized on the tail and body [38]. Unfortunately sensitive tests are not at all specific. Actually, pancreatic cancer and chronic pancreatitis are overlapping diseases.

In case of retentional jaundice, the biliary response to secretin [14] and to cholecystokinin [6] is unable to distinguish head tumors of biliary ducts from vesicular lithiasis.

The PABA-test is a tubeless digestive test, but also less sensitive than a direct study of the duodeno-pancreatic juice [9].

4.3 Tumor Markers

4.3.1 Serological Markers

4.3.1.1 Carcinoembryonic Antigen (CEA)

An elevated plasma CEA rate is found in most patients with pancreatic cancer in any stage of development. The quantity of tumor markers produced depends upon the extent of the tumor, on whether there is a pancreatic duct obstruction, on whether liver metastases exist, and also on CEA clearance by the liver. It has been demonstrated [30, 34, 45, 50] that in the advanced stage of the disease, especially with liver metastases, tumors are easily detected, whereas there is no rise in the CEA level in the early stage of pancreatic cancer. Moreover, the plasma CEA level is not very specific. On the other hand, high CEA levels have been reported to occur with other carcinomas and nonmalignant diseases [19], as well as in the case of hepatic insufficiency, benign disorders of the liver, biliary obstruction and metastases of other sites of origin [24, 26, 30].

The plasma CEA rise observed in the advanced stage of pancreatic cancer could be explained by the incapability of the liver to eliminate CEA, rather than by a rapid tumor growth or an excessive production of the antigen. In contrast, the normal levels of CEA observed in the early stages of the malignant process can be explained by the hepatic uptake of CEA. Barkin et al. [2] did a follow-up study on the plasma CEA levels in patients who had been treated for pancreatic cancer. They conclude the following: a) The CEA level is lower in nonjaundiced patients. b) A surgical resection implies a fall in the CEA level. There is no correlation between CEA and survival rates. c) The CEA level increases progressively in advanced metastatic carcinomas of the pancreas. d) Radiotherapy alone or combined with a 5-FU infusion does not change the CEA level in patients with an unresectable tumor.

The presence of CEA in pancreatic juice is an aid in diagnosing pancreatic cancer [11, 28, 43, 46]. Di Magno et al. [11] believe that among the secretory parameters, after cholecystokinin stimulation, enzymatic and bicarbonate outputs show higher correspondence to cancer than do CEA levels. For other authors [43], a rise of the CEA level in plasma and pancreatic juice is a strong probability of cancer.

4.3.1.2 Pancreatic Oncofoetal Antigen (POA)

In 1974, Banwo et al. [1] reported the existence of a fetal antigen in patients with pancreatic carcinoma. Three years later, Hobbs et al. [23] proved that this oncofetal antigen was different from CEA, alpha-fetoprotein, and other antigens or plasma proteins. Gelder et al. [20] showed that the oncofetal antigen was a glycoprotein (mol. wt. = 800000) which exists in both the fetal and the tumor pancreas, whereas it no longer exists in the normal adult pancreas. However, the oncofetal antigen is not specific, since high levels are found in sera from patients affected by pancreatic cancer as well as in other malignant or benign conditions. With a selected threshold value of 14 ng/ml of serum the specificity is relatively high (90%) but the sensitivity is low (47%) [32]. In conclusion, the elevated oncofetal antigen level in pancreatic juice would have a specificity and a sensitivity of 79% [41].

4.3.1.3 Alpha Fetoprotein (AFP)

The sensitivity (33%) and the specificity (71%) of the increase in concentration of serum alpha-fetoprotein are insufficient to be of use in diagnosing carcinoma of the pancreas [32, 37].

4.3.1.4 Galactosyltransferase Isoenzyme II (GT II)

In 1978, Podolsky et al. [36] underlined the presence of an isoenzyme of galactosyltransferase (GT II) in the serum of cancer patients. They found GT II in the sera of 165 of 232 patients suffering from various cancers. GT II was not found in a control group of 58 patients, 15 of whom had chronic or acute pancreatitis. In 1981, Podolsky et al. [37] showed that serum-GT II was the most sensitive seromarker (67%) for pancreatic cancer, twice as sensitive as CEA (34%).

For Bellart et al. [3], the galactosyltransferase activity assay discriminates between chronic pancreatitis and pancreatic cancer in only 50% of cases. Owing to its difficult assay and its lack of specificity, this test is not frequently used.

4.3.1.5 Lactoferrin and Trypsin

Lactoferrin has been isolated from the pancreatic juice of patients operated upon for calcifying chronic pancreatitis [16, 18]. Nevertheless, the specificity of lactoferrin in chronic pancreatitis was established from the study of a very small number of carcinomas of the pancreas. An increase in the lactoferrin content in pancreatic juice does not rule out the possibility of pancreatic cancer [35]; this rise may be correlated with lesions of combined pancreatitis, either surrounding the tumor or in the parenchyma distal to a stenosis of Wirsung's duct.

The level of trypsin is high in normal people, low when there is pancreatic cancer, and variable in the case of chronic pancreatitis [16, 17].

4.3.1.6 Carbohydrate Antigen 19-9 (CA 19-9)

Carbohydrate antigen 19-9 is isolated by means of a monoclonal antibody. It consists of a migratory mucin-like glucoprotein. Its glucide component makes it similar to the Lewis blood-type antigens. CA 19-9 appears to be a pancreatic tumor marker of great value [10, 39, 48]. The preliminary results of a multicentered French study are encouraging. Issued from monoclonal antibody technology, CA 19-9 can be used not only in the diagnosis of pancreatic cancer (assays of serum and pancreatic

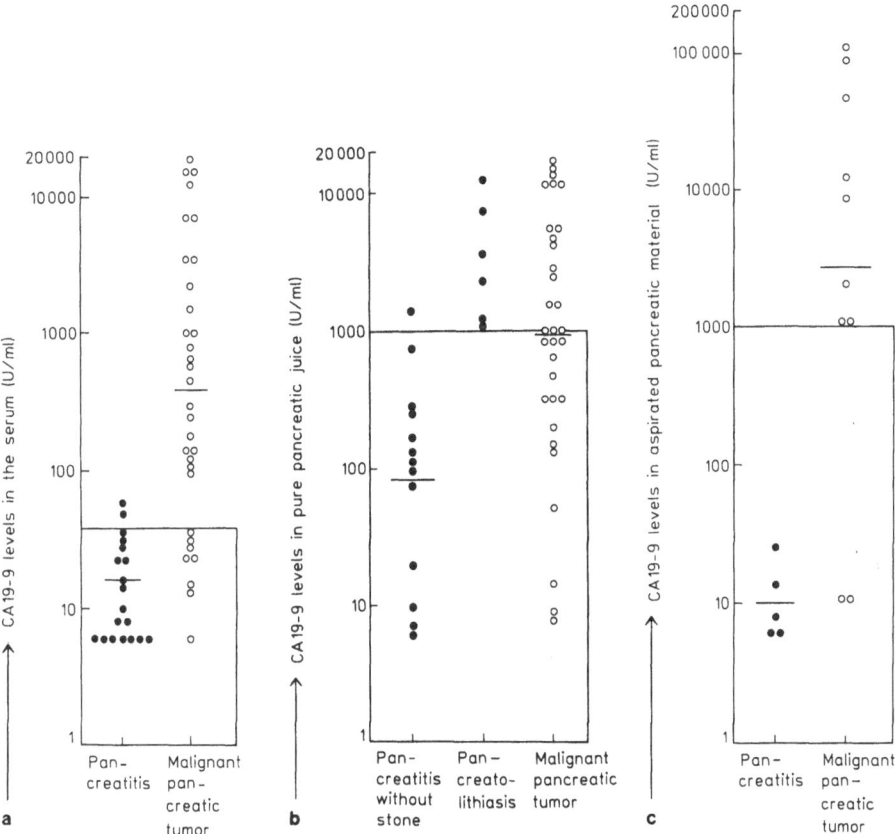

Fig. 4.1 a–c. Data from Tatsuta et al. [47]. **a** CA 19-9 levels in the serum of patients with malignant pancreatic tumors and pancreatitis. Horizontal bars indicate mean values and shading indicates the normal range. **b** CA 19-9 levels in pure pancreatic juice from patients with malignant pancreatic tumors and patients with pancreatitis with and without pancreatolithiasis. Horizontal bars indicate mean values and shading indicates the normal range. **c** CA 19-9 levels in pancreatic materials obtained by aspiration biopsy of the pancreas from patients with malignant pancreatic tumors and pancreatitis. Horizontal bars indicate mean values and shading indicates the mean range

juice), but also in a systematic appraisal of a high-risk population. Venot et al. [49] reports that in the case of an isolated pancreatopathy, an elevated CA 19-9 level indicates a neoplasm, whereas a low level is consistent with a benign pancreatic condition. More prospective studies are required to clarify the exact value of this new marker, especially as in a recently reported study [33], the specificity of CA 19-9 (0.84) tested on 102 patients with malignant or benign gastrointestinal or pulmonary diseases, was not proved to be higher than the specificity of CEA (0.90).

Nevertheless, a recent study of Tatsuta et al. [47] shows interesting results (Fig. 4.1). According to these authors the combination of the CA 19-9 assay and the cytologic study of specimens obtained by percutaneous fine-needle aspiration biopsy of the pancreas increase the diagnostic rate to 100%.

4.3.1.7 Other serological markers

The use in the field of diagnosis of new markers developed from samples of pure pancreatic juice [25, 44] remains to be defined.

4.3.2 Antitumor Immunity

A leukocyte adherence inhibition assay (LAI) with tumor pancreatic samples has been suggested in order to diagnose early pancreatic cancer [21, 41]. Goldrosen et al. [21] had positive results for this procedure in 11 of 12 patients with localized carcinomas, in ten of 12 patients with a liver free of metastases, and in 21 of 36 patients with liver metastases. These same authors proposed an inhibition assay of the migratory leukocytes obtained from normal subjects in the presence of patients' sera. Sensitivity appears to be lower. The false-positives of both tests seem to be rare (less than 5%). Whatever the technique used, the clinical significance of this test is yet to be confirmed.

In conclusion, at the present time there is no specific marker of carcinoma of the pancreas. The lack of specificity in the field of symptomatology is an even stronger argument for finding a marker which would permit early diagnosis and detection of recurrence.

References

1. Banwo O, Versey J, Hobbs JR (1974) New oncofetal antigen for human pancreas. Lancet 1: 643-645
2. Barkin JS, Kalser MH, Kaplan R, Redlhammer D, Heal A (1978) Initial levels of CEA and their rate of change in pancreatic carcinoma following surgery, chemotherapy and radiation therapy. Cancer 42: 1472-1476
3. Bellart M, Vion A, Colombel JF, Cortot A, Paris JC, Montreuil J (1985) L'activité galactosyl + transférase sérique n'est pas un bon marqueur tumoral de cancer du pancréas. Gastroenterol Clin Biol 9: 205 A
4. Braganza JM, Howat MT (1972) Cancer of the Pancreas. Clinics in Gastroenterology 1: 219-237
5. Braganza JM, Howat MT (1980) Tumeurs du pancréas exocrine: in H. Sarles et MT Howat. Le Pancréas Exocrine, Paris 463-495
6. Burton P, Evans DG, Harper AA, Howat MT, Oreesky S, Scott JE, Varley H (1960) A test of pancreatic function in man based on the analysis of duodenal contents after administration of secretin and pancreozymin. Gut 1, 111-124
7. Cancer of the pancreas task force: Staging of cancer of the pancreas. Cancer 1981, 47, 1631-1637
8. Collure WD, Burns GP, Schenk WG (1974) Clinical, pathological and therapeutic aspects of carcinoma of the panceas. Am J Surg 1974, 128, 683-689
9. Delchier JC, Soule JC (1983) BT-PABA test with plasma PABA measurements: Evaluation of sensitivity and specificity. Gut 24: 318-325
10. Del Villano BC, Brennan S, Brock P, Bucher C, Liu V, McClure M, Rake B, Space S, Westrick B, Schoemaker H, Zurawski VR (1983) Radio-immunometric assay for a monoclonal antibody-defined tumor marker CA 19-9. Clin Chem 29: 549-552
11. Di Magno EP, Malagelada JR, Moertel CG, Go VLW (1977) Prospective evaluation of the pan-

creatic secretion of immuno-reactive carcino-embryonic antigen, enzyme and bicarbonate in patients suspected of having pancreatic cancer. Gastroenterology 73: 457–461

12. Di Magno EP, Malagelada JR, Taylor WP, Go VLW (1977) A prospective comparison of current diagnostic tests in pancreatic cancer. N Engl J Med 297: 737–742

13. Dreiling DA (1951) Studies in pancreatic function, in the use of the secretin test in the diagnosis of tumors in and about the pancreas. Gastroenterology 18: 184–196

14. Dreiling DA, Hollander F (1948) Studies in pancreatic function, preliminary series of clinical studies with secretin test. Gastroenterology 11: 714–729

15. Dreiling DA (1970) The early diagnosis of pancreatic cancer. Scan J Gastroenterol (suppl) 6: 115–122

16. Estevenson JP, Sarles M, Figarella C (1975) Lactoferrin in the duodenal juice of patients with chronic pancreatitis. Scand J Gastroent 10: 327–330

17. Fedail SS, Harvey RF, Salmon PR, Brown P, Read AE (1978) Trypsin and lactoferrin levels in pure pancreatic juice in patients with pancreatic disease. Gut 20: 983–986

18. Fedail SS, Salmon PR, Harvey RF, Brown P, Read AE (1978) The value of pure pancreatic juice trypsin in the differential diagnosis of pancreatic disease. Gastroenterology 74: 1154

19. Fitzgerald PJ, Fortner JG, Watson RC, Schwartz MK, Sherlock P, Cubilla AL, Schottenfeld D, Miller D, Winauer SJ, Lightdale CJ, Leidner SD, Nisselbaum JS, Menendez-Bodet CJ, Poleski MH (1978) The value of diagnostic aids in detecting pancreatic cancer. Cancer 41: 868–879

20. Gelder FB, Reese CJ, Moossa AR, Hall T, Hunter R (1978) Purification, partial characterization, and clinical evaluation of a pancreatic oncofetal antigen. Cancer Res 38: 313–324

21. Goldrosen MH, Dashmahapatra K, Jenkins D, Howell JC, Arbuck SG, Moore MC, Douglas HO (1981) Microplate leucocyte adherence inhibition (LAI) assay in pancreatic cancer: Detection of specific antitumor immunity with patient's peripheral blood cells and serum. Cancer 47: 1614–1619

22. Gullick MD (1959) Carcinoma of the pancreas. Medicine 38: 47–84

23. Hobbs JR, Knapp ML, Branfoot AC (1979) Oncofetal pancreatic antigen (OPA), its frequency and localization in humans (Abstract N° 1) VIIth Mtg. International Society for Oncodevelopmental Biology and Medicine. London, Sept 1979 (Abstract)

24. Khoo SK, Mackay IR (1973) Carcino-embryonic antigen in serum in disease of the liver and pancreas. J Clin Path 26: 470–475

25. Klavins JW (1981) Tumor markers of pancreatic carcinoma. Cancer 47: 1597–1601

26. Lurie BB, Loewenstein MS, Zamcheck N (1975) Elevated carcino-embryonic antigen levels and biliary tract obstruction. J Amer Med Assn 233: 326–330

27. Malagelada JR (1979) Pancreatic cancer. An overview of epidemiology clinical presentation and diagnosis. Mayo Clin Proc 34: 459–467

28. Molnar IG, Vandevoorde JP, Gitnick GL (1976) CEA levels in fluids bathing gastro-intestinal tumors. Gastroenterology 70: 513–515

29. Moore TL, Kupchik HZ, Marcon N, Zamcheck N (1971) Carcino-embryonic antigen assay in cancer of the colon and pancreas and other digestive tract disorders. Amer J Digest Dis 16: 1–7

30. Moore T, Dhar P, Zamcheck N, Keeley A, Gottlieb L, Kupchik HZ (1972) Carcino-embryonic antigen(s) in liver disease. Clinical and morphological studies. Gastroenterology 63: 88–94

31. Moossa AR (1982) Pancreatic cancer: Approach to diagnosis selection for surgery and choice of operation. Cancer 50: 2689–2698

32. Moossa AR, Levin B (1981) The diagnosis of "early" pancreatic cancer: the University of Chicago experience. Cancer 47: 1688–1697

33. Olsson NO, Crimet-Montange D, Martin F (1985) Valeur diagnostique d'un nouveau marqueur sérique des cancers digestifs humains: l'antigène carbohydrate 19.9 (CA 19-9). Comparaison avec l'antigène carcino-embryonnaire. Gastroentérol Clin Biol 9: 206–211

34. Ona FV, Zamcheck N, Dhar P, Moore T, Kupchik H (1973) Carcino-embryonic antigen (CEA) in the diagnosis of pancreatic cancer. Cancer 31: 324–327

35. Pignal F, Benque A, Bouisson M, Arany Y, Ribet A (1984) Lactoferrine et cancer du pancréas. Gastroentérol Clin Biol 8: 982

36. Podolsky DK, Weiser MM, Isselbacher KJ, Cohen AM (1978) A cancer-associated galactosyltransferase isoenzyme. N Engl J Med 299: 703–705

37. Podolsky DK, McPhee MS, Alpert E, Warshaw AL, Isselbacker KJ (1981) Galactosyl transferase isoenzyme II in the detection of pancreatic cancer: comparison with radiologic, endoscopic and serologic tests. N Engl J Med 304: 1313–1318

38. Reber HA, Tweedie JH, Austin JL (1981) Pancreatic secretions as a clue to the presence of pancreatic cancer. Cancer 47: 1646-1651
39. Ricolleau G, Kremer M, Curtet C, Fumoleau P, Douillard JY, Le Mevel B, Le Bodic L, Chatal JF (1983) Intérêt diagnostique comparé au radio-immunodosage de l'antigène carcino-embryonnaire et de l'antigène CA 19-9 isolé par un anticorps monoclonal. Gastroentérol Clin Biol 7: 25 A
40. Russo AJ, Douglass HO, Leveson SH, Howell JH, Holyoke ED, Harvey SR, Chu TM, Goldrosen MH (1978) Evaluation of the micro-leukocyte adherence inhibition assay as an immunodiagnostic test for pancreatic cancer. Cancer Res 38: 2023-2026
41. Schmiegel WH, Becker WM, Arnot R, Hamann A, Sohendra N, Jessen K, Classen M, Thiele HG (1981) Pancreatic oncofetal antigen in pancreatic juice. Partial chemical characterization and diagnostic application of a pancreatic cancer associated antigen. Scand J Gastroenterol 16: 1033-1040
42. Schwartz SS, Ziedler A, Moossa AR, Kuku JF, Rubenstein AM (1978) A prospective study of glucose tolerance insulin, C-Peptide, N-Glucagon responses in patients with pancreatic carcinoma. Dig Dis Sci 23: 1107-1114
43. Sharma MP, Gregg JA, Loewenstein MS, McCabe RP, Zamcheck N (1976) Carcinoembryonic antigen (CEA) activity in pancreatic juice of patients with pancreatic carcinoma and pancreatitis. Cancer 38: 2457-2461
44. Shimano T, Loor RM, Papsidero LD, Kuriyama M, Vincent RG, Nemoto T, Holyoke ED, Berjian R, Douglass HO, Chu TM (1981) Isolation, characterization and clinical evaluation of a pancreas cancer-associated antigen. Cancer 47: 1602-1613
45. Skarin AT, Delwiche R, Zamcheck N, Lokich JJ, Frei E (1974) Carcino-embryonic antigen: clinical correlation with chemotherapy for metastatic gastrointestinal cancer. Cancer 33: 1239-1245
46. Tatsuta M, Yamamura M, Yamamoto R (1983) Significance of carcino-embryogenic antigen levels and cytology of pure pancreatic juice in diagnosis of pancreatic cancer. Cancer 52: 1880-1885
47. Tatsuta M, Yamamura H, Iishi H, Ichii M, Noguchi S, Yamamodo R, Okuda S (1985) Values of CA 19-9 in the serum, pure pancreatic juice and aspirated pancreatic material in the diagnosis of malignant pancreatic tumor. Cancer 56: 2669-2673
48. Venot J, Vincent D, Clement MN, Beck C (1984) Evaluation d'un marqueur tumoral du pancréas. Résultats préliminaires. La Presse Méd 13: 440-441
49. Venot J, Vincent D, Canard JM, Larnant A, Descottes B (1985) Pathologie pancréatique et CA 19-9. Gastroentérol Clin Biol 9: 204 A
50. Zamckeck N, Moore TL, Dhar P, Kupchik H (1972) Immunologic diagnosis and prognosis of human digestive tract cancer. Carcino-embryonic antigens. New Engl J Med 286: 83-86

5 Morphological Examinations

J.-M. Bruel, F.-M. Lopez, P. Lopez, T. Narboni, and C. Raffanel

Direct examinations of the pancreas have been substituted for indirect ones – whose sensitivity was very poor. Some are invasive (endoscopic retrograde cholangiopancreatomography, angiography). However, pancreatic exploration has benefited from the availability of imaging procedures (ultrasonography, CT). These have quite a high sensitivity and specificity, and therefore always come prior to the invasive procedures. In most cases, clinical examinations of cancer of the pancreas reveal an advanced tumor which is incurable. This cancer must be diagnosed from less suggestive symptoms; hence, more emphasis must be placed on morphological examinations.

5.1 Conventional Roentgenograms

The usual examinations – abdominal plain films and barium studies of the upper gastrointestinal tract – cannot at present be considered of value in diagnosing carcinoma of the pancreas. However, without clinical presenting symptoms which suggest a pancreatic cancer, these examinations are frequently used, and we must be able to recognize the diverse findings that can lead to a diagnosis of pancreatic mass.

5.1.1 Abdominal Plain Films

The following findings on abdominal plain films reveal the loco-regional involvment of an advanced carcinoma:
1. Contiguous invasion: displacement or amputation of the gastric air sac, enlarged gallbladder, splenomegaly by segmental portal hypertension
2. Ascites due to peritoneal carcinosis, lymphatic obstruction, or extravasation of the pancreatic juice subsequent to a rupture of the pancreatic ducts [244]; this may also be correlated with an inflammatory pathology [49, 211].

   Although calcification indicates an inflammatory pathology in 95% of cases [52], it does not rule out with certainty a benign or malignant tumor process. Actually, a carcinoma may develop from a chronic pancreatitis, it may be the origin of a distal pancreatitis, or a pancreatic tumor may become calcified (cystadenoma, cystadenocarcinoma, lymphangioma) [13, 48, 76, 109, 213, 219].

5.1.2 Upper Gastrointestinal Tract

A systematic upper gastrointestinal barium examination is of little value for the diagnosis of pancreatic cancer and is used either in an asymptomological occurrence or – in some rare cases – to evaluate the relation of a cancer with the stomach and the duodenum. The efficiency of radiology of the pancreatic mass depends upon whether the mass is localized in the head or in the body and tail of the pancreas.

Cephalic tumor induces gross abnormalities in the duodenum: enlargement, rounded angles, displacement in profile. Its characteristics are focused abnormalities of a borderline defect (image of a reversed 3 on the right margin of D 2) [70], or stenosis (Fig. 5.1), and changes in the mucosal relief, with a disorganization of the structures and a squamous or spicular aspect. A reflux into Wirsung's duct or the biliary ducts is rarely observed [73].

The efficiency of barium examination is still limited [59, 148]. It can be significantly improved through the use of double contrast and by duodenal hypotony [127, 128, 160, 180, 208].

Carcinoma of the body and tail of the pancreas can be diagnosed by signs of extrinsic compression and/or invasion, mainly in the gastric wall: anterior displacement and impression on the posterior wall [35, 52, 256], displacement toward the upper greater antral curvature, defects essentially in the greater curvature of the stomach and in the posterior wall, indicating a parietal invasion [35]. Even more exceptional are

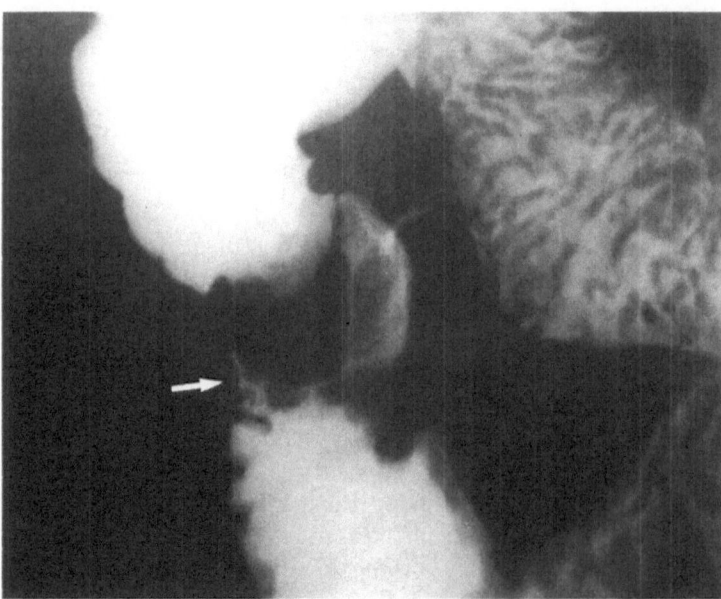

Fig. 5.1. Gastrointestinal tract examination for cancer of the head of the pancreas. *Arrow* shows extrinsic and intrinsic stenosis caused by peripheral infiltration of second duodenum wall

gastric or esophageal varices caused by segmental portal hypertension [132, 195, 268].

At the present time, abdominal plain films and barium examinations are not of great value in detecting pancreatic cancer because of (a) their low diagnostic value, (b) the late appearance of radiological signs, except in the case of pancreatic cancer with a juxtaduodenal site of origin, (c) their lack of specificity in differentiation between chronic pancreatitis and cancer, and (d) the fact that endoscopy prevails in the case of mucosal invasion.

5.2 Ultrasonography and Computerized Tomography

Ultrasonography and computerized tomography are the only examinations which allow direct morphological study of the pancreas.

5.2.1 Ultrasonography (US)

To save time in the examination, it is better to perform it with a real-time scanner, but in some cases it is preferable to use a manual scanning unit, which allows a global view of large anatomical regions [83].

An examination with ultrasonography is easy and painless and can be repeated, and gives information on the shape, size, and structure of the pancreas and at the same time, hepaticobiliary and locoregional assessment.

5.2.1.1 Ultrasound Findings in the Pancreas

Changes in Shape and Size

The study of the pancreatic area is based upon recognition of the vascular landmarks: splenic vein in the back, superior mesenteric artery, superior mesenteric vein, inferior vena cava, and aorta. The shape and size of the pancreas are estimated according to these landmarks. If a modification in shape or size goes along with a displacement of these landmarks, it is easily determined. Otherwise, the estimation is more difficult to perform (Fig. 5.2).

Classical sizes are 25 mm in diameter for the head and 15 mm for the body of the pancreas [47]. Due to a large variability from one patient to another, an increase in size, specially moderate, is difficult to evaluate. For Weill [280], diameters of more than 34 mm for the head and body of the pancreas and 24 mm for the isthmus are to be considered pathological. These values are arguable since they vary according to the series and to the author [102, 161].

The pancreas may be globally enlarged, either because of a voluminous tumor or because of a cephalic tumor associated with upper pancreatitis. The pancreatic

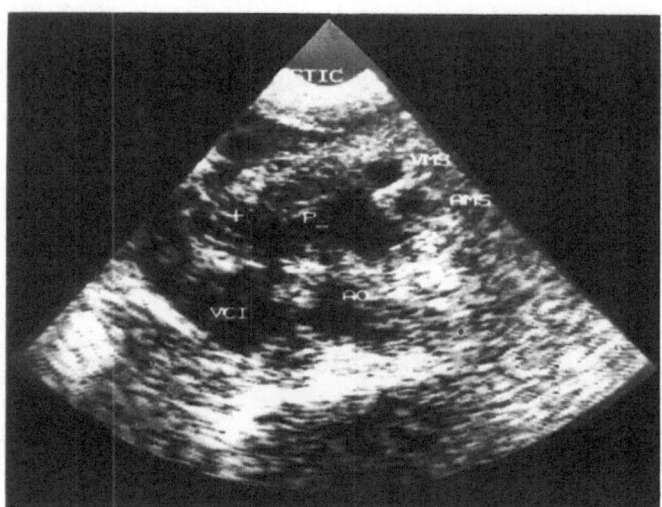

Fig. 5.2. Ultrasound displays peripancreatic vascular landmarks in cancer of the pancreatic head. *VMS* superior mesenteric vein; *AMS* superior mesenteric artery; *VCI* inferior vena cava; *AO* aorta; *P* enlarged, hypoechogenic head of pancreas

mass can be focalized and is detected by the prominence of a margin which generally appears when the tumor diameter is at least 2 cm [50].

Changes in Parenchymal Structure

In a normal subject the echogenicity of the pancreatic tissue (defining the echostructure) is homogeneous. In general, it is equal or more often greater than that of the liver [280]. It is no longer exceptional, thanks to technical advances in ultrasound examination, to visualize a nondilated Wirsung's duct ($\leqslant 2$ mm) [73, 175, 206, 280].

Pancreatic cancer may also be detected from isolated anomalies in echogenicity (Fig. 5.3). These are usually some focalized lesions, globally hypoechogenic in comparison with normal parenchyma, and frequently scattered with highly intense echos. A few cases of hyperechogenic nodules have been reported, but they remain rare (3%) [152, 175, 283]. Moreover, a malignant neoplasm, whatever its size or echogenicity, may appear as an upper dilatation of Wirsung's duct, nearly always noticeable on an ultrasonogram [73, 164, 266, 282] (Fig. 5.4).

Limitations of Ultrasound

When a morphological abnormality exists (especially a mass of large volume displacing the vascular landmarks) sometimes ultrasonography does not help to differentiate between a pancreatic lesion and a juxtapancreatic lesion (adenopathy, renal and suprarenal tumor).

When an ultrasonogram shows a pancreatic lesion, the anomalies of shape and/or echogenicity have no histopathological specificity [1, 189, 247]. As for a dilated

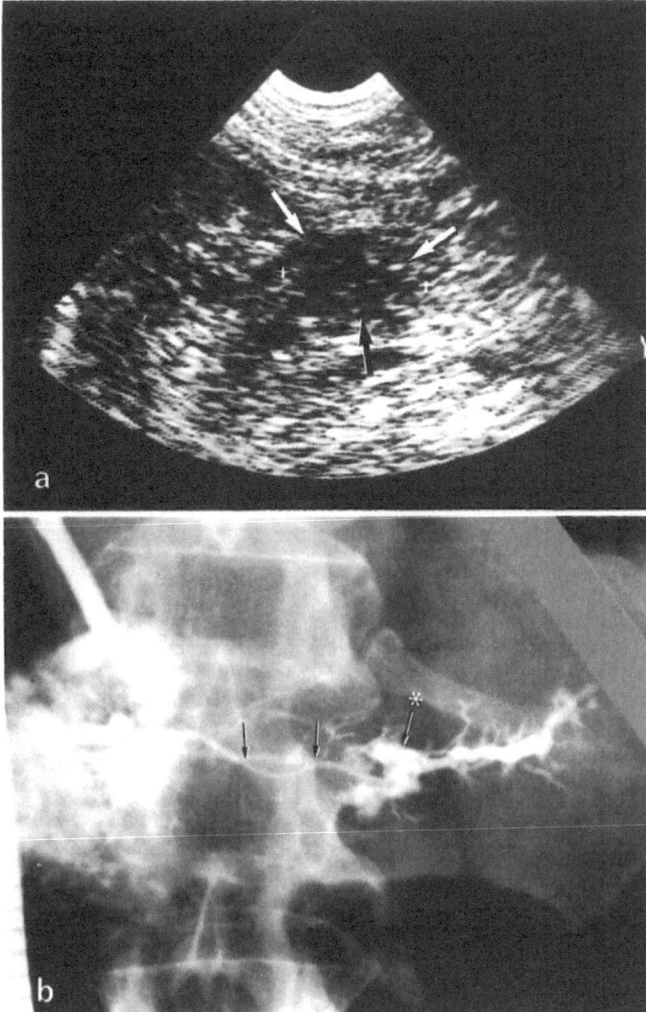

Fig. 5.3a, b. Cancer of body of the pancreas. **a** Ultrasound displays abnormalities in echogenicity, heterogeneous hypoechogenicity and slight enlargement of the body *(arrows)*. **b** Retrograde roentgenography shows stenosis along 3 cm of Wirsung's duct *(plain arrows)* and moniliform dilatation caused by distal pancreatitis *(arrow with asterisk)*

Wirsung's duct, it does not predict the type of lesion since it is also a sign of chronic pancreatitis.

5.2.1.2 Extrapancreatic Ultrasound Signs

An ultrasound semiology of the carcinoma of the pancreas must always include the study of the regional and general extension of the lesion.

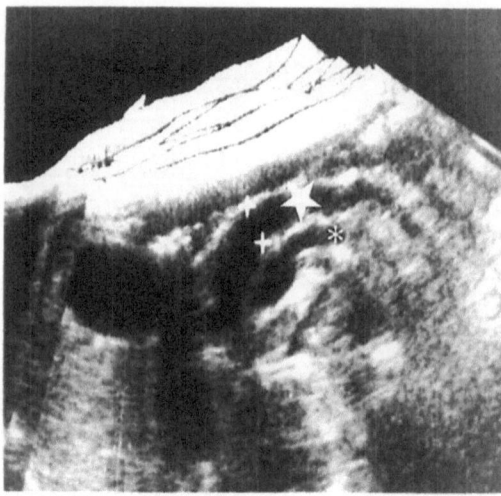

Fig. 5.4. Cancer of the pancreatic head. Ultrasound shows dilatation of Wirsung's duct distal to pancreatic head cancer and *(star)* ventral to the splenic vein *(asterisk)*

Liver and Biliary Ducts

The biliary ducts affected by pancreatic cancer are dilated. At an advanced stage of the disease, this dilatation occurs in all of the biliary ducts: intrahepatic and extrahepatic biliary ducts [166, 179, 243] (Fig. 5.5). In its early course, dilatation can be limited to the common hepatic duct and then to the common bile duct [196, 248]. It is associated with direct symptoms, at times easily identifiable, whether in the case of pancreatic mass (Fig. 5.6) or pedicular adenopathies.

The study of the biliary ducts leads to the search for liver metastases required for characterization. They can be single or multiple, and of variable echogenicity – hypoechogenic, mixed (possibly "bull's eye"), or hyperechogenic. When they are peripheral, they discretely change the margins. Yet, these metastases are difficult to assess with ultrasound when they are small or associated with a significant dilatation of the biliary ducts.

Lymph Node Metastases (Adenopathies)

Celiomesenteric adenopathies appear as generally hypoechogenic tissue masses in contact with the large vascular trunks (superior mesenteric artery, celiac trunk, aorta, and inferior vena cava) and are usually difficult to differentiate from the local extension of the pancreatic mass itself.

Because they disrupt the regional echoanatomy, in particular that of the hepatic pedicle, pedicular adenopathies are sometimes difficult to recognize. However, their recognition is fundamental to the diagnosis of jaundice.

Major Vessels

Ultrasonography allows detection of a vascular displacement or invasion by a pancreatic mass, especially at the levels of the splenic vein (Fig. 5.7) and the superior

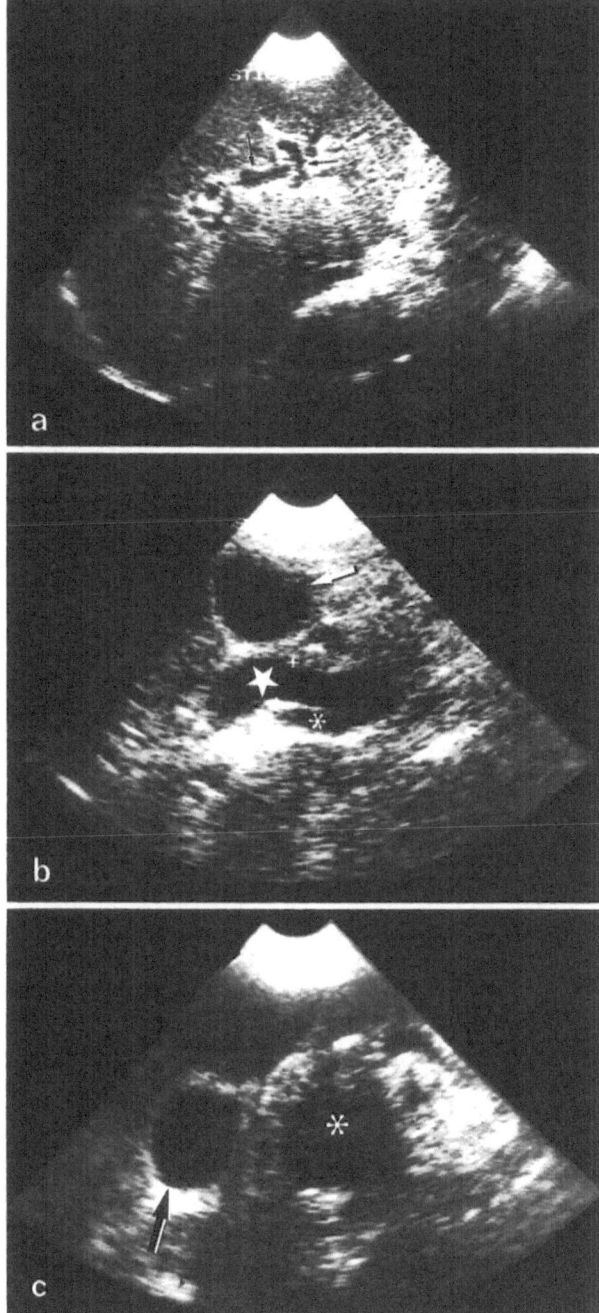

Fig. 5.5 a–c. Demonstration of dilated biliary ducts in cancer of the pancreatic head by ultrasound. **a** *Arrows* show dilated intrahepatic biliary ducts (subhilum transverse section). **b** Dilated extrahepatic biliary ducts: large gallbladder *(arrow)*; common bile duct *(star)* sectioned along its longitudinal axis in front of the portal vein *(asterisk)*. **c** Dilated common bile duct *(arrow)* and visualization of tumor mass *(asterisk)*

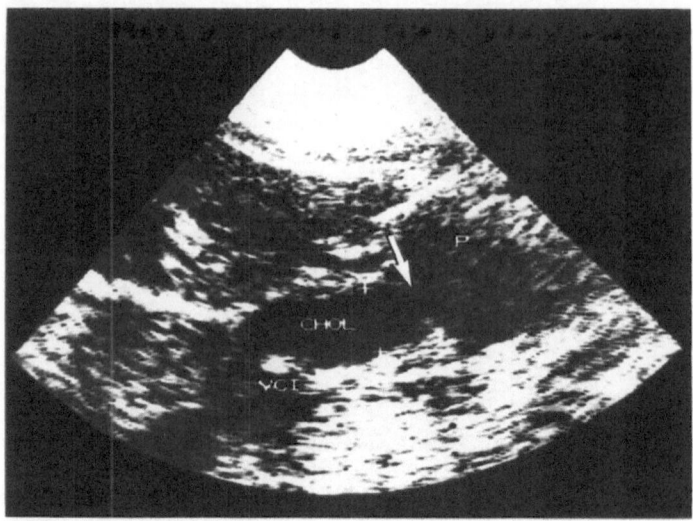

Fig. 5.6. Dilated biliary ducts in cancer of the pancreatic head, demonstrated by ultrasound: common bile duct *(chol)*, sectioned along longitudinal axis; direct image of tumor obstruction in lower common bile duct *(arrow)*, in front of inferior vena cava *(VCI)*

mesenteric vein, and secondarily on the mesenteric artery, the aorta, or the inferior vena cava [131, 175, 277].

Ascites

It is very easy to show a peritoneal liquid effusion, by ultrasonography, but this finding does not help to specify the pancreatic lesion.

5.2.2 Computerized Tomography (CT)

CT is rapidly becoming the method of choice to visualize the pancreas and its surrounding anatomy. At one time, it was used essentially to study transformations in the shape of the pancreas, but recent advances in technology permit an intrapancreatic approach to the lesions by means of a dynamic computed tomography of its vascular composition.

5.2.2.1 CT findings in the Pancreas

Changes in Size and Contour

Except for the irregular and vague limits of the pancreas that is globally invaded by cancer (Fig. 5.8) [262], lesions that alter the pancreas are represented by masses localized either in the head (Fig. 5.9) the body, or the tail of the pancreas. They are rec-

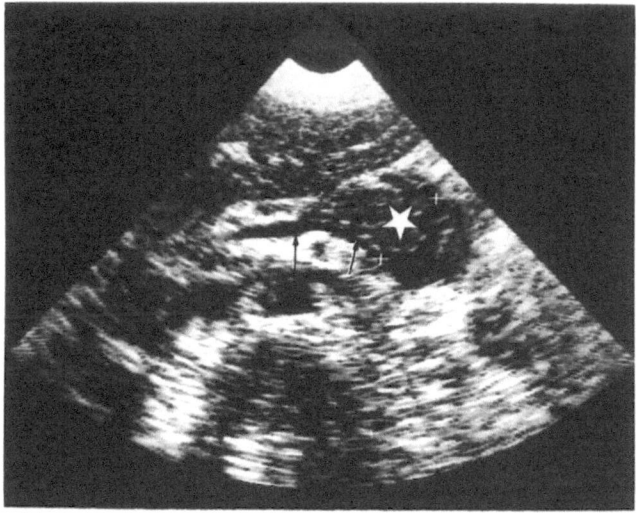

Fig. 5.7. Ultrasound demonstrates the relation of cancer of the pancreas tail to the major peripancreatic vessels. Hypoechogenic mass in tail of pancreas *(star)* encases splenic vein and displaces it posteriorly *(arrows)*

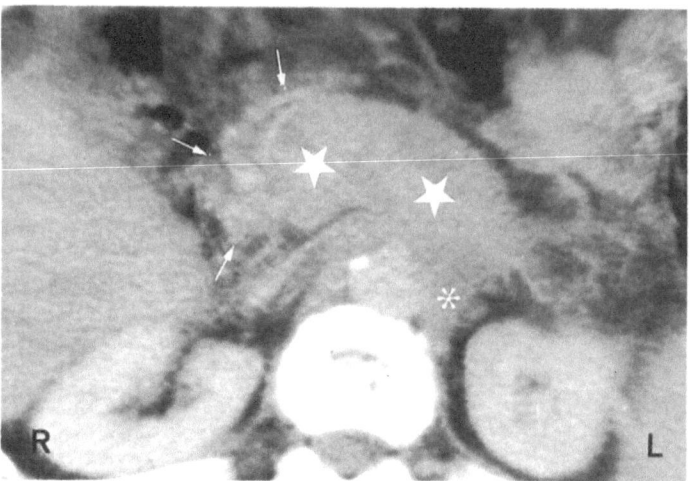

Fig. 5.8. Changes in size and contour of body and head of pancreas due to cancer, shown on CT scan. Enlargement of body and head area *(stars);* heterogeneous density with irregular, poorly defined margins *(arrows);* periaortic infiltration *(asterisk)*

ognized by a CT scan in comparison with the normal pancreas, whose size has been established either in the absolute or in relation to the adjacent vertebral structures [101, 150, 250, 259].

The tumor contours make the normal lobulation of the pancreatic margins disappear (Fig. 5.10): in this particular instance, such lesions are exceptionally equal to

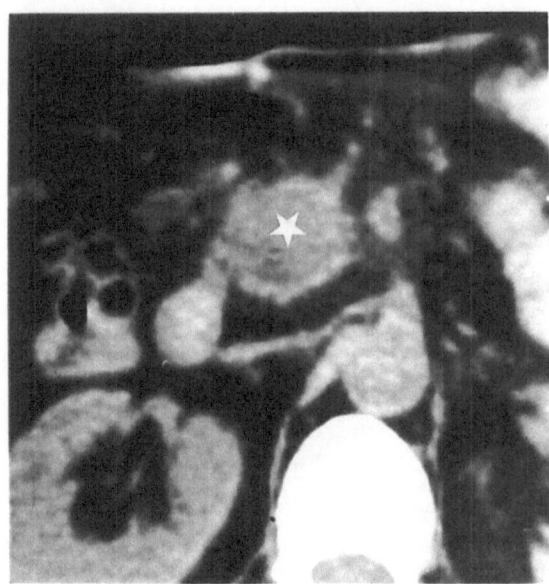

Fig. 5.9. Changes in size and contour of pancreas due to cancer of pancreas head, shown on CT scan. Note globular aspect of head, with enlarged frontal and sagittal diameters *(star)*

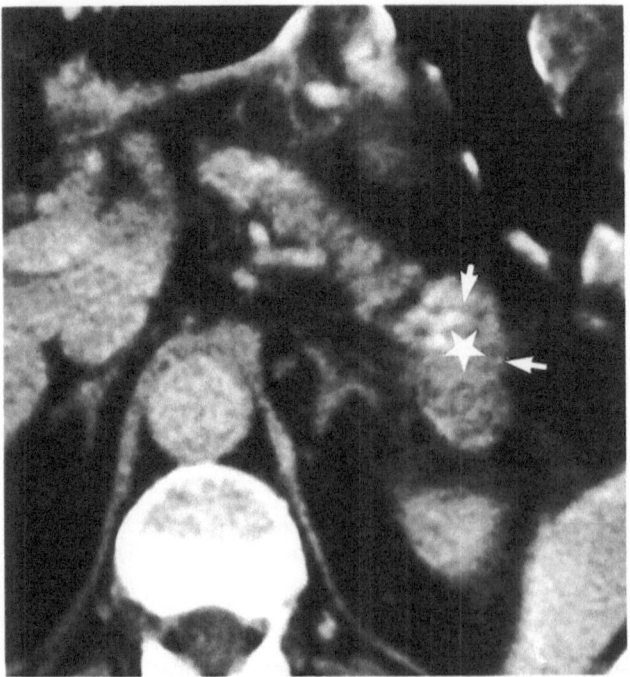

Fig. 5.10. Changes in contour of pancreas due to cancer of pancreas tail, shown on CT scan. Small caudal mass *(star)* modifies shape and causes disappearance of normal lobulations *(arrows)*

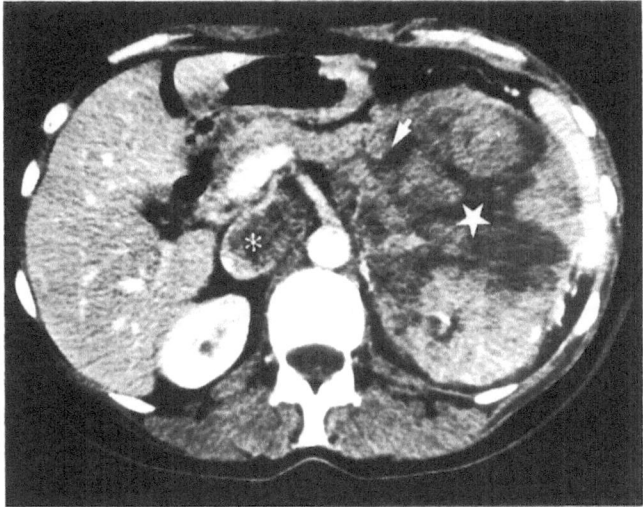

Fig. 5.11. CT scan shows a voluminous heterogeneous mass *(star)* with posterior development, but which seems to be linked to body and tail of the pancreas *(arrow)*. In fact, it is a malignant tumor in the left suprarenal gland (adenoma or carcinoma of adrenal cortex) with thrombosis of the inferior vena cava *(asterisk)*

or less than 15 mm in diameter. In contrast, it is sometimes difficult to confirm the pancreas as the site of origin of very large tumors which have infiltrated the peripancreatic fatty space and disrupted the relationships or the morphology of the adjacent organs (Fig. 5.11).

For lesions of average size, the difficulties linked to the morphological analysis depend upon the intrapancreatic localization of the lesion. For the head of the pancreas, the estimation of an increased volume which prompts a correct identification of the duodenal surroundings by intraluminal contrast medium is not easy, because measurement of the vertical diameter may be a problem, whereas an increase in the anteroposterior diameter is frequently obvious. To these morphological data, one must add the signs of the extrapancreatic changes, in particular, those of the bile ducts.

Cancers in the uncinate process are identified by the displacement of the superior mesenteric vein and artery, whose fatty cuff has disappeared (Fig. 5.12). The study of the margins of the body of the pancreas, in particular when there is little peripancreatic fat, requires identification of the body of the stomach by intraluminal contrast medium.

The tail of the pancreas has a variable topography in comparison with the rest of the gland; the caudal extremity is usually above the body and head of the pancreas, but it is sometimes situated on the same plane or, even more rarely, below. Therefore multiple joint thin cross sectioned scans are required to study the entire tail of the pancreas. Jejunum opacification differentiates between a cluster of loops and an anterior spreading of the mass. Some tumors with posterior spreading may develop behind the splenic pedicle and are then difficult to differentiate from suprarenal and left renal tumors [33]. Moreover, caudal tumors with "exopancreatic" in-

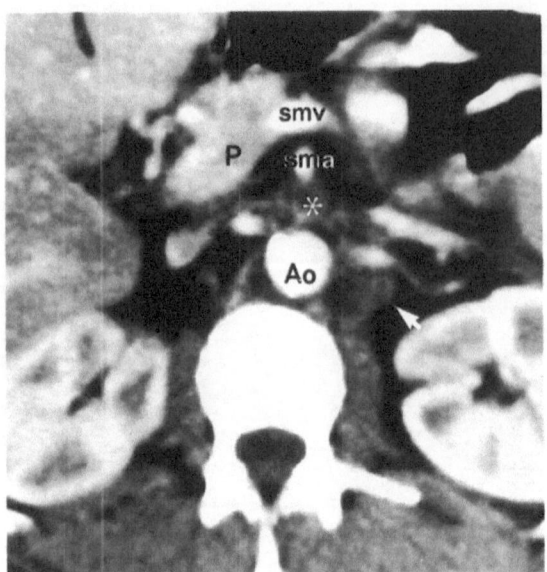

Fig. 5.12. Angioscan showing cancer of the uncinate process. Mainly extrapancreatic tumor excrescence *(asterisk)* with encasement of superior mesenteric pedicle, and latero-aortic lymph node enlargement *(arrow)* can be seen. *P* pancreas; *smv* superior mesenteric vein; *sma* superior mesenteric artery; *Ao* aorta

vasion can produce images of isolated round nodules, misleading an accessory spleen (Fig. 5.13). Therefore an angiodynamic computed tomography is indispensible even for a morphological analysis.

Alterations of the Attenuation Values Prior to and After Vascular Enhancement (Angiodynamic CT)

More than half of all pancreatic tumors are isodense without any vascular enhancement [100, 193, 250, 262, 263, 271]. A tumor may not be perceived if it does not change the outlines of the pancreas. It is important, to do angiodynamic CT in order to search for a heterogenicity in the pattern after intake of contrast medium [269, 271]. This technique requires high-resolution machines capable of realizing slices in less than 5 s [170].

Two technical modes are possible: rapid seriography along the plane of section previously chosen; seriography with sequential incrementation of 3- to 5-mm. The first mode gives a good tomographical and dynamic study of different vascular and parenchymatous times. It is well-suited to the detection of strictly intrapancreatic lesions, discernible only by anomalies in their vascular composition. The disadvantage of this method is that it necessitates as many boli as pancreatic section planes. Sequential displacement permits a more complete study of the gland and its vascular axes, and is suited to the detection of extrapancreatic effects of a significantly large lesion (Fig. 5.14).

Cancer of the pancreas is normally hypovascularized and appears on angioscans as a moderately hypodense area in relation to normal parenchyma [170, 258] (Fig. 5.15). In certain cases one finds clearly hypodense liquid areas (Fig. 5.16), usually interpreted as necrotic areas. These images could also correspond to pseu-

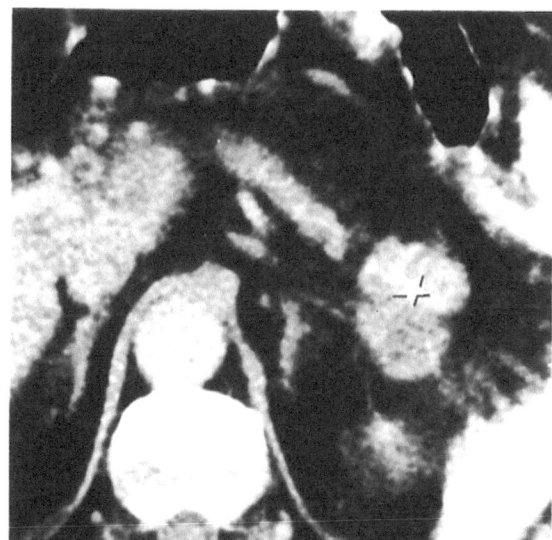

Fig. 5.13. Angioscan of the pancreas. Tumor *(star)* seems to be isolated on this slice, and only a series of slices can demonstrate the connection to the tail, and thus differentiate from an accessory spleen

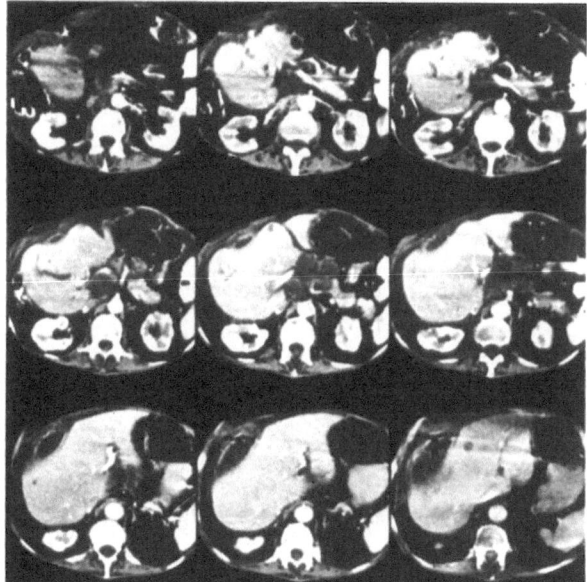

Fig. 5.14. Sequential angioscans of the pancreas, showing cancer of the body and head with locoregional invasion and liver metastases

docysts in relation to a secondary pancreatitis [15, 33, 60, 100, 134, 193, 232, 250, 258, 262, 263, 293].

A large number of pancreatic cancers affect the duct of Wirsung. Although the CT scan of this duct in its normal state is usually difficult to visualize, dilation of the duct is almost always spotted [15, 135, 142] (Fig. 5.17). On the slices without any vascular enhancement the fatty cavities between the pancreas and the splenic pedicle can suggest a dilated Wirsung's duct [292]. However, if this dilatation is a sign of

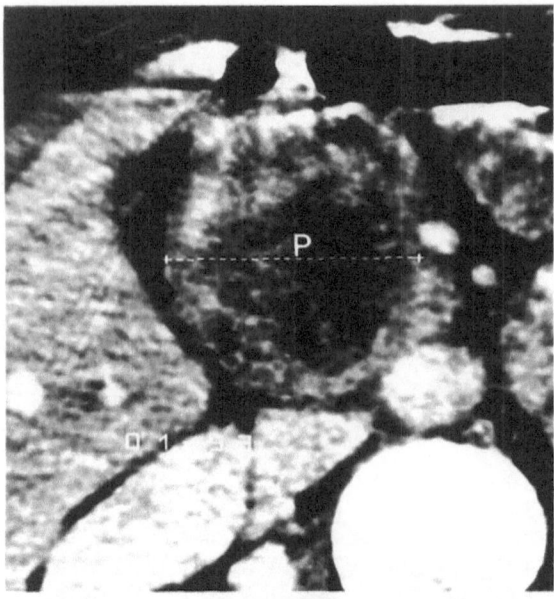

Fig. 5.15. Angioscan of pancreas following i. v. injection of contrast medium, showing a heterogeneous mass in the head of the pancreas *(P)*

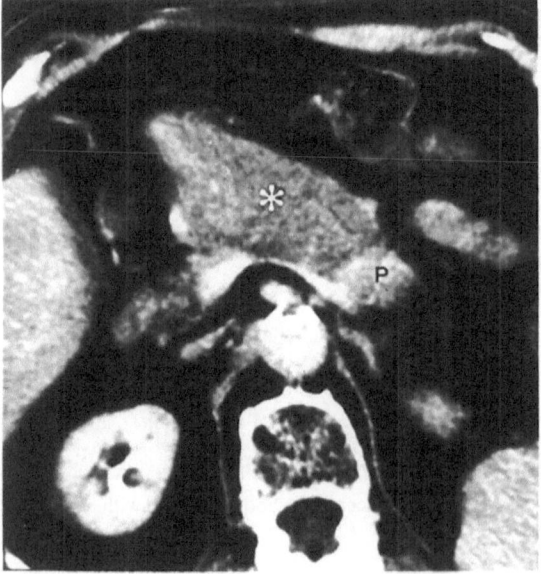

Fig. 5.16. Angioscan showing cancer of pancreas body. After i. v. injection of contrast medium a hypodense, liquid-like mass is seen *(asterisk);* the area of the pancreas around the tumor has a normal density *(P)*

pancreatic pathology, it has no histological value, as it can also be found in chronic pancreatitis [64, 68]. Hypodense areas indicating pseudocysts of the upper pancreatitis can coexist with this dilatation. Moreover, a round, hypodense zone in the head of the pancreas can correspond to the low part of the dilated common bile duct, above a tumor adjacent to the bile duct as in ampullary carcinoma [15].

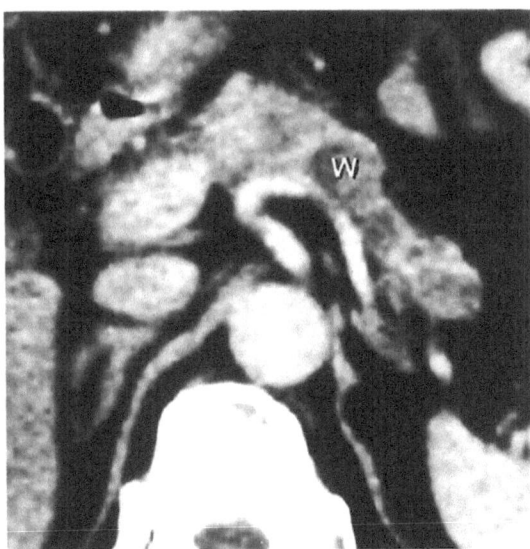

Fig. 5.17. CT scan showing Wirsung's duct *(W)* dilated distal to cancer of the isthmus

Limitations of CT

Direct and indirect findings of pancreatic cancers are related to fibrosis of the tumor stroma reaction. This fibrosis is a histopathological component common to chronic pancreatitis and pancreatic carcinoma. These signs are thus histologically nonspecific, all the more since distal pancreatitis is frequent in pancreatic cancer.

5.2.2.2 Extrapancreatic Findings by CT

Semiological CT of pancreatic cancer always integrates a study of regional and general extension of the lesions.

Involvement of Liver and Biliary Ducts (Fig. 5.18)

Dilatation of Biliary Ducts. CT easily identifies a dilatation of the intrahepatic biliary ducts as linear images, treelike, hypodense, converging towards the hilum, and not enhanced by an injection of vascular contrast medium (differential diagnosis with the veins) [149, 226, 249].

When the dilatation of the extrahepatic biliary ducts (hepatic bile duct, gallbladder, and cystic duct) is obvious, a CT scan demonstrates this dilatation. The assessment of an enlarged gallbladder poses no problem; the dilatation of the vesicular infundibulum, of the right, left, and common hepatic ducts at the level of the hilum, can show up as juxtaposed images of hydric tonality. At times, these give the aspect of divided cystic lesions. On the other hand, the dilatation of the common bile duct must be pursued along its entire length, and the number of slices involving the dilated common bile duct is of relevance in diagnosis of the obstruction [214].

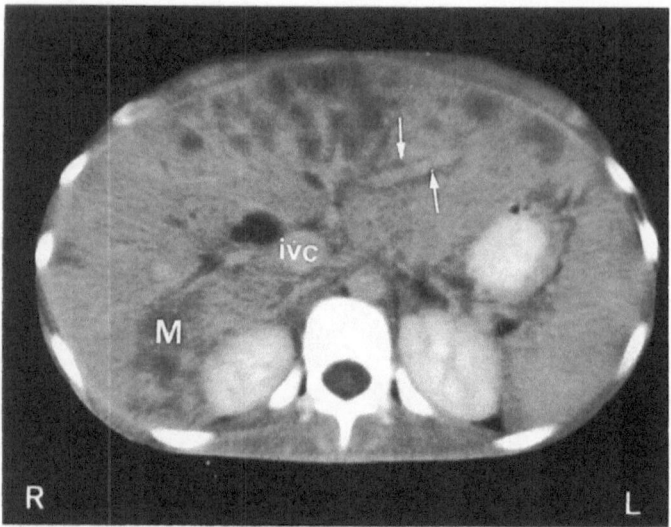

Fig. 5.18. Angioscan showing dilatation of intrahepatic biliary ducts *(arrows)* and liver metastases *(M)* filling the interhepatorenal space and displacing inferior vena cava *(IVC)* anteriorly

Direct symptoms of the obstruction, whether it consists of a pancreatic mass or a pedicular hepatic extension, are usually recognizable on CT scan [89, 110, 169].

Liver Metastases. Angiographic CT is required to visualize liver metastases [74, 240]. This constitutes a fundamental element of the characterization of the pancreatic lesion, although metastases of both pancreas and liver or even bifocal determinations of a malignant lymphoma are not exceptional [165, 241, 295].

Adenopathies

Adenopathies (Fig. 5.19) visible in the form of isolated nodules or multiple cyclic outlines filling in the fatty spaces between the pancreas and the major juxtapancreatic or retroperitoneal vessels [165, 193, 232, 250, 263]. It is often difficult to make a clear differentiation between the pancreatic mass itself and its satellite adenopathies.

Lesions of the Major Vessels

The "angioscan" recognizes lesions of vascular obstruction (Figs. 5.19 and 5.20) through direct signs in arterial attacks, and through direct and indirect symptoms (collateral circulation) in venous attacks.

The splenic pedicle is usually time impaired with involvement of the pancreas body or tail. The previous opacification of the splenic artery, at the time of the early "angioscan", can then appear encased in the pancreatic mass, as well as stenotic or amputated.

Direct symptoms of impairment of the splenic vein include amputation or ste-

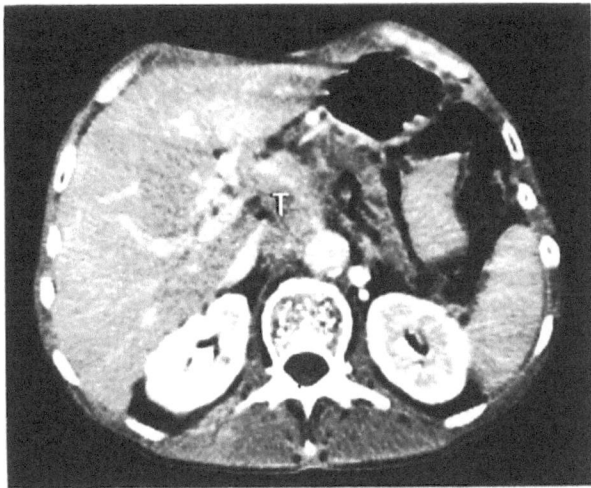

Fig.5.19. Angioscan showing lymph nodes and major vessels invaded by cancer of the isthmus. Note voluminous tumor mass *(T)* with locoregional extension; difficulty lies in differentiation of the lesion from its satellite adenopathies

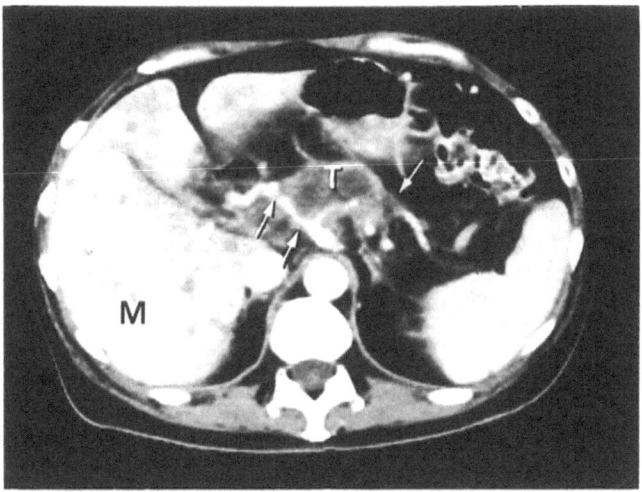

Fig.5.20. Angioscan showing invasion of the major vessels by cancer *(T)* of pancreas body. Note retroperitoneal invasion and vascular encasement *(arrows)*, and liver metastases *(M)*

nosis accompanied by segmental portal hypertension, collateral circulation in the area of the left gastric vein (gastric varices) [36, 158, 182, 184] and along the great curvature of the stomach (large right gastroepiploic vein), enlargement of the spleen, in which surrounding triangular zones of splenic infarct may appear, as hypodensity area after vascular enhancement [39]. Superior mesenteric pedicular invasion is visible in corporal lesions or in the uncinate process [99, 250, 258, 262].

Ascites

The presence of an effusion of intraperitoneal fluid poses no problems for CT but it permits no characterization of the pancreatic lesion.

5.2.3 Value and Limitations of Ultrasonography and Computerized Tomography in Diagnosis of Pancreatic Cancer

The semiological findings of US and CT in pancreatic cancer show the importance of these two methods in discovering lesions whose clinical expression is polymorphic, and which develop from an organ that cannot be explored by other than relatively invasive morphological procedures.

Ultrasonic and CT techniques and technology are stabilized at present. Minimally, an ultrasound unit produces a diagnostic scan with a real-time scanner unit, and a CT installation permits routine angiodynamic studies with short scanning times, elevated cadence, and if possible sequential incrementation.

Theoretically, a relatively overall approach to these two methods should take into account the following: technical and technological problems regarding the examiner's expertise, the sampling of the series studied, the percentage of normal cases, the percentage of interpretable tests, and lastly, the type, size, and localization of the pancreatic lesions.

The operator's skill plays a leading part in echography and consists as much in minimizing the number of uninterpretable examinations – which, depending upon the author vary from 7% to 20% [6, 72, 117, 133, 162, 177, 218, 222, 234], as in being able to recognize the limitations of the method with respect to the localization of the lesion in the head, body, or tail of the pancreas. If the rules for CT are followed and fast scanners are available for angioscans, a satisfactory study of the pancreas is almost always possible [78, 133, 249, 271].

An analysis of the scientific literature demonstrates the extreme difficulty in determining the respective value of each technique. This is due to the heterogenicity of the basis criteria and also to the unequal accuracy of the various machines used in each series. For example, some studies take into account the intrapancreatic localization of cancer, others do not, and the staging of the cancer is not always considered. Another point is that not all protocols can be superimposed upon one another; for instance, the use of fast angioscans is not systematic. Finally, the statistical evaluations carried out also pose a problem in their interpretation. They do not always employ the same elements, and the number of cases of several series seems too small for a satisfactory analysis.

Overall, however, taking these reservations into account, CT gives a more precise diagnosis (85%–94%), with a highly predictive negative value (93%) than does US (accuracy of 70%–90%, predictive negative value 86%) [6, 10, 31, 41, 50, 60, 67, 78, 101, 117, 136, 145, 162, 163, 183, 217, 218, 226, 249, 259, 265, 278, 284, 294].

CT scanning alone is capable of achieving an accurate diagnosis of pancreatic cancer in 84% of cases, according to Freeny and Lawson [73], whereas it is rarely possible to count on ultrasonic explorations alone in a patient suspected to have cancer of the pancreas.

Many authors point out the value of performing both tests. However, taking all these observations into account, *CT scanning must take prominence in the search for pancreatic cancer.*

5.3 Exploration of Bile Ducts and Wirsung's Duct

5.3.1 Cholangiography

5.3.1.1 Lesional Aspects

There is often a considerable dilatation of the biliary ducts in pancreatic cancer. All of the intrahepatic biliary ducts are dilated, and this is generally accompanied by a dilatation of the extrahepatic biliary ducts as well.

The common bile duct, whose diameter can reach many centimeters, has an obstruction that is often characteristic. This is chiefly seen in its topography at the level of the upper duodenum rather than in its morphology. The blockage is total, with an overall rounding of the extremity of the duct in more than 50% of cases. When the obstruction is incomplete and the stenosed segment can be filled with contrast material, there are no specific malignant stenosis, and irregular stenoses are more frequent [69, 125, 151, 197, 205] (Fig. 5.21).

The appearance of the dilated biliary duct can be deceptive. Actually, the metastatic hilar extension can entail an isolated dilatation of the intrahepatic biliary ducts, and even aberrant segmental dilatations [45, 73, 95]. This dilatation can be accompanied by displacement and compression of the intrahepatic biliary ducts, which evoke metastases [72].

5.3.1.2 Usable Techniques

Intravenous cholangiography is useful, and it is further improved by exceptionally slow perfusion techniques [2, 45, 95, 286]. At the present time, the opacification of a particular part of a dilated biliary branch without the possibility of performing a morphological analysis is of no interest.

Direct opacification of the biliary ducts can be achieved by transhepatic puncture with an inframillimetric needle (Chiba needle) [9, 54, 62, 63, 88, 106, 207, 215, 216, 227] or after catheterization via the jugular vein [90, 104, 239]. Transhepatic cholangiography is easier the greater the dilatation. However, the use of this technique is limited by the rather high risk of complications (3.40%) [106]. These are most commonly choleperitonitis, hemoperitoneum, and infection, with death occurring in 0.14% of cases [106]. Moreover, this technique cannot be used in the case of serious coagulation problems [45, 73, 90, 239]. Needle puncture of the biliary

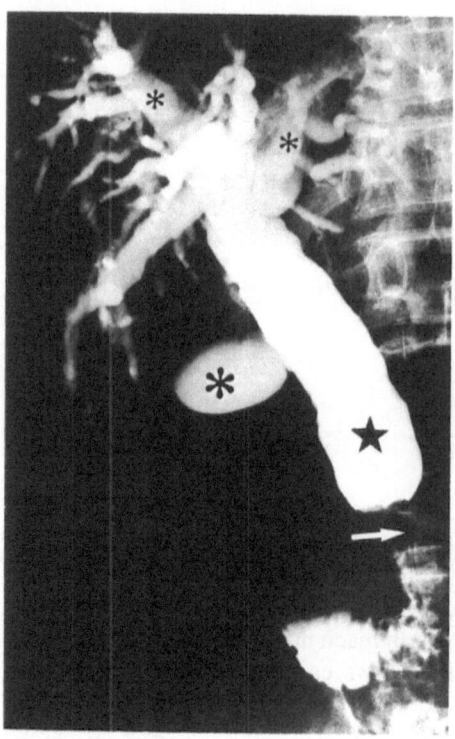

Fig. 5.21. Transparietal cholangiography in pancreas head cancer shows dilatation of common bile duct *(star)*, gallbladder *(large asterisk)*, and intrahepatic biliary ducts *(small asterisk)* in front of a filiform tumor stenosis in lower part of the common bile duct *(arrow)*

ducts can be carried out by a technically more complex route through the jugular vein, normally avoiding any peritoneal penetration; the transjugular method can also be used in the case of coagulation problems [45, 69, 72, 95, 159, 197]. The administration of contrast medium by such techniques shows evidence of the whole dilated intrahepatic biliary ducts; the left ducts are usually not opacified when the patient is in dorsal decubitus [62, 144].

Investigation aims at the total opacification of the hepatic common bile duct, which sometimes requires prior evacuation of the biliary ducts and always involves changing the position of the patient. This allows partial opacification of the common bile duct and the enlarged gallbladder [73, 88, 187, 215, 220].

Finally, these techniques of direct approach permit the development of an interventional radiology for the biliary ducts [27, 51, 61, 73, 121, 220, 231, 264].

5.3.2 Endoscopic Retrograde Cholangiopancreatography (ERCP)

With ECRP one can study the effect of the pancreatic cancer both on the pancreatic ducts and on the main bile duct. Moreover, cannulation of the pancreatic duct allows for cytology of the pancreatic juice samples obtained by aspiration.

Preliminary endoscopy makes one aware of the possible gastroduodenal side effects of pancreatic cancer [84, 137, 228, 233, 289].

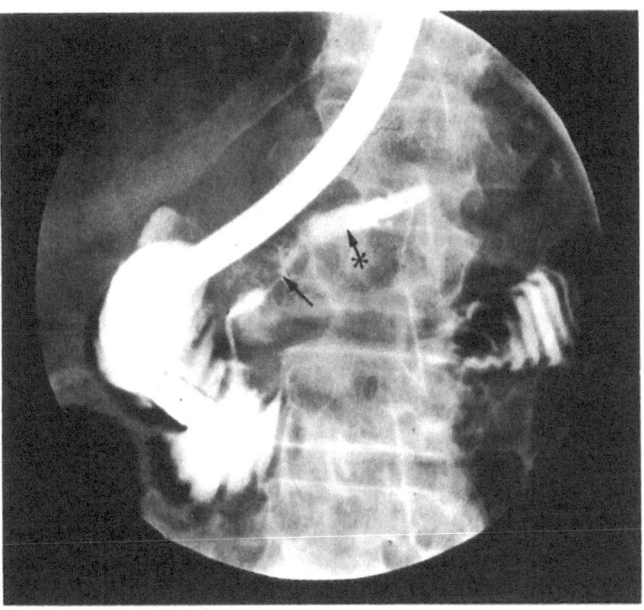

Fig. 5.22. Roentgenography of Wirsung's duct in cancer of the isthmus of the pancreas; stenosis of Wirsung's duct *(plain arrow)*, with dilatation of upper part *(arrow with asterisk)* and normal lower part

5.3.2.1 Pancreatic Anomalies

The most frequently encountered lesions are those of the major pancreatic ducts [73, 84, 103, 202] (Fig. 5.22). These lesions are more easily demonstrated when they are situated on the duct of Wirsung or its principal collaterals. The demonstration of lesions at the level of the distal branches is difficult, as their opacification is usually incomplete [71, 73, 228, 267].

The pancreatic ducts are most often the site of a complete obstruction or encasement [71, 73, 84, 140, 202, 228, 270]. An obstruction appears as a complete cutoff, usually irregular or eccentric, situated on the pancreatic duct and associated with proximal parenchyma opacification: classically, the main duct on the papillary side of the point of encasement has a normal appearance in pancreatic cancer as opposed to chronic pancreatitis, where it is generally irregular [4, 71, 138, 235, 251]. The encasement is short and irregular, with a large upper dilatation of the duct and an abrupt transition from the healthy zone [73, 86, 235]. Occasionally, it can entail a diffuse encasement of all the ducts [73, 84, 270].

Tumor cavities are much rarer (5%). These correspond to necrotic zones communicating with the excretory ducts. Their contours are usually irregular, while pseudocysts normally have regular outlines [3, 37, 71, 73, 77, 84, 86, 134, 139, 151, 233, 252, 257, 270].

Peripheral lesions appear as intraparenchymatous defect images that can cut off the collaterals (see Fig. 5.3). They are seen only exceptionally and should not be searched for systematically, due to the risks of iatrogenic pancreatitis [17, 159]

caused by parenchymography. The search for these lacunar zones is facilitated by a CT scan performed immediately after ERCP [80, 129]. The use of the nonionized surfactant HCO has been recommended to enhance the visualization of the paren-chyma and to diminish the risks of secondary pancreatitis [173].

These various signs are not specific to adenocarcinoma and can be found as well in the course of a chronic pancreatitis [21, 44]. The preoperative diagnosis is made even more difficult in that pancreatic cancer often coexists with chronic pancreatitis (associated or secondary pancreatitis) [85].

5.3.2.2 Anomalies of the Common Bile Duct and Intrahepatic Biliary Ducts

Cancer of the head of the pancreas can compress or invade the common bile duct. There is a stenosis - usually abrupt and not very extensive, with a large upper dila-tation - or a complete stenosis (type V of Caroli) [73, Guien and Thowat in 245]. The topography of the lesion is a very important element in its diagnosis: obstruction or stenosis at the level of the superior margin of the pancreas [8, 23, 97]. Neither the lack of selective opacity of the common bile duct (a failure rate of 10%–20% [172] when evaluated by the best teams) nor the particular difficulty due in certain cases to spreading to the papilla, should not be considered indicative of a total obstruc-tion of the common bile duct.

Cancers of the head of the pancreas are occasionally the origin of bifocal le-sions, with attacks on the pancreatic ducts and the common bile duct [52, 221]. The "double-duct" sign is considered by some authors to be quasi-characteristic of pan-creatic head cancer. However, chronic pancreatitis can also produce bifocal lesions with no image specificity [15, 73, 75, 221, 224].

Metastastic pedicular adenopathies are the origin of the images of extrinsic compression or cephalad occlusions of the main biliary duct [46]. Hepatic metas-tases can compress, repress, or amputate the intrahepatic biliary ducts [264].

5.3.2.3 Pancreatic Cytology by ERCP

The possibility of direct withdrawal of pure pancreatic juice, notably after brushing, by endoscopic catheterization of the papilla, has renewed interest in cytological di-agnosis of pancreatic cancer [19, 56, 93, 141, 147, 192, 210]. Indeed, up until now, the juice was taken at the level of the duodenum and had consequently a cellular con-tent that was extremely varied and denatured by the digestive enzymes activated in the duodenum.

The technique consists of a simple procedure that can be coupled with a func-tional and radiological study of the pancreas. The contrast medium is rapidly drain-ed into the duodenum and the introduction of the catheter is done after the intrave-nous injection of secretin at 1 U/kg. The pancreatic juice is then extracted starting at the 10th min and up until the 30th min, at 10-min intervals. Cytology is done im-mediately, or after conservation at 0 °C for several hours [19, 141]. The procedure usually consists of centrifugation before spreading and staining, and certain authors use a method which filters the fluid through a Millipore filter [18].

The results of cytological study appear to correlate well with the topography of pancreatic tumors: 67% positive results for head tumors and 33% for body and tail tumors [56]. When pancreatic cancer is suspected, cytology of the pancreatic juice should be performed even if the roentgenography of Wirsung's duct is normal.

In addition to indirect findings of extrinsic compression and/or gastroduodenal invasion by advanced pancreatic head cancer, preliminary endoscopy may show a periampullary invasion, in which case it is very difficult - virtually impossible - to catheterize the papilla; however, a histological diagnosis remains possible by means of direct biopsy [73, 137, 228, 289].

5.3.3 Value and Limitations of Cholangiography and ERCP in Diagnosis of Pancreatic Cancer

Opacification of the biliary ducts is one possible way of diagnosing an obstructive jaundice. It is very effective in demonstrating a ductal dilatation [90, 207]. However, owing to the risks involved [106], ultrasonography and CT scanning are preferable being both effective and nonaggressive.

Direct opacification of the biliary system defines the level of the obstruction. However, there is practically no possibility of characterization of the obstruction [69, 125, 159, 197, 205]. Therefore, interventional radiology is used in conjunction with external biliary drainage realized by ERCP [27, 45, 51, 61, 73, 95, 121, 228, 231, 276]. The accuracy of roentgenography of Wirsung's duct during ERCP depends both on the approach to opacification and on cytology. Even if certain aspects of the radiopaque pancreatic duct are indicators of cancer of the pancreas, there is no specific semiology for this cancer. Only the existence of malignant cells proven by cytology has a formal diagnostic value. A negative cytological report (25%–50% of the cases) is of no value [56, 94, 107, 192, 285].

A cytological examination of pancreatic juice permits the definitive assessment of cancer in 54%–75% of cases [17, 56, 107, 192, 285, 289]. A combination of cytology and roentgenography gives a positive diagnosis in more than 85% of cases [96], but is somewhat limited with regard to contraindications, risks, and failures.

The prevention of incidents and complications that occur in 1.2%–3% of cases [17, 20, 198, 296] depending strictly upon the expertise of the operator, requires the careful selection of patients and several technical measures. Complications are infectious diseases, occasionally duodenal perforations and necrosing cholecystitis, and above all acute pancreatitis, which occurs in 1%–2% of cases. The morbidity associated with this examination is estimated to be 2%–3%, whereas the mortality is 1/1000.

The failures are due in part to anatomical conditions (inaccessible duodenum, intradiverticular papilla) and in part to technical conditions; e.g., the impossibility of absolute catheterization of the papilla (2%–10%) or a fault in selective catheterization (85%–92% success for Wirsung's duct, 70%–85% success for the common bile duct).

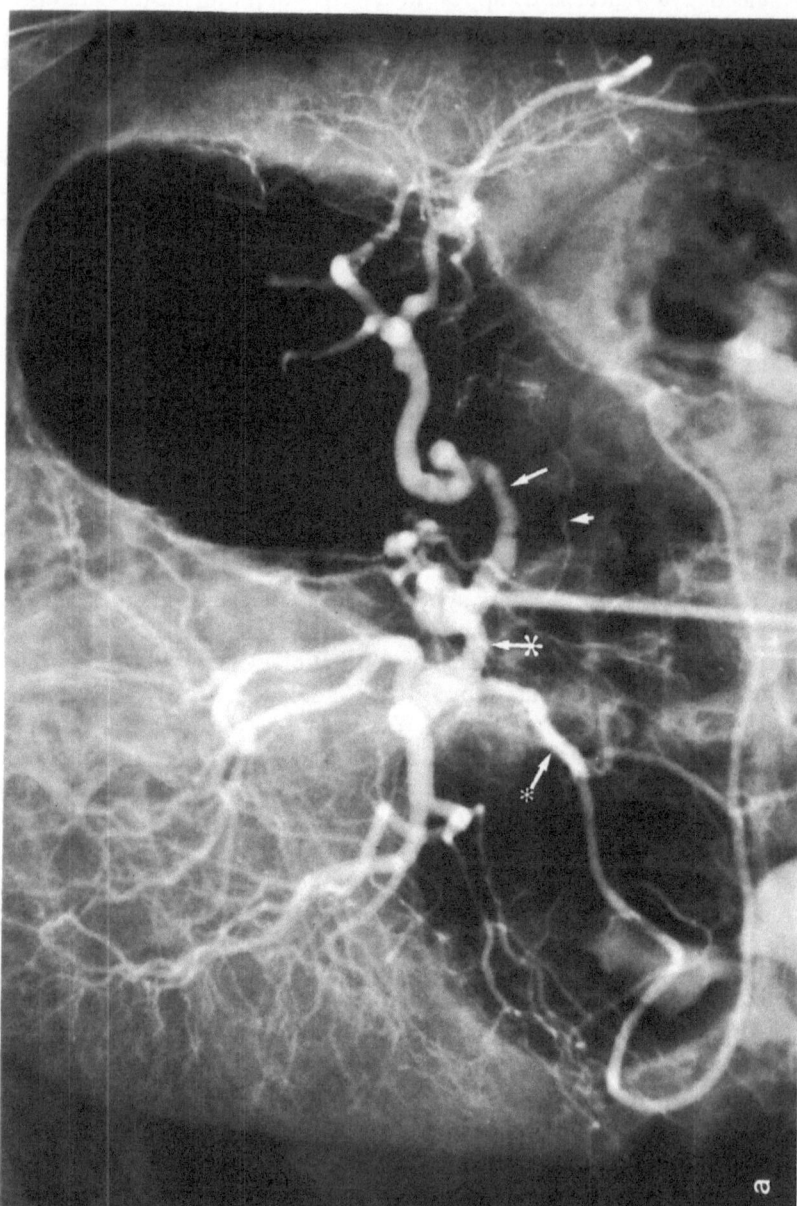

Fig. 5.23a, b. Arterioportography of the celiac trunk in advanced cancer of the pancreas body. **a** Arterial opacification time: infiltration of splenic artery (*arrow*), hepatic artery (*arrow with large asterisk*) and gastrointestinal artery (*arrow with small asterisk*), and extension to intrapancreatic arteries (*arrowhead*)

5.4 Angiography

Though pancreatic angiography was long the best technique in the detection of pancreatic lesions, it present role in the diagnosis of pancreatic cancer has diminished through the expansion of techniques that are less invasive and just as successful.

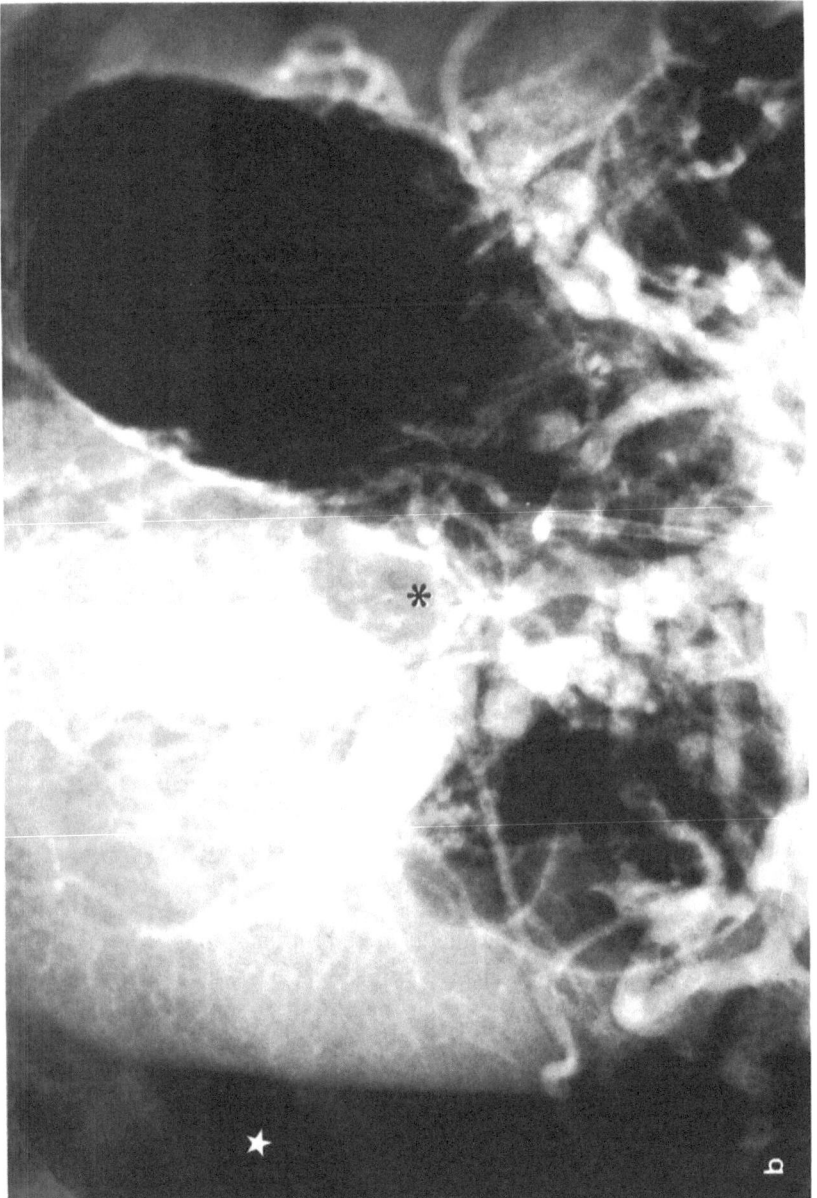

Fig. 5.23 b Venous return time: obstruction of splenoportal confluent *(asterisk)* with collateral circulation; hepatoparietal detachment by ascites *(star)*

Pancreatic angiography is based upon selective - or better still, hyperselective - celiomesenteric arteriography [12, 22, 25, 28, 115, 116, 199, 200, 201, 203, 204].

Arterioportographical findings of very advanced pancreatic cancer pose no diagnostic problem (Fig. 5.23). Along with signs of segmental portal hypertension due to complete obstruction in front of the splenic vein, possibly extensive, are associated symptoms of arterial stretching and invasion of the celiac trunk branches and superior mesenteric artery.

Segmental lesions of the major contiguous pancreatic trunk vessels are often found in cancer of the pancreas. Venous involvement [30, 92, 167, 174, 238] usually manifests as total obstruction along with segmental portal hypertension. The splenic vein is the most frequently affected [82, 236], with the superior mesenteric vein usually implicated early in the development of cancer of the uncinate process [11].

Invasion of the juxtapancreatic arterial trunks proceeds to encasements, occasionally irregular and extensive, with potential displacement [82, 92, 174, 186].

These venous and arterial signs are not at all specific and can be found just as easily in chronic pancreatitis as in pancreatic cancer [14, 24, 29, 113, 123, 143, 154, 155, 181, 225, 230, 242, 274]. Nevertheless, once a lesion has been discovered or identified, such vascular findings become a fundamental part of the preoperative assessment [16, 55, 112, 113, 130, 146, 168, 178, 191, 246, 260, 267], providing information on the difficulties of resection. At the same time, celiomesenteric arteriography attempts to define the hepatic extension of the pancreatic lesion.

A detailed semiology of intrapancreatic arterial lesions in pancreatic cancer has been established in numerous studies [7, 28, 30, 53, 92, 111, 114, 115, 174, 176, 201, 229, 237, 275]. The goal is to detect small intrapancreatic cancer and to allow its differentiation, in these focal lesions, from a chronic pancreatitis.

For arteries of small and medium caliber, the principal criteria are encasement, total obstruction and angulation (Fig. 5.24). Cancer of the pancreas is usually hypovascularized and can appear as a focal defect in the parenchymatous phase.

As far as neovascularization is concerned, it is difficult to differentiate from a disease of the small arterioles. This is because the vessels are too small to be analyzed by in vivo arteriography and their overall incidence is much less than has been supposed.

Findings of arterial lesions are supported by nonspecific and fibrous histological lesions (reaction of the stroma in cancer of the pancreas and aggressive fibrosis in chronic pancreatitis). Chronic pancreatitis is otherwise often associated with cancer; under these conditions intrapancreatic arterial findings do not permit differentiation between cancer and chronic pancreatitis [14, 146]. Selective venography performed with a portal catheter does not permit more specific findings in the case of pancreatic cancer.

5.5 Laparoscopy

Laparoscopy has lost its importance in comparison with the previously mentioned examinations. It is rarely done for pancreatic cancer. Located retroperitoneally, the pancreas is not - as the liver is - directly visible by laparoscopy.

Certain technical artifices [188] permit inspection of the pancreas through the lesser omentum in about 60% of cases. Guided cytological aspiration is therefore possible, but remains, in spite of this, very rare.

In the course of pancreatic cancer laparoscopy can provide certain information [212]:

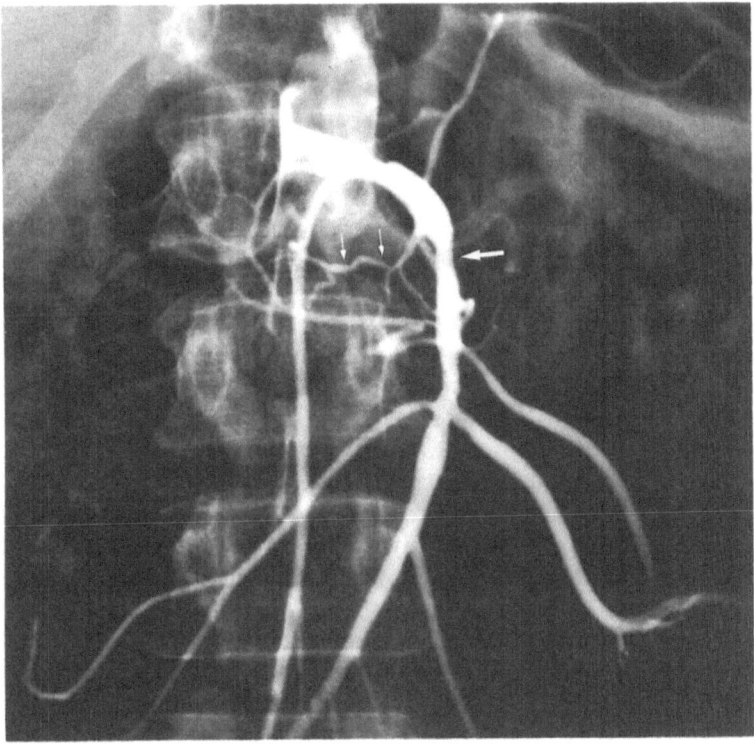

Fig. 5.24. Superior mesenteric arteriography in cancer of the pancreas body: infiltration and stenosis of intrapancreatic arterioles *(small arrows);* encasement of the superior mesenteric artery *(large arrow)*

1. Direct signs: only a bulging of the gland visible from behind the peritoneum can be considered a direct sign; it is nevertheless not specific, as it can also be observed in chronic pancreatitis.
2. Indirect signs are caused by the occasional compression of the tumor mass.
   a) Biliary involvement leads to gallbladder dilatation associated with a greenish cholestatic liver.
   b) Venous involvement causes segmental portal hypertension.
   c) Lymphatic invasion produces highly visible ectasia at the level of the liver and mesentery.
3. Specific signs are neoplasms that are directly visible: these are hepatic and peritoneal metastases, of which the latter can be revealed only by laparoscopy. This investigation then permits a biopsy of these structures, revealing adenocarcinomas whose pancreatic origin is rarely recognized by the pathologist.

   In conclusion, laparoscopy does not add a great deal to the other tests. It is an invasive method whose benefits are disproportionate to its drawbacks.

5.6 Percutaneous Needle Biopsy

5.6.1 Method

Various approaches have been proposed for guiding a fine-needle aspiration biopsy of the pancreas [87]. At the present time, by means of opacification of the pancreatic ducts (wirsungography) [38, 185] or of the vascular network (pancreatic angiography) [57, 209], some more systematic methods such as ultrasonography [40, 105, 122, 253, 272, 273] and CT [66, 98, 101, 108] predominate. These techniques give information on the target, on the contiguous pancreatic lesions, and on the puncture route.

Under CT control, projections of the face and profile (radiological mode), along with axial slices, permit one to determine the points of entry, the route of biopsy, and the depth of the target [223]. New slices permit location of the extremity of the needle with respect to the target.

Control through ultrasound can be done by standard transducers enveloped in a sterile pocket or by ones specially made for guided and sterilized aspirations [105, 291]. The guiding is done by adapting the angulation of the needle to the plane of the beam, and sometimes directly locates the moving extremity of the needle.

Diverse adaptations have been made in an attempt to facilitate the biopsy itself, to augment the yield and diminish the risks. Fine needles are used [124, 190], with various profiles occasionally conical (to obtain tissue samples), whose reduced length improves the guidance. The sample yield is increased by performing an up-and-down aspiration within the lesion [26]. An extemporaneous examination of the slides after rapid staining reduces the risk of acellular withdrawals by repetitive aspirations. Under these optimal conditions, a spreading on a thick slide is given to the cytologist.

5.6.2 Diagnostic Accuracy

The diagnostic accuracy of needle aspiration depends in part on the samples and the operator's skills, and in part on the conditions of the examination and the cytologist's skills. These problems have been detailed in a previous chapter on anatomopathology.

The numerous fine-needle aspiration biopsy series of the pancreas reported in the literature indicate the popularity of this technique [26, 57, 91, 105]. One must be critical of the results, depending both on the series and on the type of patient examined. Some concern only patients *proven to have* cancer of the pancreas and the rate of positive cytological diagnoses ranging from 70%–90% is not remarkable, but these series are more theoretical than practical and the large number of inconclusive results must be taken as false negatives.

It is more interesting to consider the results of a series of patients who are *suspected* of having pancreatic cancer. As it is very difficult to confirm with certainty a nonmalignant cyst, not a great deal can be found in the literature. Therefore, the great value of fine-needle aspiration lies in the histological results, since there are a very few number of false positives, and in the fact that it carries very little risk.

Most authors have reported accidents. Infectious complications (gram-negative septicemia) [66], inflammation (acute pancreatitis) [26, 58, 185] and perforations [26] (hemoperitonitis, choleperitonitis) have been reported from time to time. There is only one case report of a malignant seeding of the tract after fine-needle biopsy [65], and this risk in other domaines (lung, prostate cancer) is negligible.

5.7 Magnetic Resonance

Some MR images have shown interesting morphological distinctions [254, 261, 281]. The results are very dependent upon the synchronization between the images and the respiratory and cardiac rhythms.

In theory, magnetic resonance allows a direct approach to the vascular axes, more precise tissue characterization, and the use of "contrast media", some of which could be specific, but the sensitivity and specificity of this technique for cancer of the pancreas have not actually been proved.

5.8 Morphological Diagnosis of the Principal Varieties of Pancreatic Tumors

5.8.1 Adenocarcinoma

Pancreatic adenocarcinoma is clinically a lesion with a particular polymorphism. Medical imaging must assess or eliminate, to a greater or lesser extent with difficulty, a likely pancreatic cancer.

5.8.1.1 Positive Diagnosis

Direct Signs

Whatever the clinical symptoms, the first techniques to use in looking for direct signs of pancreatic cancer are ultrasonography and CT for they allow a global abdominal and, in particular, a pancreatic hepatobiliary, approach [135, 146, 191, 222]. They can demonstrate the mass that is altering the pancreatic contours, which is easily recognized, but it is still difficult to determine the site of origin of voluminous tumors in the upper abdomen (see Fig. 5.11).

More frequently and earlier, ultrasound and CT scans try to recognize a cancer of the pancreas before it can deform the contours of the gland. A positive diagnosis rests, at this stage, on defined anomalies of pancreatic pattern; ultrasound and CT may fail here, the former because it is often difficult to differentiate an area which is hypoechogenic overall from the normal echogenic tissue, the latter because the hypovascularization of the lesion rapidly disappears in the CT scan after venous injection of contrast medium.

Indirect Signs

Indirect signs are easily discernible by ultrasound and CT scans during the course of pancreatic cancer. But other imaging techniques often intervene: angiography and biliopancreatic duct opacification are often necessary to complete the etiological and pretherapeutic workup of a lesion recognized by ultrasound and CT scan.

In other instances, ERCP [79] will more likely be used to assess or invalidate a diagnosis of a small cancer of the pancreas, if there are suspicious results from ultrasound or CT scan, if there are liver metastases but a normal pancreatic image, or even if there is a simple radioclinical discrepancy with regard to the pancreas.

5.8.1.2 Differential Diagnosis

Differential diagnosis is the formal affirmation of a pancreatic cancer and is indispensible to therapeutic management. When morphological explorations discover a pancreatic tumor, it is essential to differentiate between pancreatic cancer and a node of chronic pancreatitis. Even the histological characterization is difficult [135].

There is no specific radiological semiology for pancreatic cancer, even considering hyperselective angioscans or ERCP. The demonstration of a pancreatic tumor with locoregional spreading and/or metastases to the liver leads to a presumption equal to a formal diagnosis. Yet this link is not specific for a primary pancreatic cancer, as there is an invasion of the pancreatic, juxtapancreatic, and hepatic regions by extrapancreatic neoplasm. The importance of such a distinction remains negligible, either because the primary cancer has already been defined or because a laparotomy is envisaged.

When the tumor is not very developed, in particular when it is intrapancreatic, and if a formal diagnosis is indispensible to indicate or contraindicate surgery, it is determined by histological and/or cytological samples, taken by ultrasound- and CT-scan-guided aspiration or by brushing during ERCP [185, 190, 192].

In the case of a negative or inconclusive cytological result and if the clinical suspicion of pancreatic cancer remains very strong, the solution is surgical exploration, and often serial study of the resected tissue. In other instances, only clinical evolution permits a quasi-definitive diagnosis.

A pancreatic nodule can correspond to lesions other than cancers of the pancreas, nodules of pancreatitis, or metastasis. The discovery of a hypervascularized (pancreatic) tumor must make one suspect, even with the lack of endocrine indicators, an endocrine pancreatic tumor – an islet-cell tumor or an especially nonfunctional nesidioblastoma.

Occasionally, in a patient treated for chronic pancreatitis and followed up, further troubles make one suspect cancer of the pancreas. The confirmation of chronic pancreatitis without cancer always requires histological checks, frequently intraoperative, and will be reinforced only through its evolution.

5.8.2 Cystadenocarcinoma

The radiological picture of cystadenocarcinoma is based upon the pathological features of cystic tumors of the pancreas. The criteria of classification are the presence or absence of malignant cells in benign cystadenomas on the one hand, and in malignant cystadenocarcinomas on the other hand. However, this classification is not satisfactory [118], as it confuses two different cystic disorders under the same term of cystadenoma. Compagno and Oertel [42, 43] proposed a classification distinguishing between the two large groups of cystic tumors: serous microcystic adenomas - always benign - and mucinous macrocystic tumors - malignant (cystadenocarcinoma) or potentially malignant (mucinous cysts) -. These two groups differ through multiple anatomopathological features [42, 43, 119, 120], some are macroscopic, and are radiologically predominant during diagnosis [126] (Table 5.1).

Under these conditions, the radiological descriptions given prior to 1978 must be reviewed. At the present time, the problem no longer lies in the search for vascularized anomalies, hypothetically revealing malignancy, but rather in the detection of specific features of microcystic adenomas on the one hand, and of cystadenoma or cystadenocarcinoma on the other.

5.8.2.1 Positive Diagnosis

The conventional examinations for cystadenocarcinoma, as for adenocarcinoma, are of little interest at present. In 10%-15% of these tumors there are some calcifications [43, 109, 194, 219], the morphology and topographical distribution of which is

Table 5.1. Morphological Characteristics of cystic tumors (from Itai et al. [126])

	Serous cystadenoma	Mucinous cystadenoma and cystadenocarcinoma
External appearance	Well-encapsulated ovoid or multinodular mass	Well-encapsulated, round or lobulated; (locally invasive)[a]
Cystic portion No. and size of cysts	Multilocular (innumerable), 0.1-0.2 cm cysts usually located in the periphery	Unilocular or multilocular; often one large cyst with smaller daughter cysts along its internal surface
Content	Thin and clear, no mucin	Thick, mucoid, cloudy brown, or hemorrhagic and necrotic
Solid portion	Central stellate septa with trabeculae and a smooth outer wall; honeycomb appearance	Dominant fibrous wall (0.2-1.5 cm) with papillary projections and/or convolutions
Calcification	Often ("sunburst")	Occasionally (small)

[a] = Occasionally noticed in over malignancy

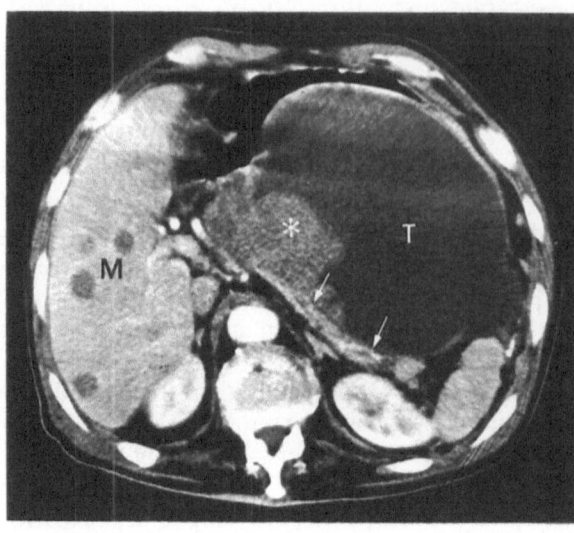

Fig. 5.25. Angioscan showing pancreatic cystadenocarcinoma. Voluminous cyst *(T)* displaces splenic vessels to the back *(arrows)*. Note vegetative formation on inside *(asterisk)* and hypodense, cystlike liver metastases *(M)*

better detected by means of CT. Baryum studies of the gastrointestinal tract could allow definition of the effects of a pancreatic tumor syndrome, which are important relative to the advanced stage of the tumor.

Ultrasonography shows voluminous cystic, uni- or multilocular lesions which have some intracystic echogenic areas related to septation and nodular tumor excrescences [34, 73, 76, 81, 288].

CT shows a cystic component mass. These cystic elements are generally multiple and end up in a septate cystic lesion [34, 81, 126, 288]. There are some occurrences of calcification, rarer than with serous cystadenoma. They appear like amorphous peripheral calcifications. The intratumor septae are enhanced after administration of contrast medium and follow the solid tumor wall, which is itself frequently hypervascularized (Figs. 5.25 and 5.26).

The arteriographical picture [32, 81, 118, 279] of cystadenocarcinoma is one of a voluminous cystic lesion where indirect features of displacement and stretching prevail and with parenchymatous signs of hypovascularized lesions. These signs are always associated with peri- or intracystic hypervascularized areas, evaluated on parenchymal and arteriolar arterioportography.

Ultrasonography, CT and angiography can show, as for pancreatic adenocarcinoma, some signs of local, regional, or metastatic (particularly hepatic) extension of the tumor (see Figs. 5.25 and 5.26).

5.8.2.2 Differential Diagnosis

The radioclinical picture of cystadenocarcinoma may falsely lead to other diagnoses. However, one must contrast the usual clinical cases with the lesions that appear exceptionally.

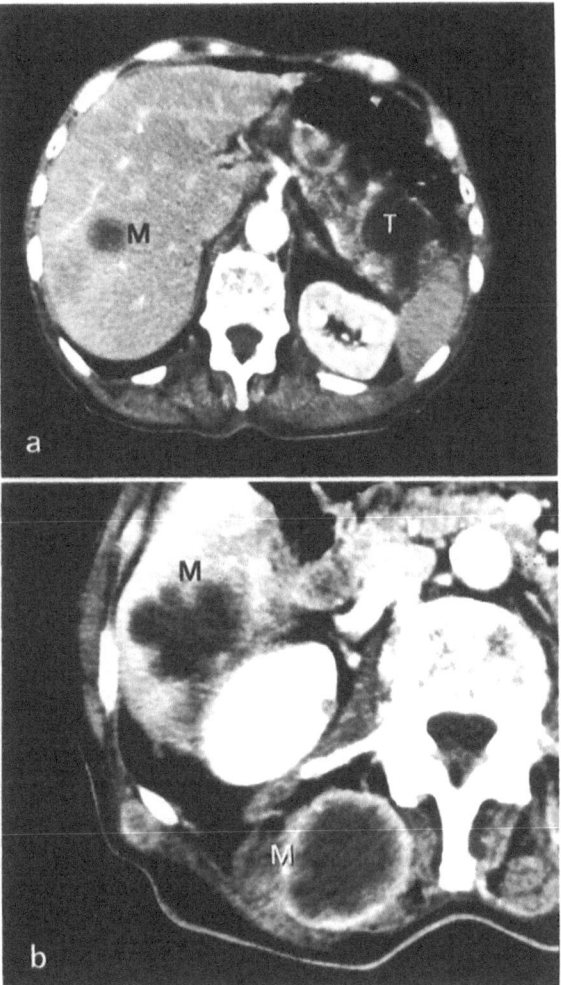

Fig.5.26a, b. Angioscan of pancreatic cystadenocarcinoma. **a** Polylobate cystic mass in tail of pancreas *(T)*. **b** Metastases *(M)* with hypervascularized corona and hypodense center, in liver and posterior lumbar wall

Practically, assessment of the pancreatic origin of a voluminous cystic or necrotic lesion of the left upper abdomen remains difficult, even if it changes all of the anatomical pancreatic relationships. There must be evidence of a continuation between the lesion and the contiguous pancreas (isthmus or body of the pancreas), and the adjacent anatomical structures such as the spleen, the left suprarenal, the superior pole of the left kidney, and the straight part of the stomach must be identified.

A more or less necrosed voluminous lesion of the pancreas, whether an adenocarcinoma or an endocrine pancreatic tumor [81], can give ultrasonographic, scanographic, and angiographic signs very difficult to differentiate from those given by a cystadenocarcinoma [87, 134].

Moreover, it is important not to confuse a cystadenocarcinoma, with its cystic appearance, with a pancreatic pseudocyst [118, 126, 153]. The demonstration of a very thick and hypervascularized wall in an a priori pseudocystic lesion is very suspicious [5, 118].

Exceptionally, one must be very careful in diagnosing less common lesions, even in the presence of benign serous cystadenomas of macrocystic appearance, of cystic lymphangiomas, or of hydatic cysts which have been reported from studies to be possibly isolated from the pancreas.

5.9 Radiological Invasion Workup

The anatomical environment of the pancreas and the venous splanchnic drainage show different steps in the course of pancreatic cancer. In fact, it can be divided into three stages: invasion by contiguity, invasion of the liver, and distant systemic invasion. These stages can be paradoxically dissociated: for instance, a systemic invasion may be confirmed without the apparent existence of liver metastases.

Classically, it is contiguous invasion which distinguishes three main clinical forms of pancreatic cancer: the jaundiced type in head cancer, the painful solar type in body cancer, and the tumoral type in cancer of the tail of the pancreas.

While techniques such as ultrasonography, and particularly CT scanning (Figs. 5.27 and 5.28), show better locoregional invasion of the biliary ducts and the hilum of the liver for head tumors, of the splanchnic region (and the mesentery root) for tumors of the isthmic region and of the uncinate process, and of the pararenal area and the spleen for tail cancer, angiography plays an important role in the detection of vascular invasion [168, 191]. These invasions do not all have the same significance; infiltration of the large retroperitoneal vessels and to the mesenteric axes is more damaging than infiltration of the splenic axis, which is more frequently found.

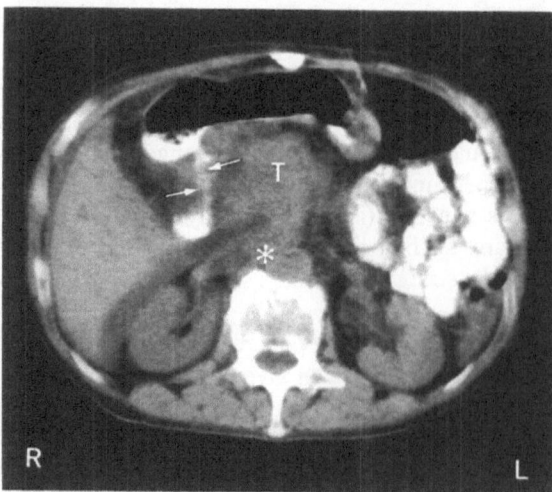

Fig. 5.27. CT scan showing locoregional extent of cancer of the body and head of the pancreas. Note stenosis *(arrows)* and duodenal invasion by the pancreatic tumor mass *(T)* and retroperitoneal lymph node metastases *(asterisk)*

Segmental portal hypertension created by venous invasion can be identified by the existence of collateral circulation, splenic infarction, and ascites. This peritoneal effusion can have several origins, in particular, it can be provoked by an upper pancreatic lesion or a peritoneal metastastic spreading. These distinctions are more evident in the analysis of pancreatic juice rather than on radiographic examination.

The search for hepatic metastases (see Fig. 5.28) is performed nowadays first by means of ultrasonography, which as a general rule obviates the need for other further investigations of patients affected by disseminated metastases to the liver. CT scanning is at present the most sensitive method [156, 157, 171, 240] in the search for liver metastases. However, the diagnosis of integrity of the liver or of a hepatic lobe

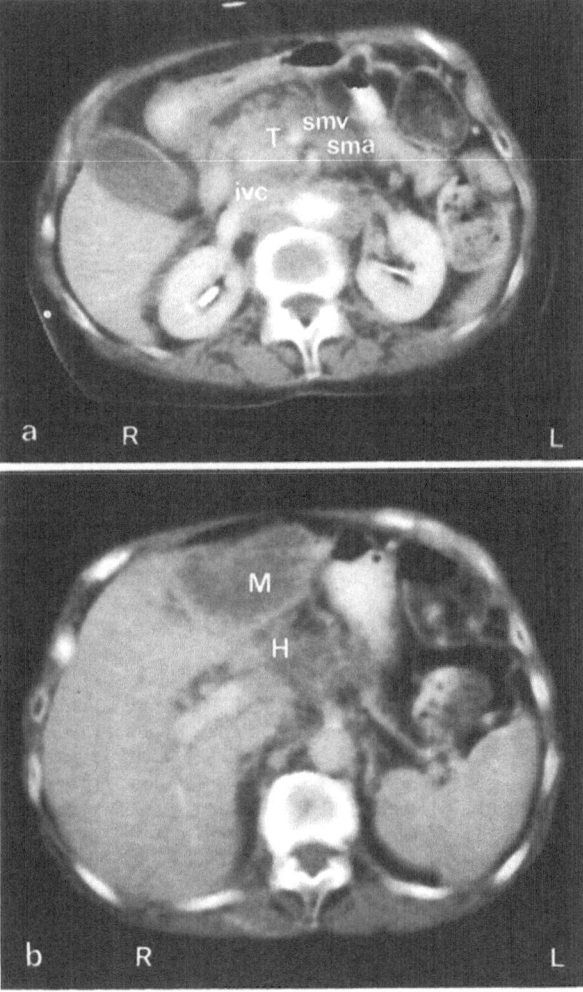

Fig. 28a, b. Angioscan showing extrapancreatic tumor extension in cancer of the body and tail of the pancreas. **a** Large nonhomogeneous, poorly defined tumor excrescence *(T)* encasing the aorta *(Ao)*, inferior vena cava *(ivc)*, and superior mesenteric vessels *(smv, sma)*. **b** Extension to hepatic hilum *(H)*, and hypervascularized metastases *(M)* in left lobe of liver

must never be definitive, because numerous metastases, particularly when they are small, can remain undetected, as has been shown by Smith et al. [255]. That is to say that certain of these metastases can only be seen either directly or by means of intraoperative ultrasound at laparotomy.

Finally, the extent of systemic invasion is seen on clinical examination, by means of a chest radiograph and sometimes by a thoracic CT scan, which is more precise than the normal thorax films, while the pleuropulmonary bases are generally more clearly seen through an abdominal scan. A brain scan is sometimes performed.

References

1. Ackerman NB, Aust JC, Brendenberg CE et al. (1976) Problems in differentiating between pancreatic lymphoma and anaplastic carcinoma and their management. Ann Surg 184: 705-708
2. Allen WMC (1969) A Cholangiographie par perfusion dans les cas d'échec de la cholangiographie. Br J Radiol 42: 347-350
3. Anacker H, Weiss HD, Kramann B, Rupp N (1974) Experience with endoscopic retrograde pancreatography. AJR 122: 375-384
4. Anacker H, Weiss HD, Kramann B (1977) Endoscopic retrograde pancreaticocholangiography (ERCP). Springer, Berlin Heidelberg New York
5. Araki T, Ohtomo K, Itai Y, Iio M (1982) Demonstration of septa in cystic lesions. Comparison study by computed tomography and ultrasound. Clin Radiol 33: 325-329
6. Arger PH, Mulhern CB, Bonavita JA et al. (1979) An analysis of pancreatic sonography in suspected disease. J Clin Ultrasound 7: 91-97
7. Ariyama J, Shirakabe H, Ikenobe H (1976) Angiographic diagnosis of pancreatic carcinoma. Stomach Intestine 11: 1605-1618
8. Ariyama J, Shirakabe H, Ikenobe H, Kurosawa A, Owman T (1977) The diagnosis of the small resectable pancreatic carcinoma. Clin Radiol 28: 437-44
9. Ariyama J, Shirakabe M, Ohaslh K, Roberts GM (1978) Experience with percutaneous transhepatic cholangiography using the Japanese needle. Gastro Intest Radiol 2: 359-365
10. Barlin J, Vinning D, Miale A Jr, et al. (1977) Computerized tomography diagnostic ultrasound and radionuclide scanning. Comparison of efficacy in diagnosis of pancreatic carcinoma. JAMA 238: 2040-2042
11. Baron MG, Mitty HA, Wolf BS (1967) The arteriographic appearance of carcinoma of the uncinate process of the pancreas. AJR 101: 649
12. Baum S, Roy R, Finkelstein AK, Blakemore WS (1965) Clinical application of selective celiac and superior mesenteric arteriography. Radiology 84: 279-295
13. Becker WF, Welsh RA, Pratt HS (1965) Cystadenoma and cystadenocarcinoma of the pancreas. Ann Surg 161: 845-863
14. Benko G (1970) Problems of differential diagnosis in angiography of the pancreas. Radiol Clin 39: 334
15. Berland LL, Lawson TL, Foley WD, Geenen JE, Stewart ET (1981) Computed tomography of the normal and abnormal duct: correlation with pancreatic ductography. Radiology 141: 715-724
16. Bernardino ME, Barnes AP (1982) Imaging the pancreatic neoplasm. Cancer 40: 2681-2688
17. Bilbao MK, Dotter CT, Lee TG, Katon RM (1976) Complications of endoscopic retrograde cholangio-pancreatography (ERCP) - A study of 10000 cases. Gastroenterology 70: 314-320
18. Bitoun A, De Saint Laurent P, Bagnel C, Bagnel JC, Brenier JJ (1979) Cytologie du liquide pancrétique recueilli par cathétérisme endoscopique du canal de Wirsung. Gastroenterol Clin Biol 3: 795-802
19. Blackstone MO, Cockerham L, Kirnser JB et al. (1977) Intraductal aspiration for cytodiagnosis in pancreatic malignancy. Gastrointest. Endosc 23: 145-147

20. Blackwood WD, Vennes JA, Silvis SE (1973) Postendoscopy pancreatitis and hyperamylasuria. Gastrointest Endosc 20: 56-58
21. Block MD, Schuman BH, Weckstein MC (1975) Interpretative problems in endoscopic retrograde cholangiopancreatography. Am J Surg 129: 29-33
22. Boijsen E, Olin T (1965) Meeting of Scandinavian Association for Medical Radiology 1961. Acta Radiol [Suppl] (Stockh) 235
23. Boijsen E, Tylin U (1972) Vascular changes in chronic pancreatitis. Acta Radiol (Stockh) 12: 34-48
24. Boijsen E, Ekerman CA, Olin T (1966) Selective pancreatic angiography. Br J Radiol 39: 481
25. Bookstein JJ, Oberman HA (1966) Appraisal of selective angiography in localizing islet cell tumors of the pancreas. Radiology 86: 682-685
26. Bret PM (1984) La ponction percutanée du pancréas à l'aiguille fine. In: Actualités chirurgicales. 85ème Congrès Français de Chirurgie. II. Chirurgie abdominale et digestive (2e partie). Masson, Paris, p 893
27. Brooks JR, Culebras JM (1976) Cancer of the pancreas: palliative operation. Whipple procedure or total pancreatectomy. Am J Surg 131: 516-520
28. Bruel JM (1974) Peut on encore demander en 1974 une artériographie pour explorer le pancréas? Bilan critique - Perspectives d'avenir. Medical dissertation, University of Montpellier
29. Bucheler E, Boldt I, Frommholdt M, Kauger C (1971) Die angiographische Diagnostik der Pancreastumoren und der Pancreatitis. RöFo 195: 726
30. Buranasiri S, Baum S (1972) The significance of the venous phase of celiac and superior mesenteric arteriography in evaluating pancreatic carcinoma. Radiology 102: 11-20
31. Burger J, Blavenstein VW (1974) Lument aspects of ultrasonic scanning of the pancreas. AJR 116: 406-412
32. Busilacchi P, Rizzatto G, Bazzocchi M, Boltro E, Candiani F, Ferrari F, Giuseppetti GM, Mirk P, Rubaltelli L, Volterrani L, Zappasodi F (1982) Pancreatic cystadenocarcinoma: diagnostic problems. Br J Radiol 55: 558-561
33. Callen PW, Breiman RS, Korobkin M, et al. (1979) Carcinoma of the tail of the pancreas: an unusual CT appearance. AJR 133: 135-137
34. Carrol B, Sample WF (1978) Pancreatic cystadenocarcinoma: CT body scan and gray scale ultrasound appearance. AJR 131: 339-341
35. Chait H, Faegenburg DH (1960) Illusory neoplasms of the stomach and duodenum as a manifestation of carcinoma of the pancreas. Radiology 74: 771-777
36. Clark KE, Foley WD, Lawson TL et al. (1980) CT evaluation of oesophageal and upper abdominal varices. J Comput Assist Tomogr 4: 510-515
37. Classen M, Anacker H, Stadelmann O, et al. (1975) The diagnosis of tumors of the papilla of Vater and of the pancreas by endoscopic radiologic cholangiopancreatography (ERCP). In: Anacker M (ed) Efficiency and limits of radiologic examination of the pancreas. Thieme, Stuttgart
38. Clouse ME, Gregg J, MacDonald DJ, Legg MA (1977) Percutaneous fine needle aspiration biopsy of pancreatic carcinoma. Gastrointest Radiol 2: 67-71
39. Cohen BA, Mitty HA, Mendelson DS (1984) Computed tomography of splenic infarction. J Comput Assist Tomogr 8 (1): 167-168
40. Cohen MM (1979) Early diagnosis of pancreatic cancer using ultrasound and fine needle aspiration cytology. Am Surg 45: 715-717
41. Cohen MM, Switzer PJ, Cooperberg PL (1979) Sensitivity of ultrasonography in the diagnosis of pancreatic cancer. Can Med Assoc J 120: 453-455
42. Compagno J, Oertel JE (1978) Microcystic adenomas of the pancreas (glycogen rich cystadenomas). A clinicopathologic study of 34 cases. Am J Clin Pathol 69: 289-298
43. Compagno J, Oertel JE (1978) Mucinous cystic neoplasm of the pancreas with overt and latent malignancy (cystadenocarcinoma and cystadenoma). A clinicopathologic study of 41 cases. A J Clin Pathol 69: 573-580
44. Cotton P (1977) ERCP. Gut 18: 316-341
45. Croisille M, Les méthodes d'exploration radiologique du foie. EMC, Paris, Radiodiagnostic IV, 33510 A 10, 4-1-12
46. Cubilla AL, Fortner J, Fitzgerald PJ (1978) Lymph node involvement in carcinoma of the head of the pancreas area. Cancer 41: 880-887

47. De Graaf CS, Taylor KJW, Simons BD, Rosenfield AJ (1978) Gray-scale echography of the pancreas. Re-evaluation of normal size. Radiology 129: 157-161
48. Dodds WJ, Margolin FR, Goldberg HI (1969) Cavernous lymphangioma of the pancreas. Radiol Clin Biol 38: 267-270
49. Donowitz M, Kerstein MD, Spiro HM (1974) Pancreatic ascites. (Baltimore) Medicine 53: 183-195
50. Doust BD (1975) Ultrasonic examination of the pancreas. Radiol Clin North Am 13: 467-478
51. Dubreuil A, Bonneville B, Winckel P (1979) Drainage percutané transhépatique des voies biliaires. Nouv Presse Med 8: 862-864
52. Eaton SB, Ferrucci JT Jr (1973) Radiology of the pancreas and duodenum. Saunders, Philadelphia 261-265
53. Eisenberg H (1973) Pancreatic angiography. In: Hilal SK (ed) Small vessel angiography: imaging, morphology, physiology and clinical applications. Mosby, St Louis, pp 405-433
54. Elias E, Hamlyn AN, Jain S, et al. (1976) A randomized trial of percutaneous transhepatic cholangiography versus endoscopic retrograde cholangiography for bile duct vizualization in obstructive jaundice. Gastroenterology 71: 439-444
55. Elliott IF (1981) Current concepts in pancreatic imaging. Surg Clin North Am 61 (1)
56. Endo Y, Morii T, Tamura H, et al. (1974) Cytodiagnosis of pancreatic malignant tumors by aspiration under direct vision using duodenal fiberscope. Gastroenterology 67: 944-951
57. Evander A, Imse I, Lunderquist A, Tylen U, Akerman M (1978) Percutaneous cytodiagnosis of carcinoma of the pancreas and bile duct. Ann Surg 188: 90-92
58. Evans WK, Chia-Sing HO, McLoughlin MJ, Liang-Che-Tao (1981) Fatal necrotizing pancreatitis following fine needle aspiration biopsy of the pancreas. Radiology 141: 61-62
59. Eyler W, Clark M, Rian RL (1962) An evaluation of roentgen signs of pancreatic enlargement. JAMA 181: 967-971
60. Fawcitt RA, Forbes WSC, Isherwood I et al. (1978) Computed tomography in pancreatic disease. Br J Radiol 51: 1-4
61. Feduska NJ, Dent TC, Lindenauer SM (1971) Results of palliative operations of carcinoma of the pancreas. Arch Surg 103: 330-334
62. Ferrucci JT Jr, Wittenberg J (1977) Refinements in chiba needle transhepatic cholangiography. AJR 129: 11-16
63. Ferrucci JT Jr, Wittenberg J, Sarno RA, Dreyfuss JR (1976) Fine needle transhepatic cholangiography: a new approach to obstructive jaundice. AJR 127: 403-407
64. Ferucci JT Jr, Wittenberg J, Black EB, Kirkpatrick RH, Hall DA (1979) Computed body tomography in chronic pancreatitis. Radiology 130: 175-182
65. Ferrucci JT, Wittenberg J, Margolies MN, Carey RW (1979) Malignant seeding of the tract after thin needle aspiration biopsy. Radiology 130: 345-346
66. Ferrucci JT, Wittenberg J, Mueller PR, Simeone JF, Harbin WP, Kirkpatrick RH, Taft PD (1980) Diagnosis of abdominal malignancy by radiologic fine needle aspiration biopsy. AJR 134: 323-330
67. Filly RA, Freimanis AK (1970) Echographic diagnosis of pancreatic lesions. Ultrasound scanning techniques and diagnostic findings. Radiology 96: 575-582
68. Fishman A, Isikoff MB, Barkin JS, Friedland JT (1979) Significance of a dilated pancreatic duct on CT examination. AJR 133: 225-227
69. Fleming MP, Carlson HC, Adson MA (1972) Percutaneous transhepatic cholangiography: the differential diagnosis of bile duct pathology. AJR 116: 327-336
70. Forstberg N (1938) Characteristic duodenal deformity in cases of different kinds of perivaterial enlargement of pancreas. Acta Radiol (Stockh) 19: 164-173
71. Freeny PC, Ball TJ (1978) Evaluation of endoscopic retrograde cholangiopancreatography and angiography in the diagnosis of pancreatic carcinoma. AJR 130: 683-691
72. Freeny PC, Ball TJ (1981) Endoscopic retrograde cholangiopancreatography (ERCP) and percutaneous transhepatic cholangiography (PTC), in the evaluation of suspected pancreatic carcinoma. Diagnostic limitation and contemporary roles. Cancer 47: 1666-1678
73. Freeny PC, Lawson TL (1982) Radiology of the pancreas. Springer, Berlin Heidelberg New York
74. Freeny PC, Anatonovic R, Gutierrez OH et al. (1976) Diagnosis effectiveness of infusion hepatic angiography. Röfo 124: 534-541
75. Freeny PC, Bilbao MK, Katon RM (1976) "Blind" evaluation of endoscopic retrograde chol-

angiopancreatography (ERCP) in the diagnosis of pancreatic carcinoma: the "double duct" and other signs. Radiology 119: 271-274

76. Freeny PC, Weinstein CJ, Taft DA, Allen FM (1978) Cystic neoplasms of the pancreas: new angiographic and ultrasonography findings. AJR 131: 795-802

77. Freeny PC, Ball TJ, Ryan J (1979) Impact of new diagnostic imaging methods on pancreatic angiography. AJR 133: 619-624

78. Freeny PC, Marks WM, Ball TJ (1982) Impact of high resolution computed tomography of the pancreas on utilisation of ERCP and angiography. Radiology 142: 35-39

79. Frick MP, Feinberg SB, Goodale RL (1982) The value of endoscopic retrograde cholangiopancreatography in patients with suspected carcinoma of the pancreas and indeterminate computed tomographic results. Surg Gynecol Obstet 155: 177-182

80. Frick MP, O'Leary JF, Salomonowitz E (1984) Stoltenberg P, Hutton S, Gedgaudas E (1984) Pancreas imaging by computed tomography after endoscopic retrograde pancreatography. Radiology 150: 191-194

81. Friedman AC, Lichtenstein JE, Dachman AH (1983) Cystic neoplasms of the pancreas. Radiological-pathological correlation. Radiology 149: 45-50

82. Frihmann-Dahl J (1961) Radiology in tumors of the pancreas. Clin Radiol 12: 73

83. Frija J, Vadrot D, Laval-Jeantet M (1983) Le pancréas normal et pathologique en échographie et en scanner. EPU

84. Fukumoto K, Nakajima M, Murakami K, Kawai K (1974) Diagnosis of pancreatic cancer by endoscopic pancreatocholangiography. Am J Gastroenterol 62: 210-223

85. Gambill E (1971) Pancreatitis associated with pancreatic carcinoma. A study of 26 cases. Mayo Clin Proc 46: 174-177

86. Garabedian M, Shanozad M (1975) Pancreatography in the diagnosis of carcinoma of the pancreas. Med Clin North Am 59: 239-246

87. Gold J, Rosenfield AT, Sostman D, Burrel M, Taylor KJW (1978) Non functioning islet cell tumor of the pancreas: radiographic and ultrasonic appearance in two cases. AJR 131: 715-717

88. Gold RP, Casarella WJ, Stern G, Seaman WB (1979) Transhepatic cholangiography: the radiological method of choice in suspected obstructive jaundice. Radiology 133: 39-44

89. Goldberg HI, Filly RA, Korobkin M et al. (1978) Capability of CT body scanning and ultrasonography to demonstrate the status of the biliary ductal system in patients with jaundice. Radiology 129: 731-737

90. Goldman ML, Gonzales AC, Galambos JT, Gordon IJ, Oen KT (1978) The transjugular technique of hepatic venography and biopsy, cholangiography and obliteration of oesophagal varices. Radiology 128: 325-331

91. Goldstein HM, Zornoza J (1978) Percutaneous transperitoneal aspiration biopsy of pancreatic masses. Dig Dis 23: 840-843

92. Goldstein HM, Neiman HL, Bookstein JJ (1974) Angiographic evaluation of pancreatic disease. A further appraisal. Radiology 112: 275-282

93. Goodale RL, Condie RM, Dresselt TD et al. (1979) A study of secretoryproteins, cytology and tumor site in pancreatic cancer. Ann Surg 189: 340-344

94. Goodale RL, Gajl-Peizalska A, Dresselt T, Samuelson J (1981) Cytologic studies for the diagnosis of pancreatic cancer. Cancer 47: 1652-1655

95. Grellet J, Viguier AC, Goverou M, Piekarski SD, Curet P, Weissman A (1980) Cancer du pancréas. EMC Paris, Radiodiagnostic IV, 33653 A10, 6, 1980.

96. Gudjonsson B, Spiro HM (1978) Biopsy techniques in the diagnosis of pancreatic cancer. Gastroenterology 75: 726-728

97. Guien C, Amatte R (1971) Valeur diagnostique et étude comparative des signes radiologiques des techniques standard dans les affections du pancréas. Acta Gastroenterol Belg 34: 115-121

98. Haaga JR, Alfidi RJ (1976) Precise biopsy localization by computed tomography. Radiology 118: 603-607

99. Haaga JR, Alfidi RJ (1977) Computed tomographic scanning of the pancreas. Radiol Clin North Am 15: 367-376

100. Haaga JR, Alfidi RJ, Zelch MG et al. (1976) Computed tomography of the pancreas. Radiology 120: 589-595

101. Haaga JR, Alfidi RJ, Havrillaa TR, Tubbs R, Gonzales L, Meaney TF, Corsi MA (1977) Definite role of CT scanning of the pancreas. Radiology 124: 723-730

102. Haber K, Freimanis AK, Asher MN (1976) Demonstration and dimensional analysis of the normal pancréas with gray-scale echography. AJR 126: 624–628
103. Hall TJ, Cooper M, Gugles RG, Levin B, Sdinner DB, Moossa AR (1977) Pancreatic cancer screening. Analysis of the problem and the role of radionucleide scanning. Am J Surg 134: 544–548
104. Hanafee WN, Rosch J, Weiner M (1970) Transjugular opacification of the biliary duct system. Radiology 94 (2): 429–432
105. Hancke S, Holm HH, Koch F (1975) Ultrasonically guided percutaneous fine needle biopsy of the pancreas. Surg Gynecol Obstet 140: 361–364
106. Harbin WP, Mueller PR, Ferrucci JT (1980) Transhepatic cholangiography: complications and use patterns of the fine needle technique. A multi institutional survey. Radiology 135: 15–22
107. Harfield ARW, Smithies A, Wilkins R, Levy AJ (1976) Assessment of endoscopic retrograde cholangiography (ERCP) and pure pancreatic juice cytology in patients with pancreatic diseases. Gut 17: 14–21
108. Harter LP, Moss AA, Goldberg HI, Gross BH (1983) CT guided fine needle aspirations for diagnosis of benign and malignant disease. AJR 140: 363–367
109. Haukohl RS, Melamed A (1950) Cystadenoma of the pancreas: a report of two cases showing calcification. AJR 63: 234–245
110. Havrilla TR, Haaga JR, Alfidi RJ, et al. (1977) Computed tomography and obstructive biliary disease. AJR 128: 765–768
111. Hawkins IF Jr, Kaude JV, MacGregor A (1975) Priscoline and epinephrine in selective pancreatic angiography. Radiology 116: 311–321
112. Hemmingsson A, Jacobson G, Lindgren PG, Lonnerholm T, Loreluis Nordgren CE (1982) Radiologic assessment of resectability carcinoma of the head of the pancreas. Acta Radiol [Diagn] (Stockh) 23
113. Hepp J, Moreaux J, Bismuth V, Hernandez C (1966) L'intéret de l'artériographie sélective dans la chirurgie pancréatique. Ann Chir 20: 465
114. Herlinger H, Finley DBL (1978) Evaluation and follow-up of pancreatic arteriograms. A new role for angiography in the diagnosis of carcinoma of the pancreas. Clin Radiol 29: 277–284
115. Hernandez C, Morin G, Ecarlat B (1965) L'embol pulsé en artériographie sélective digestive. Presse Méd 73: 2889
116. Hernandez C, Ecarlat B, Bismuth V (1967) L'artério-portographie des affections pancrétiques. J Radiol 48: 327
117. Hessel SJ, Siegelmann SS, MacNeil BJ et al. (1982) Prospective evaluation of computed tomography and ultrasound of the pancreas. Radiology 143: 129–133
118. Hingrat JY, Le Neel JC, Charles JF, Cousin C, Lenne Y (1980) Cystadénomes ou plutôt adénomes microkystiques et kystes mucineux du pancréas. J Chir 117 (6–7): 369–375
119. Hodgkinson DJ, Remine WH, Weiland LM (1978) Pancreatic cystadenoma. A clinicopathologic study of 45 cases. Arch Surg 113: 512–519
120. Hodgkinson DJ, Remine WH, Weiland LH (1978) A clinicopathologic study of 21 cases of pancreatic cystadenocarcinoma. Ann Surg 188: 679–684
121. Hoevels J, Lunderguist A, Ihse I (1978) Percutaneous transhepatic intubation of bile ducts for combined internal-external drainage in preoperative and palliative treatment of obstructive jaundice. Gastrointest Radiol 3: 23–31
122. Holm MH, Pedersen JF, Kristensen JK, Rasmussen SN, Jensen F (1975) Ultrasonically guided percutaneous puncture. Radiol Clin North Am 13: 493–503
123. Honjo I, Susuki T, Yoshitomi G (1968) L'artériographie pancréatique, sa valeur dans les cancers du pancréas. Lyon Chir 64: 587
124. Isler RJ, Ferrucci JT, Wittenberg J, Mueller PR, Simeone JF, van Sonnenberg E, Hall DA (1981) Tissue score biopsy of abdominal tumor with a 22-gauge cutting needle. AJR 136: 725–728
125. Isley JK, Schauble JF (1962) Interpretation of the percutaneous cholangiogram. AJR 88: 772–777
126. Itai Y, Moss AA, Ohtomo K (1982) Computed tomography of cystadenoma and cystadenocarcinoma of the pancreas. Radiology 145: 419–425
127. Jacquemet P (1966) Diagnostic précoce des tumeurs pancréatiques par la duodénographie hypotonique. J Electr 47: 264
128. Jacquemet P, Liotta D, Mallet-Guy P (1965) The early radiological diagnosis of diseases of the

pancreas and ampulla of vater: Elective exploration of the ampulla of vater and the head of the pancreas by hypotonic duodenography. Thomas, Springfield

129. Jaffe MH, Glazer GM, Amendola MA, Nostrant T, Wilson JAP (1984) Endoscopic retrograde computed tomography of the pancreas. J Comput Assist Tomogr 8 (1): 63-66

130. Jafri SZM, Aisen AM, Glazer GM, Weiss A (1984) Comparison of CT and angiography resectability of pancreatic carcinoma. AJR 142: 525-529

131. Johnson CC, Baggentoss AH (1949) Mesenteric vascular occlusion. Study of 99 cases of occlusion vein. Mayo Clin Proc 65: 45-47

132. Johnston F, Myers RT (1973) Etiologic factors and consequences of the splenic vein obstruction. Ann Surg 177: 736-739

133. Kamin PD, Bernardino ME, Wallace S, Bao-Shan Jing (1980) Comparison of ultrasound and computed tomography in the detection of pancreatic malignancy. Cancer 46: 2410-2412

134. Kaplan JO, Isikoff MB, Barkin J, Livingstone AS (1980) Necrotic carcinoma of the pancreas: the "pseudo-pseudocyst" J Comput Assist Tomogr 4: 166-167

135. Karasawa E, Goldberg HI, Moss AA, Federle MP, Stuart SL (1983) CT pancreatogram in carcinoma of the pancreas and chronic pancreatitis. Radiology 148: 489-493

136. Karp W, Lunderguist A, Tylen U, et al. (1980) Angiography and ultrasound examination in the evaluation of pancreatic lesions. Acta Radiol Diagn (Stockh) 21: 169-176

137. Kasugai T, Kuno N, Aoki I, et al. (1971) Fiberduodenoscopy: analysis of 353 examinations. Gastrointest Endosc 18: 9-16

138. Kasugai T, Kuno N, Kizu M, et al. (1972) Endoscopic pancreatography II. The pathologic endoscopic pancreatocholangiogram. Gastroenterology 63: 227-234

139. Kasugai T, Kuno N, Kizu M (1973) Endoscopic pancreatocholangiography with special reference to manometric method. Med J Aust 2: 717-725

140. Kawanishi H, Pollard HM (1979) Endoscopic evaluation of cancer of the pancreas. Semin Oncol 6: 309-317

141. Kawanishi M, Sell JE, Pollard HM (1975) Combined endoscopic pancreatic fluid collection and retrograde pancreatography in the diagnosis of pancreatic cancer and chronic pancreatitis. Gastrointest Endosc 22: 82-85

142. Kazam E, Whalen JP (1979) Computed tomography. In: Margulis AR, Burhenne HJ (eds) Alimentary tract radiology, vol 3. Mosby, St Louis, pp 72-122

143. Kieny R, Warter P, Japy C, Fontaine R (1965) Aspects angiographiques dans les affections pancréatiques. J Radiol 46: 867

144. Kittredge RD, Baer JW (1975) Percutaneous transhepatic cholangiograph. Problems in interpretation. AJR 125: 35-46

145. Koehler R, Anderson RE (1980) Computed angiotomography. Radiology 137: 843-845

146. Kolmannskog F, Schrumpf E, Bergan A, Larsen S (1982) Diagnostic value of computed tomography in pancreatic carcinoma; a comparison with other radiologic methods. Acta Radiol [Diagn] (Stockh) 23

147. Kozu T, Endoscopic collection of intraductal pure pancreatic juice and its applications to the cytodiagnosis in endoscopy of pancreatography.

148. Kreel L (1967) The pancreas. Newer radiological methods of investigation. Postgrad Med 43: 14-23

149. Kreel L (1980) Computed tomography of pancreatic tumors. In: Kawai K (ed) Early diagnosis of pancreatic cancer. Igaku-Shoin, New York, pp 89-104

150. Kreel L, Haertel M, Katz D (1977) Computed tomography of the normal pancreas. J Comput Assist Tomogr 1: 290-299

151. Kruse A, Thommesen P, Frederiksen P (1978) Endoscopic retrograde cholangiopancreatography in pancreatic cancer and chronic pancreatitis. Scand J Gastroenterol 13: 513-517

152. Kunzmann A, Bowie JD, Rochester D (1979) Texture patterns in pancreatic sonograms. Gastrointest Radiol 4: 353-357

153. Laing FC, Gooding GAW, Brown T, Leopold GR (1979) Atypical pseudo-cysts of the pancreas: an ultrasonographic evaluation. J Clin Ultrasound 7: 27-33

154. Lamarque JL, Ginestie JF, Combes C, Senac JP (1972) Aspects artériographiques des cancers du pancréas et des pancréatites. Confrontations sémiologiques et radioanatomiques, à propos de 70 cas confirmés chirurgicalement et histologiquement. Ann Radiol (Paris) 15: 697

155. Lamarque JL, Bruel JM, Senac JP (1974) L'artériographie dans le bilan des affections pancréatiques; étude critique à propos de 200 cas. IX Congrès de Radiologie de Culture Latine, Venice

156. Lamarque JL, Bruel JM, Dondelinger R, Vendrell B, Pelissier O, Rouanet JP, Michel JL, Boulet P (1979) The use of iodolipids in hepatosplenic computed tomography. J Comput Assist Tomogr 3: 21-24
157. Lamarque JL, Bruel JM, Rouanet JP (1983) La détection précoce du cancer secondaire du foie. Valeur, limite et indication de l'échographie, de la scanographie, de l'artériographie. Rev Fr Gastroenterol 185: 49-51
158. Lamonte CS, Decosse JJ, McPeak CJ (1962) Carcinoma of the pancreas presenting with gastrointestinal bleeding. JAMA 180: 974-976
159. Lang EK (1978) Percutaneous transhepatic cholangiography. Radiology 112: 283-290
160. Laufer I (1979) Double contrast gastrointestinal radiology with endoscopic correlation. Saunders, Philadelphia
161. Laval-Jeantet P, Gardeur P, Taboury J, Monnier JP, Bigot JM (1976) Anatomie échographique du pancréas normal. J Radiol 57: 149-155
162. Lawson TL (1978) Sensitivity of pancreatic ultrasonography in the detection of pancreatic disease. Radiology 128: 733-736
163. Lawson TL, Irami SK, Stock M (1978) Detection of pancreatic pathology by ultrasonography and endoscopic retrograde cholangiography. Gastrointest Radiol 3: 335-341
164. Lawson TL, Berland LL, Foley WD, et al. (1982) Ultrasonic visualization of the pancreatic duct. Radiology 144: 865-871
165. Lee JKT, Stanley RJ, Melson GL et al. (1979) Pancreatic imaging by ultrasound and computed tomography. A general review. Radiol Clin North Am 16: 105-117
166. Lee TG, Henderson SC, Ehrlich R (1977) Ultrasound diagnosis of common bile duct dilatation. Radiology 124: 793-797
167. Lemaitre G, L'Herminie C, Rembert A, Delhay J (1972) Le retour veineux mésentérique supérieur au cours de l'hypertension portale. J Radiol 53: 311-316
168. Levin DC, Wilson R, Abrams HL (1980) The changing role of pancreatic arteriography in the era of computed tomography. Radiology 136: 245
169. Levitt RG, Sagel SS, Stanley RJ, et al. (1977) Accuracy of computed tomography of the liver and biliary tract. Radiology 124: 123-128
170. Levitt RG, Stanley RJ, Sagel SS, Lee JTK, Weyman PJ (1982) Computed tomography of the pancreas: three second scanning versus 18 second scanning. J Comput Assist Tomogr 6 (2): 259-267
171. Lewis E, Aufderheide JF, Bernardino ME, Barnes PA, Thomas JL (1982) CT detection of hepatic metastases with ethiodized oil emulsion 13. J Comput Assist Tomogr 6: 1108-1114
172. Liguory C, Coffin JC (1977) Cathétérisme endoscopique rétrograde des voies biliaires. Rev Prat 27: 3629-3639
173. Liguory CL, Canard JM, Sahel J (1984) Endoscopic digestive diagnostique. EMC Estomac Intestin, 9013, B10 3
174. Lunderquist A (1965) Angiography in carcinoma of the pancreas. Acta Radiol [Suppl] (Stockh): 235
175. MacCain AH, William A, Berkmann, Bernardino ME (1984) Pancreatic sonography: past and present. J Clin Ultrasound 12: 325-332
176. Mackie CR, Lu CT, Noble HG, Cooper MJ (1979) Prospective evaluation of angiography in the diagnosis and management of patients suspected of having pancreatic cancer. Ann Surg 189: 11-17
177. Mackie CR, Bowie J, Cooper MJ et al. (1978) Prospective evaluation of gray-scale ultrasonography in the diagnostic of pancreas cancer. Am J Surg 136: 575-581
178. Mackie CR, Moossa AR, Franck PM (1980) The place of angiography in the diagnosis and management of pancreatic tumors. In: Moossa AR (ed) Tumors of the pancreas. Williams and Wilkins, Baltimore, 355-380
179. Malini S, Sabel J (1977) Ultrasonography in obstructive jaundice. Radiology 123: 429-433
180. Mallet GP, Jacquemet P (1967) Résultats comparatifs de la duodénographie hypotonique et des autres techniques d'exploration radiologique du pancréas. J Radiol 48: 352
181. Margulis AR (1973) Neoplasms of the pancreas. In: Margulis AR, Burhenne HJ (eds) Alimentary tract roentgenology, vol 2. St Louis
182. Marks LJ, Weingarten B, Gerst GB (1952) Carcinoma of tail of pancreas associated with bleeding gastric varices and hyperplenism. Ann Intern Med 37: 1077-1079

183. McCormack LR, Seat SG, Strum WB (1977) Pancreatic carcinoma. Survival following detection by ultrasonic scanning. JAMA 238: 240-241
184. McDermott WV Jr (1980) Portal hypertension secondary to pancreatic disease. Ann Surg 152: 147-149
185. McLoughlin MJ, Ho GS, Langer B, McHattie J, Tao LL (1978) Fine needle aspiration biopsy of malignant lesions in and around the pancreas. Cancer 41: 2413-2419
186. Meaney TF, Winkelman E, Sullivan BM, Brown CH (1963) Selective splanchnic arteriography in the diagnosis of pancreatic tumours. Cleve Clin Q 30: 193
187. Merba MJ, Kiss J (1971) Percutaneous transhepatic cholangiography experience with 106 examinations. J Can Assoc Radiol 22: 22-29
188. Meyer-Burg J, Zieller V, Kirstaedter I, Palme G (1973) Peritonoscopy in carcinoma of the pancreas. Report of 20 cases. Endoscopy 5: 86-90
189. Mittlestaedt C, Leopold GR (1977) B-scan ultrasound of the liver, the gallbladder and pancreas. Int Surg 62: 277
190. Mitty HA, Efremidis SC, Yeh HC (1981) Impact of the fine needle biopsy on management of patients with carcinoma of the pancreas. AJR 137: 1119-1121
191. Moossa AR (1982) Pancreatic cancer; approach to diagnosis selection for surgery and choice of operation. Cancer 50: 2689-2698
192. Morii T, Endo Y, Ebara M, Tatsuta M, Okuda S, Tamura H (1974) Diagnosis of pancreatic cancer by pancreatography and cytology with duodenal fiberscope (Abstr). In: XIth International Cancer Congress, Florence. Excerpta Medica, Amsterdam
193. Moss AA, Kressal HY (1977) Computed tomography of the pancreas. Dig Dis 22: 1018-1027
194. Mozan AA (1951) Cystadenoma of the pancreas. Am J Surg 204: 214
195. Muhletaler C, Gerlock AJ Jr, Goncharenko V et al. (1979) Gastric varices secondary to splenic vein occlusion. Radiographic diagnosis and clinical significance. Radiology 132: 593-598
196. Muhletaler CA, Gerlock AJ Jr, Fleischer AC et al. (1980) Diagnosis of obstructive jaundice with nondilated bile ducts. AJR 134: 1149-1152
197. Mujahed Z, Evans JA (1966) Percutaneous transhepatic cholangiography. Radiol Clin North Am 4: 535-545
198. Nebel OT, Silvis SE, Rogers G, Sugawa C, Maldelstam P (1975) Complications associated with endoscopic retrograde cholangiopancreatography. Results of the 1974 A/SG/E. Surg Gastrointest Endosc 22: 34-36
199. Nebesar RA, Pollard JJ (1965) Advances in abdominal angiography. Postgrad Med 37: 504-512
200. Nebesar RA, Pollard JJ (1967) A critical evaluation of selective and superior mesenteric angiography in the diagnosis of pancreatic diseases, particular malignant tumor: facts and "artefacts". Radiology 89: 1017-1027
201. Nebesar RA, Pollard JJ, Edmunds UH Jr, McKhann DF (1964) Indications for selective celiac and superior mesenteric angiography. Experience with 128 cases. Radiology 92: 1100-1109
202. Norton RA, Ogoshi K, Hara Y, Niwa M, Paul RE Jr, Thomas J, Fawaz K (1973) Pancreatographic abnormalities due to pancreatic cancer. Gastrointest Endos 20: 13-14
203. Odman P (1958) Percutaneous selective angiography of the coeliac artery. Acta Radiol [Suppl] (Stockh) 159
204. Odman P (1959) Percutaneous selective angiography of the superior mesenteric artery. Acta Radiol (Stockh) 51: 25
205. Ohto M, Ono T, Tsuchiya Y, Saisho H (1978) Cholangiography and pancreatography. University Park Press, Baltimore
206. Ohto M, Saotome N, Saisho H, et al. (1980) Real-time sonography of the pancreatic duct. Application to percutaneous pancreatic ductography. AJR 134: 647-652
207. Okuda K, Tanikawa K, Emura T, Kuratomi S et al. (1974) Nonsurgical percutaneous transhepatic cholangiography - diagnostic significance in medical problems of the liver. Am J Dig Dis 19: 21-36
208. Op Den Orth JO (1973) Hypotonic duodenography without the use of a stomach tube. Radiol Clin Biol 42: 173-174
209. Oscarson J, Stormby N, Sundgren R (1972) Selective angiography in fine needle aspiration cytodiagnosis of gastric and pancreatic tumors. Acta Radiol [Diagn] (Stockh) 12: 737-749
210. Osnes M, Serck Hanssen A, Myren J (1975) Endoscopic retrograde brush cytology (ERBC) of the biliary and pancreatic ducts. Scand J Gastroenterol 10: 829-831

211. Paloyan D, Skinner DB (1976) Clinical significance of pancreatic ascites. Am J Surg 132: 114-117
212. Paolaggi JA, La laparoscopie en pathologie hépatobiliaire. Encycl Méd Chir Paris. Foie pancréas 4.1.10 7008 A - 10
213. Paulino-Netto A, Dreiling DA, Barnofsky ID (1960) Relationship between pancreatic calcification and cancer of the pancreas. Ann Surg 151: 530-537
214. Pedrosa CS, Casanova R, Rodriguez R (1981) Computed tomography in obstructive jaundice. Radiology 139: 627-634
215. Pereiras R, White P, Dusol M Jr et al. (1976) Percutaneous transhepatic cholangiography utilizing the chiba university needle. Radiology 121: 219-221
216. Pereiras R, Chiprut RO, Greenwald RA et al. (1977) The "skinny" needle: a rapid, simple and accurate method in the diagnosis of cholestasis. Ann Intern Med 86: 562-568
217. Perlemitter GS (1977) Pancreas. In: Folberg BB (ed) Abdominal grayscale ultrasonography. Wiley Medical, New York, pp 168-213
218. Pietri H, Sahel J, Sarles H (1977) Diagnosis of cancer of the pancreas by echotomography, endoscopic wirsungography, arteriography and other means. In: Glass GBJ (ed) Progress in gastroenterology. Grune and Stratton, New York, pp 617-642
219. Piper CE, Remine WH, Priestley JT (1962) Pancreatic cystadenoma. Report of 20 cases. JAMA 180: 648-652
220. Plecha FR, Hugues CW, Smith ML et al. (1966) Percutaneous transhepatic cholangiography. Arch Surg 92: 672-676
221. Plumley TF, Rohrmann CA, Freeny PC, Silvenstein FE, Ball JT (1982) Double duct sign reassessed significance in endoscopic retrograde cholangiopancreatogram. AJR 138: 31-35
222. Pollock D, Taylor KJW (1981) Ultrasound scanning in patients with clinical suspicion of pancreatic cancer. Cancer 47: 1662-1665
223. Poos C (1983) Application de la scanographie à la radiologie d'intervention. Medical dissertation, University of Strasbourg
224. Ralls PW, Hallis J, Renner I, Juttner H (1980) Endoscopic retrograde cholangiopancreatography in pancreatic disease. A reassessment of the specificity of ductal abnormalities in differentiating benign from malignant disease. Radiology 134: 347-352
225. Ranniger K, Saldino RM (1966) Arteriographic diagnosis of pancreatic lesions. Radiology 86: 470
226. Raptopoulos V, Schellinger D (1979) Imaging of the pancreas with computed tomography. Computed Tomography 3: 37-47
227. Redeker AJ, Karvountzis GG, Richman RM et al. (1975) Percutaneous transhepatic cholangiography: an improved technique. JAMA 231: 386-387
228. Reuben A, Cotton PB (1979) Endoscopic retrograde cholangiopancreatography in carcinoma of the pancreas. Surg Gynecol Obstet 148: 179-184
229. Reuter SR (1975) Superselective pancreatic angiography. In: Anacker H (ed) Efficiency and limits of radiologic examination of the pancreas. Thieme, Stuttgart, pp 149-158
230. Reuter SR, Redman HC, Bookstein JJ (1970) Differential problems in the angiographic diagnosis of carcinoma of the pancreas. Radiology 96: 93
231. Ring EJ, Oleaga JA, Freiman DB, Husted JW, Lunderquist A (1978) Therapeutic application of catheter cholangiography. Radiology 128: 333-338
232. Robbins AH, Gerzof SG, Pugatch RD (1979) Newer imaging techniques for the diagnosis of pancreatic cancer. Semin Oncol 6: 332-343
233. Roberts-Thomson IC (1977) Endoscopic retrograde pancreatography. Analysis of the normal pancreatogram and changes which are associated with chronic pancreatitis and pancreatic carcinoma. Med J Aust 2: 793-796
234. Rohmer P, Bagni A, Manzoni JM, Weill F (1982) Etude sémiologique et statistique comparative. Ultrasons et scanographie des affections pancrétiques. J Radiol 63: 535-542
235. Rohrman CA Jr, Silvis SE, Vennes JA (1976) The significance of pancreatic ductal obstruction in differential diagnosis of the anormal endoscopic retrograde pancreatogram. Radiology 121: 311-314
236. Rosch J, Herfort K (1962) Contribution of splenoportography to the diagnosis of diseases of the pancreas. Acta Med Scand 251: 1971
237. Rosch J, Holman DC (1975) Superselective arteriography of the pancreas. In: Anacker H (ed)

Efficiency and limits on radiologic examination of the pancreas. Thieme, Stuttgart, pp 159-167
238. Rosch J, Judkins MP (1968) Angiography in the diagnosis of pancreatic disease. Semin Roentgenol 3: 296-309
239. Rosch J, Lakin PC, Antonovic R, Dotter CT (1973) Transjugular approach to liver biopsy and transhepatic cholangiography. N Engl J Med 289: 227-231
240. Rosch J, Freeny PC, Antonovic R et al. (1976) Infusion hepatic angiography in diagnosis of liver metastases. Cancer 38: 2278-2286
241. Rumancik WM, Megibow AJ, Merton A, Hilton S (1984) Metastatic disease to the pancreas. Evaluation by computed tomography. J Comput Assist Tomogr 5: 829-834
242. Sammons BP, Neal MP, Armstrong RM Jr, Hager HG (1967) Ten years experience with celiac and upper abdominal superior mesenteric arteriography. AJR 101: 345
243. Sample WF, Sarti SA, Goldstein LI et al. (1978) Gray-scale ultrasonography of the jaundiced patient. Radiology 128: 719-725
244. Sankaran S, Sugawa C, Walt AJ (1979) Value of endoscopic retrograde pancreatography in pancreatic ascites. Surg Gynecol Obstet 148: 185-192
245. Sarles H (1980) Le pancréas exocrine. Flammarion, Paris, p 21
246. Sati T, Saitoh Y, Koyama K, Watanable K (1968) Presperative determination of operability in carcinomas of the pancreas and periampullary region. Ann Surg 168: 876-886
247. Schwartz THR, William GMR (1983) Bile duct obstruction secondary to lymphomatous involvement of the pancreas. J Clin Ultrasound 11: 391-394
248. Shanser JD, Korobkin M, Goldberg HI et al. (1978) Computed tomographic diagnosis of obstructive jaundice in the absence of intrahepatic ductal dilatation. AJR 131: 389-392
249. Sheedy PF II, Stephens DH, Hattery RR et al. (1977) Computed tomography of the pancreas. Radiol Clin North Am 15: 349-366
250. Sheedy PF II, Stephens DH, Hattery RR, MacCarty RL (1977) Computed tomography in the evaluation of patients with suspected carcinoma of the pancreas. Radiology 124: 731-737
251. Silvis SE, Schuman BM (1977) Benig conditions of the pancreas. In: Stewart ET, Vennes JA, Greenen JE (eds) Atlas of endoscopic retrograde cholangiopancreatography. Mosby, St Louis
252. Silvis SE, Rohrmann CA, Vennes JA (1973) Diagnostic criteria for the evaluation of the endoscopic pancreatogram. Gastrointest Endosc 20: 51-55
253. Smith EH, Bartrum RJ, Chang YC et al. (1985) Percutaneous aspiration biopsy of the pancreas under ultrasonic guidance. N Engl J Med 292: 825-828
254. Smith FW, Reid A, Hutchinson JMS, Mallard JR, Path FRC (1982) Nuclear magnetic resonance imaging of the pancreas. Radiology 142: 677-680
255. Smith TJ, Kemeny MM, Sugarbaker PH, Jones AE, Vermess H, Shawker TA, Edwards BK (1982) A prospective study of hepatic imaging in the detection of metastatic disease. Ann Surg 195: 486-491
256. Sorabella PA, Campbel WL, Seaman WB (1975) Comparative detection of pancreatic body-tail enlargement using the supine translateral and axial pancreatic views. A prospective statistical study. AJR 125: 143-153
257. Stadelmann O, Safrang L, Loffler A, et al. (1974) Endoscopic retrograde cholangiopancreatography in the diagnosis of pancreatic cancer. Endoscopy 6: 84-93
258. Stanley RJ (1980) Pancreas. Computed tomography. In: Moss AA, Goldberg HI (eds) Computed tomography, ultrasound and X-ray: an integrated approach. Masson, Paris, pp 89-105
259. Stanley RJ, Sagel SS, Levitt RG (1977) Computed tomography of the pancreas. Radiology 124: 705-712
260. Stanley RJ, Sagel SS, Evens RG (1981) The impact of new imaging methods on pancreatic arteriography. Radiology 136: 251
261. Stark DD, Moos AA, Goldberg HI et al. (1984) Magnetic resonance and CT of the normal and deseaded pancreas: a comparative study. Radiology 150: 153-162
262. Stephens DH, Hattery RR, Sheedy PF II (1976) Computed tomography of the abdomen. Early experience with the EMI body scanner. Radiology 119: 331-335
263. Stephens DH, Sheedy PF II (1979) Computed tomography. In: Margulis AR, Burhenne HJ (eds) Alimentary tract radiology, abdominal imaging. Mosby, St Louis, pp 251-274
264. Stewart ET, Vennes JA, Geenen JE (1977) Atlas of endoscopic retrograde cholangio-pancreatography. Mosby, St Louis, p 247

265. Stuber JL, Templeton AW, Bishop K (1972) Sonography diagnosis of pancreatic lesions. AJR 116: 406-412
266. Suhas G, Parulekar SG (1980) Ultrasonic evaluation of the pancreatic duct. J Clin Ultrasound 8: 457-463
267. Susuki T, Manabe T, Tani T, Tobe T (1980) Angiography and pancreatoductography in resectable carcinoma of the pancreas. Acta Radiol [Diagn] (Stockh) 21
268. Sutton JP, Yarborough DY, Richards JT (1970) Isolated splenic vein occlusion. Arch Surg 100: 623-626
269. Tada S, Fukuda K, Aoyagi Y, Avada J (1980) CT of abdominal malignancies: dynamic approach. AJR 135: 455-461
270. Takemoto T, Kasugai T (1979) Endoscopic retrograde pancreatocholangiography. Igaku-shoin, Tokyo
271. Takuya Hosoki (1983) Dynamic CT of pancreatic tumors. AJR 140: 959-965
272. Tatsuta M, Yamamoto R, Yamamura H et al. (1983) Cytologic examination and CEA measurement in aspirated pancreatic material collected by percutaneous fine needle aspiration biopsy under ultrasonic guidance for the diagnosis of pancreatic carcinoma. Cancer 52: 693-698
273. Taylor KJW, Brand MH (1979) Ultrasonic biopsy guidance in the management of patients with pancreatic cancer. J Clin Gastroenterol 1: 267-272
274. Tylen U (1973) Angiographic differentiation between inflammatory disease and carcinoma of the pancreas. Acta Radiol (Stockh) 14: 257
275. Tylen U (1973) Accuracy of angiography in the diagnosis of carcinoma of the pancreas. Acta Radiol (Stockh) 14: 449-466
276. Tylen U, Hoevels J, Vang J (1977) Percutaneous transhepatic cholangiography with external drainage of obstructive biliary lesions. Surg Gynecol. Obstet 144: 13-18
277. Walls WJ, Templeton JW (1977) The ultrasonic demonstration of inferior vena caval compression. A guide to pancreatic head enlargement with emphasis on neoplasm. Radiology 123: 165-167
278. Walls WJ, Gonzales G, Martin NL et al. (1975) B. scan ultrasound evaluation of the pancreas. Radiology 114: 127-134
279. Warter J, Walter P, Bareiss P, Sibilly A (1981) Cystadenomes du pancréas. Considérations sur leur vascularisation et les maladies qui leur sont associées. Sem Hop Paris 57 (11-12): 529-537
280. Weill F (1982) Ultrasonographie en pathologie digestive. Vigot, Paris
281. Weinreb JC, Maravilla KR, Redman HC, Nunnally R (1984) Improved MR imaging of the upper abdomen with glucagon and gas. J Comput Assist Tomogr 5: 835-838
282. Weinstein DP, Weinstein PJ (1979) Ultrasonic demonstration of the pancreatic duct: an analysis of 41 cases. Radiology 130: 729-734
283. Weinstein DP, Wolfman NT, Weinstein BJ (1979) Ultrasonic characteristics of pancreatic tumors. Gastrointest Radiol 4: 245-251
284. Whaklen JP (1979) Caldwell lecture. Radiology of the abdomen. Impact of new imaging methods. AJR 133: 587-618
285. Wilkins RA, Hatfield A (1977) Cholangio-pancreatography and pancreatic cytology in carcinoma of the pancreas. AJR 128: 747-749
286. Wise RE (1962) Intravenous cholangiography. Thomas, Springfield
287. Wittenberg J, Ferrucci JT (1979) Radiologically guided needle biopsy of abdominal neoplasms. - Who, how, where, and why? J Clin Gastroenterol 1: 273-284
288. Wolfman NT, Ramquist NA, Karstaedt N, Hopkins MB (1982) Cystic neoplasm of the pancreas: CT and sonography. AJR 138: 37-41
289. Wood RAB, Moosaa AR, Blackstone MO et al. (1976) Comparative value of four methods of investigating the pancreas. Surgery 80: 518-522
290. Wright CH, Maklad F, Rosenthal SJ (1979) Gray scale ultrasound characteristics of carcinoma of the pancreas. Br J Radiol 52: 281-288
291. Yamanaka T, et al. (1979) Differential diagnosis of pancreatic mass lesion with percutaneous fine needle aspiration biopsy under ultrasonic guidance. Dig Dis Sci 24: 694
292. Yong HO, Auh Rubenstein WA, Kneeland JB, Kazam E, Whalen JP (1984) The peripancreatic vascular arcade. A source of pitfalls for CT and ultrasound diagnoses. RSNA Scientific Program 133
293. Yuji I, Moss AA, Goldberg HI (1982) Pancreatic cysts caused by carcinoma of the pancreas. A pitfall in the diagnosis of pancreatic carcinoma. J Comput Assist Tomogr 6: 772-776

294. Yuji I, Tsutomi A, Akiri T, Masakazu M (1982) Computed tomographic appearance of resectable pancreatic carcinoma. Radiology 143: 719-726
295. Zeman RK, Washington DC, Jaffe MH, Clark LR, Paushter D, Schiebler M, Moser BE, Choyke P, Grant EG (1984) The clinical and imaging spectrum of pancreatico-duodenal nodal enlargement. RSNA Scientific program: 134
296. Zimmon DS, Falkenstein DB, Riccobono C, Aaron B (1975) Complications of endoscopic retrograde cholangiopancreatography. Analysis of 300 consecutive cases. Gastroenterology 69: 303-309

6 Present Strategies for Diagnosis

H. Baumel, B. Deixonne, A. Dubois, F. M. Lopez, and P. Lopez

The results of therapy for carcinoma of the pancreas are very poor; therefore, this chapter, generated by the desire to improve the end results, should be read from a special point of view. At present, nearly 90% of the pancreatic cancers are incurable at the time of surgical intervention [12]. In order to improve the prognosis of these cancers diagnoses must be achieved earlier.

6.1 Early Diagnosis

With the present state of art, can we really diagnose early pancreatic cancer, i. e., can we detect resectable tumors, 1–2 cm long, that may possibly be cured by the appropriate surgery? Theoretically, yes, for present techniques allow it, but in practice, no, for this cancer is asymptomatic in its early stage. The answer to this question will no doubt remain negative as long as epidemiologists are unable to define precisely a population at high risk. The epidemiological data, as previously reported, are still uncertain, in particular for local factors (pancreatitis, ductal hyperplasia, dysplasia) which would help in defining precancerous states. Besides such conditions are not easily detected, owing to the difficulty of pancreatic exploration. This is really unfortunate, for the local risk factors are by far the best epidemiological parameters of early cancer detection. We must hope for further advances in this field, in order that we may take preventive measures (elimination of some environmental factors) and – more important – efficiently survey the high risk subjects. As long as such a population is not clearly defined, we cannot contemplate submitting symptom-free groups to an invasive screening procedure involving long and expensive investigations. It has been established that the screening of more than 10000 subjects would be necessary for a case study to detect one asymptomatic cancer out of the lot [10]. For many reasons, such a program can not be carried out.

In the meantime we can at least try to make less late diagnoses. To succeed, we must better our knowledge of the first revealing symptoms of pancreatic cancer. They are generally vague and imprecise, so much so, that it appears necessary to inform the public as well as the doctors of pancreatic pathology.

6.2 Presenting Symptoms

The pancreas, as a result of its deep anatomical localization and "silent" functions, is totally ignored by most people. No patient thinks of the pancreas as the possible origin of his symptoms, though he would likely relate some signs to the liver, stomach, kidney, etc.

From another point of view, a great many doctors tend to localize many organs in the upper abdomen or in the back, forgetting that the pancreas also projects to these regions. Under these conditions, it is not surprising that the presenting symptoms alarm neither the patients, who neglect them, nor the doctors, who – blaming other organs – require symptomatic therapies and ask for investigations directed toward other targets. The weeks or even months thus lost result in a smaller chance of survival.

A campaign is necessary to inform the public about the pancreas, to assure a better knowledge of this organ, its functions, and its diseases. Medical teaching should make doctors better aware of the traps and seriousness of pancreatic cancer and should train them to ask, in the presence of certain symptoms, for earlier explorations.

Among all the symptoms of pancreatic cancer, not even one is specific for this disease; they are nearly all "borrowed" symptoms which appear late in its course. Jaundice is perhaps the most suggestive, and encourages more examinations. Unfortunately, it is a presenting symptom in only 40%–54% of cases [3, 7, 13]. A great many investigations are often necessary to determine its pancreatic origin.

The other symptoms are more frequent and more deceptive. For instance, epigastric pain is frequently taken for the pain of an ulcer and is therefore treated by antacid therapy, which may lead to a false and dangerous improvement. Pain in the back is frequently attributed to a vertebral arthrosis. A recent onset of diabetes may be interpreted as banal diabetes of the over-50 age-group. In fact, diabetes mellitus may either precede carcinoma of the pancreas or be a consequence of it [5].

In a prospective diagnostic study, Di Magno et al. [6] hold to the following five criteria:

1. Upper abdominal pain
2. Abdominal pain with nocturnal awakening or radiation of pain into the back
3. Weight loss of 10% of ideal body weight
4. Unexplained obstructive jaundice
5. Unexplained pancreatitis

When a patient presents at least two of these symptoms he or she should undergo more morphological investigations. The results of this study show the predictive value of Di Magno's criteria as 43%.

Similary, Moossa defined a suspicious-symptom index for doctors [12]:

1. Recent (less than 2 years' duration) upper abdominal and/or back pain consistent with a retroperitoneal origin
2. Recent vague upper abdominal pain (or dyspepsia) with negative gastrointestinal investigations
3. Obstructive jaundice
4. Unexplained weight loss greater than 5% of normal body weight

5. Sudden unexplained onset of diabetes mellitus in an adult without a predisposing
   cause, such as family history or obesity

Marton et al. [9] underlined that the sensitivity and specificity of such symptoms
are difficult to define clearly. Their sensitivity is globally evaluated to be 75%. Actually, most patients who harbor a carcinoma of the pancreas present at least one of
these symptoms, often two. As to their specificity, it cannot be defined, though Marton tried by applying Bayes' formula.

These symptoms frequently appear later in the course of the disease and their
value in early diagnosis is very relative. It is best to consider them "pancreatic warn-
ing lights," in order to shorten the time between the onset of the disease and diagnosis. Jaundice alone can be relevant in the case of small tumors of the head, or for
periampullary or juxtacholedochal tumors, but this is unfortunately very rare.
Diagnosis is achieved more rapidly in the presence of this symptom, within 5 weeks
or so, whereas 4 months are usually required when there is no jaundice [12].

6.3 Further Investigations

Nowadays, a great many more or less invasive and expensive explorations are possible. Thus, it is important to define the performance of each, to be able to decide
which will lead to an earlier diagnosis. Many works have tried to report their respective accuracy (sensitivity, specificity and predictive value). It is impossible at this
point to discuss them all, this have been done elsewhere (cf. chaps. 4 and 5). Some
confusion emerges from these studies, and to some extent a certain contradiction.
Here we shall just give our personal opinion on the value of these examinations and
on the strategic priorities that can lead to earlier detection of carcinoma of the pancreas.

In general, *biological examinations* do not have favorable results. As far as sero-
diagnoses and tumor marker assays are concerned, the ideal tumor marker has not
yet been defined, especially as regards an "early diagnosis." Some authors stress the
value of pancreatic function tests performed by means of duodenal intubation and
also of aspiration cytology after stimulation; but generally, the most sensitive tests
are unfortunately not always the most specific. Other authors emphasize the value
of tumor markers in the pancreatic juice. We consider these tests of little value, giv-
en the fact that most positive results concern advanced tumors. In spite of certain
studies [8, 11], several questions remain to be answered before we know if they are
truly reliable for small-tumor diagnosis.

On the whole, *morphological examinations* yield very good diagnostic results.
Nowadays, the best investigations for early diagnosis are ultrasonography (US)
and/or computerized tomography (CT), endoscopic retrograde cholangiopancreatography (ERCP), cytology, and laparotomy.

Ultrasonography is in the same class as CT. Both are noninvasive techniques
and allow a systematic gross evaluation of the organs. Moreover, they have great
predictive value as well as great diagnostic accuracy. Cancers of the head of the
pancreas are better detected by means of US, while cancers of the body and tail of

the pancreas are more likely to require CT scanning. The latter appears to be of greater overall value.

ERCP allows a ductal and cytologic-morphological study. Because it does not change the contours of the pancreas, ERCP helps in confirming the diagnosis of small intraglandular masses, otherwise only suggested or even ignored by US or CT scans. When combined with cytology, ERCP is the technique of choice in diagnosing the nature of a pancreatic mass. The limitations of this method are that it is an invasive investigation, with possible side effects, and that it sometimes fails, even in experienced hands.

Percutaneous needle aspiration is being used more and more. The findings depend on both the operator's and the cytologist's skills. Among the series reported by ten different authors [2], the average reliability of this investigation is 78%, with extremes ranging from 66% to 100%!

The comparative study of five different methods of investigation reported by Moossa and Levin [11] is interesting, for it makes a strong case of their respective sensitivity as a function of the resectability of the tumor (Fig. 6.1).

The endoscopic ultrasonography advocated by Yasuda is still used very little [4]. However, it should have a very high sensitivity in diagnosing small tumors of the head of the pancreas.

6.4 Pretherapeutic Appraisal

A pretherapeutic appraisal must be made whenever an investigation has suggested or proved a pancreatic lesion to be malignant. It should include a strict appraisal of the general well-being of the patient and a search for the extent of the tumor.

The extent can be estimated precisely only at laparotomy. However, it must be evaluated prior to any operation, particularly using US and/or CT to detect distant metastases, as their presence has great significance for decisions on therapy. Invasion by contiguity must be estimated by the search for adenopathies and the involvement of juxtapancreatic vessels. In such cases, CT and angiography are the best methods for detecting nodes and vascular invasion respectively. We feel that angiography is more helpful in this investigation than in characterizing the malignancy of a pancreatic mass. Moreover, it can give the surgeon information on possible vascular malformation.

The results of angiography and ERCP can be compared, and it is then easier to determine the contiguous invasion of the tumor. This is advised by Susuki et al. [15], who studied the resectability rates as compared with the previous data (Table 6.1). Actually, angiography gives more information of the tumor extent to the contour of the pancreas, as ERCP only permits the definition of the intra-glandular invasion.

The assay of tumor markers is not reliable enough to provide valuable information during this appraisal, but an elevated serum level does imply a voluminous tumor and extraglandular extension.

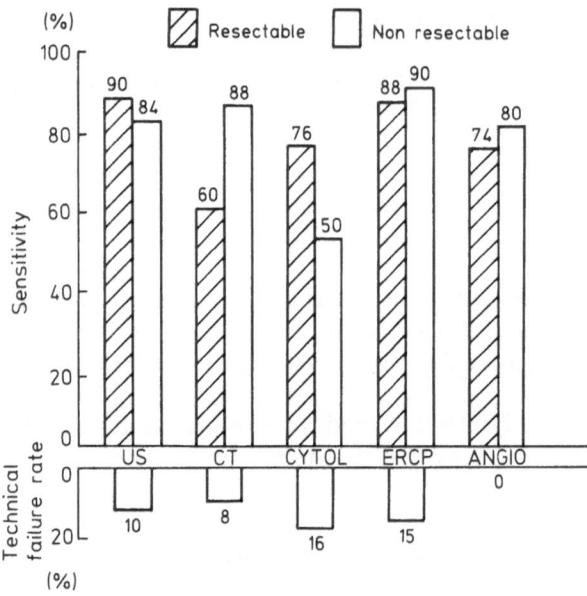

Fig. 6.1. Performance of five tests in diagnosis of resectable and nonresectable pancreatic cancer (from Moossa and Levin [11])

Table 6.1. Incidence and resectability of 37 cancers of the pancreas in relation to findings by arteriography and pancreatography (from Susuki et al. [15])

Type	Vascular invasion on arteriography	Ductal invasion on pancreatography	No. of cases	No. of resectable cases	Resectability rate (%)
Vessel-negative with duct-negative	No	No	1	1	100
Vessel-negative with duct-positive	No	Yes	4	4	100
Vessel-positive with duct-negative	Yes	No	4	2	50
Vessel-positive with duct-positive	Yes	Yes	28	5	17.8

6.5 Exploratory Laparotomy

Except when the preoperative cytodiagnosis is positive, only laparotomy can provide a definitive diagnosis. It is frequently the last step showing the gross aspect of the lesion and providing pancreatic and/or nodal samples (biopsy, needle aspiration) to determine its characteristics exactly.

When a patient cannot undergo laparotomy owing to general ill health, the operation can be replaced by a "mini-lap" or a laparoscopy, which permit the search for peritoneal or liver metastases and performance of a direct-vision biopsy. Laparoscopy is a less invasive investigation than the "mini-lap" and shortens hospitalization time [10]. This is one of its rare indications.

Even laparotomy does not always provide a definitive diagnosis. The gross estimates are not necessarily obvious, and associated pancreatitis can be at the origin of "false-negative" findings. The resected nodes themselves can be falsely negative.

Intraoperative ultrasound shows a mass or a pancreatic nodule, but is not sufficiently specific to differentiate tumor tissue from the surrounding pancreatitis. By the way, it does not allow a useful guidance for a needle punction when performed at laparotomy. A few times, a systematic intra-operative US of the pancreas showed evidence of little cancerous nodules (15 mm) [1, 14]. But these cases remain rare, and we will see later (chapter 8) that the main application of US is the characterization of the nature of the lesion itself through indirect symptoms, when they exist (invasion to the porta trunk, liver metastases), as the direct signs are more doubtful, even in the presence of a heterogeneous appearance.

Rarely, the situation remains vague in spite of the rigor of the examinations, forcing the surgeon to make a difficult decision which may appear to be abusive or insufficient. In such cases, our advice is to perform a limited left or right resection of the lesion, and to perform a histological examination of the specimen during the operation, prior to deciding which therapy to follow. These cases often concern small curable tumors; thus, even at laparotomy, it is difficult to achieve an early diagnosis. In our attempt to improve our diagnoses, we will probably increase the number of negative laparotomies as well. This is as risk we must be aware of.

6.6 Diagnostic Steps

They depend on the clinical criteria and on the performances of further investigations as well. They must be chosen relatively to their rapidity, cost and therapeutical capabilities. These are the reasons why a great deal of strategies were proposed by different authors.

In a comparative theoretical study of various diagnostic procedures, Marton imagined five different strategies applied to a hypothetical population of 10000 subjects reporting abdominal pains [9]. Though interesting, this study should be read cautiously; besides, it does not take CT into account.

Strategy 1

1. Ultrasound for any patient reporting abdominal pain
2. If US is negative, perform pancreatic function test
3. ERCP or angiography in case of abnormal US or pancreatic function test
4. If ERCP or angiography indicates a possible cancer, perform a laparotomy

Strategy 2

1. Ultrasound for any report of abdominal pain
2. ERCP or angiography when ultrasound shows abnormality
3. Laparotomy when ERCP or angiography show a potential cancer

Strategy 3

1. Apply Di Magno's clinical criteria
2. Follow strategy 1 if the patient fulfills two minor criteria

Strategy 4

1. Apply Di Magno's clinical criteria
2. Perform ERCP in patients who fulfill at least two criteria
3. Perform laparotomy if ERCP suggests a possible cancer

Strategy 5

1. Apply Di Magno's clinical criteria
2. Laparotomy right away if the patient presents at least two criteria

The results of these strategies are analyzed according to the number of positive diagnoses, the number of useless laparotomies, and the cost of the investigations (Table 6.2).

In the control group, the prevalence of pancreatic cancer is 0.01%. That is to say that 100 of 10000 subjects will have a carcinoma of the pancreas. At this point, Marton worked out how many patients will have positive or negative results and how many will undergo laparotomy using each of these strategies.

Strategy 1 is the best for positive diagnoses. However, it would lead to too many useless laparotomies. Strategy 3 provides only 69% positive diagnoses but entails fewer laparotomies and has the lowest cost. Strategies 2, 4, and 5 have intermediate results.

Marton's analysis shows that the percentage of positive laparotomies (assessing a cancer) increase for all strategies in proportion to the probability of cancer (Fig. 6.2).

In our opinion, the investigations must be chosen according to clinical criteria. With this in mind, let us consider three situations leading to three different strategies:

Strategy I: patients with jaundice alone or associated with one or more symptoms (pain, weight loss, diabetes mellitus)
Strategy II: nonjaundiced patients presenting only one of the symptoms mentioned above
Strategy III: nonjaundiced patients presenting two of the symptoms mentioned above

Table 6.2. Outcome of five strategies for detecting pancreatic cancer in a hypothetical population of 10000 patients with abdominal pain (potential morbidity or mortality due to testing or surgery not included) (from Marton et al. [9])

Strategy	Outcome No. of clinical evaluations done	No. of ultrasound tests done	No. of PFT's[a] done	No. of ERCP tests done	Total lab costs (US $)	Correctly diagnosed cancers (per 100)	No. of laparotomies with negative results	Cost of surgery (US $)
1	0	10000	8440	3266	1888500	93	317	2050000
2	0	10000	0	1560	1040000	71	149	1100000
3	10000	174	103	105	1542710	69	4	365000
4	10000	0	0	174	1543500	71	10	405000
5	10000	0	0	0	1500000	75	99	807000

[a] PFT, Pancreatic function test

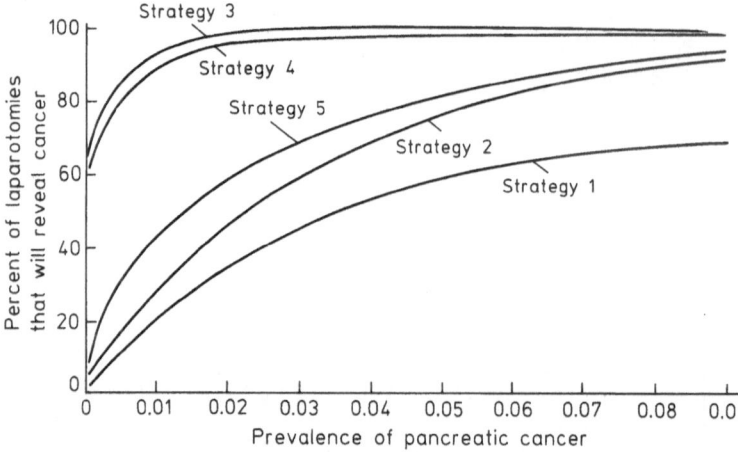

Fig. 6.2. Effect of prevalence of pancreatic cancer on the number of laparotomies with abnormal findings. As prevalence of cancer in the population under study increases there are fewer laparotomies with negative findings (from Marton et al. [9])

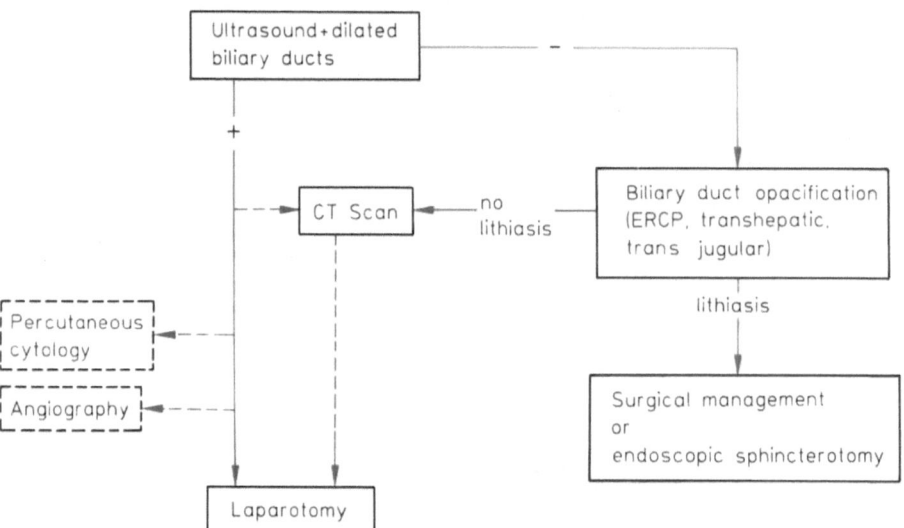

Fig. 6.3. Strategy I, for patients with jaundice and with or without pain, diabetes, and loss of weight. Pancreatic mass and enlarged gallbladder *(+);* normal pancreas and normal gallbladder *(−)*

These strategies are schematized in Figs. 6.3, 6.4, and 6.5, and can, of course, be contemplated only when laparotomy is not formally contraindicated.

The fact that biological examinations are not included in these strategies does not mean that they do not exist, but only that we do not believe them to be of primary interest for the diagnosis.

For nonjaundiced patients, laparotomy is obviously performed only when the

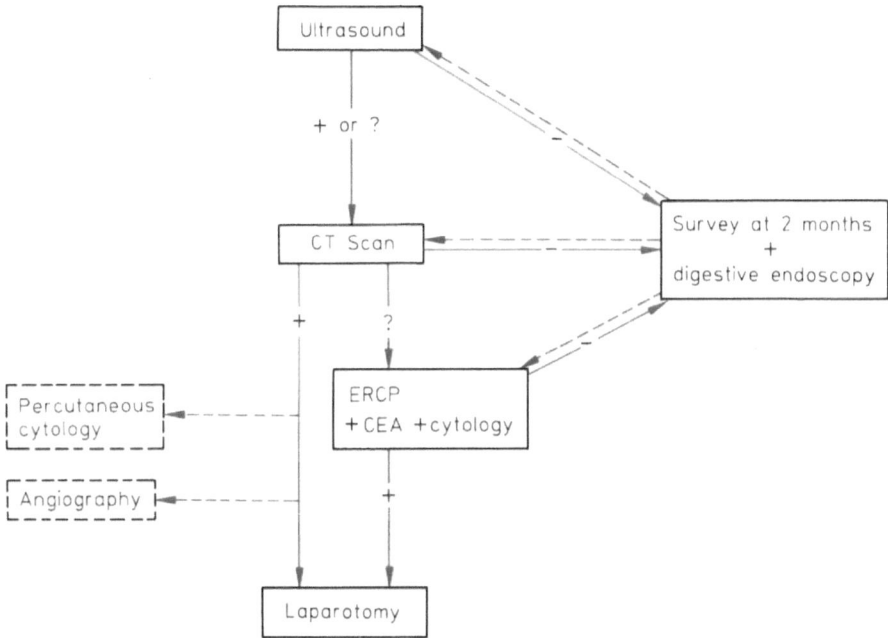

Fig. 6.4. Strategy II, for patients with no jaundice, but with one of the following: pain, diabetes, weight loss. Pancreatic mass *(+);* normal pancreas *(−);* uncertain results *(?)*

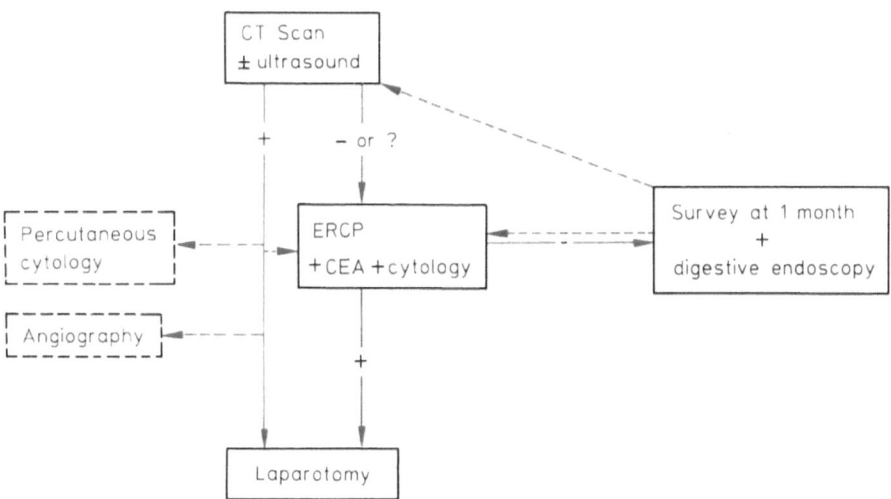

Fig. 6.5. Strategy III, for patients with no jaundice but with two of the following: pain, diabetes, weight loss. Pancreatic mass *(+);* normal pancreas *(−);* uncertain results *(?)*

nature of the lesion has been confirmed by cytology or when cancer is strongly suspected on the basis of CT and ERCP, and to avoid this way too many useless laparotomies.

6.7 Conclusion

Due to the fact that no diagnosis of asymptomatic, infraclinical cancer is possible, we must shorten the time between the onset of primary signs and the first treatment.

The strategy differs greatly depending on whether or not jaundice is present. Diagnosis of carcinoma of the head is easier and can be made earlier than for carcinoma of the body or tail of the pancreas.

The present-day techniques are globally valuable in the diagnosis of a pancreatic cancer. Morphological examinations are more reliable than biological ones. The cost and the invasive character of each examination must be taken into consideration. In these terms, US and CT appear to be the methods to perform first. In order to achieve rapid diagnoses, it is necessary that these investigations be done in specialized centers where the greatest accuracy can be expected.

The present strategies are not definitive. They will be modified according to new techniques and to a new approach to asymptomatic cancers relative to the screening of high-risk subjects, which is not yet possible.

References

1. Alexandre JH, Hernigou A, Billebaud T, Bouillot JL, Plainfosse MC (1985) Echotomographie per-opératoire du pancréas. Gastroenterol Clin Biol 9: 572–577
2. Beazley RM (1981) Needle biopsy diagnosis of pancreatic cancer. Cancer 47 (6): 1685–1687
3. Cancer of the Pancreas Task Force (1981) Staging of the cancer of the pancreas. Cancer 47 (6): 1631–1639
4. Classer M, Kawai K (1984) Frontiers of GI endoscopy. Scand J Gastroenterol. [Suppl] 102: 19
5. Cubilla AL, Fitzgerald PI (1978) Pancreas cancer (non endocrine). A review. Part 1. Clin Bull 8: 144
6. Di Magno EP, Malagelada UP, Taylor WF, et al. (1977) A prospective comparison of current diagnostic tests for pancreatic cancer. N Engl J Med 297: 727–743
7. Gambill EE (1970) Pancreatic and ampullary carcinoma: Diagnosis and prognosis in relationship to symptoms, physical findings and elapse of time as observed in 255 patients. South Med J 63: 1119–1122
8. Go VL, Taylor WF, Di Magno EP (1981) Efforts at early diagnosis of pancreatic cancer: The Mayo Clinic experience. Cancer 47 (6): 1698–1703
9. Marton KI, Rudd P, Sox HC (1980) Diagnosing pancreatic cancer. An analysis of several strategies. West J Med 133: 19–25
10. Moossa AR, Lewis MH, Mackie CR (1979) Surgical treatment of pancreatic cancer. Mayo Clin Proc 54: 468–474
11. Moossa AR, Levin B (1981) The diagnosis of early pancreatic cancer: The University of Chicago experience. Cancer 47 (6): 1688–1697
12. Moossa AR (1982) Pancreatic cancer. Approach to diagnosis, selection for surgery and choice of operation. Cancer 50 (11): 1689–2698

13. Sahel J (1983) Progrès dans le diagnostic des cancers du pancréas. Masson, Paris (Actualités Dig Med Chir, 4ème série)
14. Sigel B, Coelho JCU, Macht J, Flanigan DP, Donahue PE, Wood DK, Spigos DG (1982) Detection of pancreatic tumors by ultrasound during surgery. Arch Surg 117: 1058-1061
15. Susuki T, Imamura M. Tamura K, et al. (1979) Correlative evaluation of angiography and pancreatoductography in relation to surgery for cancer of the pancreas. Surgery 85 (6): 644-651

7 Therapeutic Management

H. Baumel and B. Deixonne

Cancer of the pancreas requires the same therapeutic management as do other cancers: surgical resection, radiation therapy, and chemotherapy are used. Additional purely symptomatological treatments have been achieved for jaundice, pain relief, or digestive stenosis. Surgical resection associated or not with radiochemotherapy is the only possible curative treatment.

7.1 Pancreatectomies

Oberling and Guerin wrote in *Le Cancer du Pancréas* (Doin, Paris, 1931), that the problem of treatment had been stationary for a long time, and at a period where surgical excision of gastric, colonic, and renal tumors was already common practice, the pancreas, because of its deep retroperitoneal and prevertebral position, seemed to be defying all attempts at operative treatment. Nevertheless, in France some surgeons (Villar in 1905, Sauvé and Desjardins in 1907, and Leriche in 1910) had already proposed techniques for pancreatectomy.

Effectively, before Whipple's report in 1935 of a pancreatoduodenectomy of the head of the pancreas in two stages with a 25-month mean survival time [81], surgical resections for pancreatic cancers remained isolated. A poor surgical environment and very high operative mortality (70% or so) were the main reasons. Nowadays, however, surgical resections are well codified interventions.

After a brief return to the anatomical basis for pancreatectomies and to the surgical approaches, we will provide a critical review of the various operative techniques.

7.1.1 Anatomical Basis for Surgery

Rouviere described the pancreas as follows: "A voluminous, full, right end, termed the head, followed by a thinner and elongated part called the body, which is linked to the head by a narrow segment, the neck, that ends up in a thin part, the tail" [69]. This does reflect the actual morphology of this gland, but we prefer, along with many other authors, to refer to the *right and left pancreas* divided by the paramedian isthmus. This bipartite view of the pancreas is reinforced not only by its anatomy, but also by its embryology, vascularization, and innervation. The exocrine drainage is ensured through the ducts of Wirsung and Santorini, frequently linked at the isthmus with a narrowing, described by Leger as a more or less poorly defined fusion of two buds, one ventral and one dorsal, its total absence being represented by the pancreas divisum [41].

We will not go any further into the pancreatic vascularization itself, but only recall its main *vascular relationships*. These often close relationships with large vessels sometimes pose problems at dissection, especially when they have been altered by an important tumor mass. Guillemin et al. are correct in reporting these relationships as one of the major surgical issues [32].

Among the venous relationships is, first of all, the splenic and mesenteric portal confluence, which presents some difficulties with the variations in inosculation of the inferior mesenteric vein, either in the splenic vein to form the splenomesenteric trunk, or at the level of the mesenteric and splenic fusion, or in the superior mesenteric vein. There are also variations of the gastrocolic trunk of Henle and the veins of the retropancreatic right process (or lamina) always cause difficulties at dissection between the mesentericoportal axis and the retrovenous pancreas (Fig. 7.1). The arteries are easier, especially the superior mesenteric artery. One must be careful in the search for the gastroduodenal artery, for it is sometimes very short and must be recognized rapidly at the superior border of the first duodenum. The superior right colic arterial relationships may be modified by a large tumor mass in the right pancreas. Variations in the arterial vascularization of the liver are frequent. Without preoperative angiography it is necessary to consider the important risk rep-

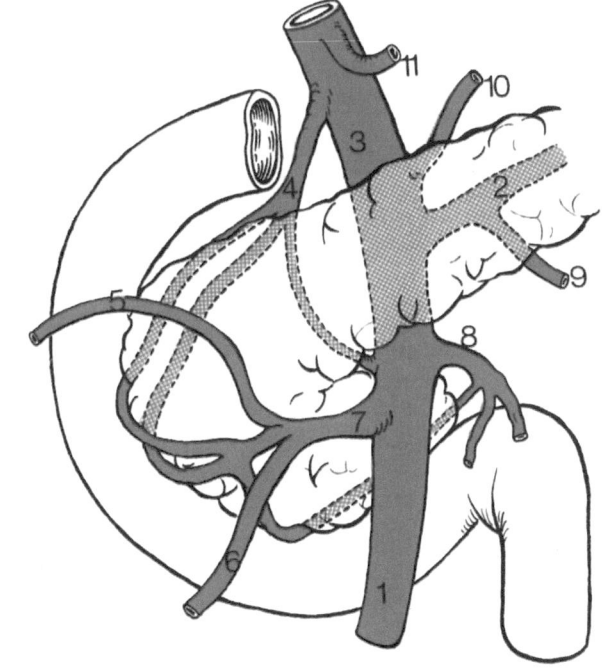

Fig. 7.1. Venous relationships of the right pancreas and the posterior portion of the neck of the pancreas. *1* Superior mesenteric vein; *2* splenic vein; *3* portal vein; *4* posterosuperior duodenal pancreatic vein; *5* right gastroepiploic vein; *6* right superior colic vein; *7* common venous trunk; *8* jejunal vein; *9* inferior mesenteric vein; *10* gastric coronary vein; *11* pyloric vein

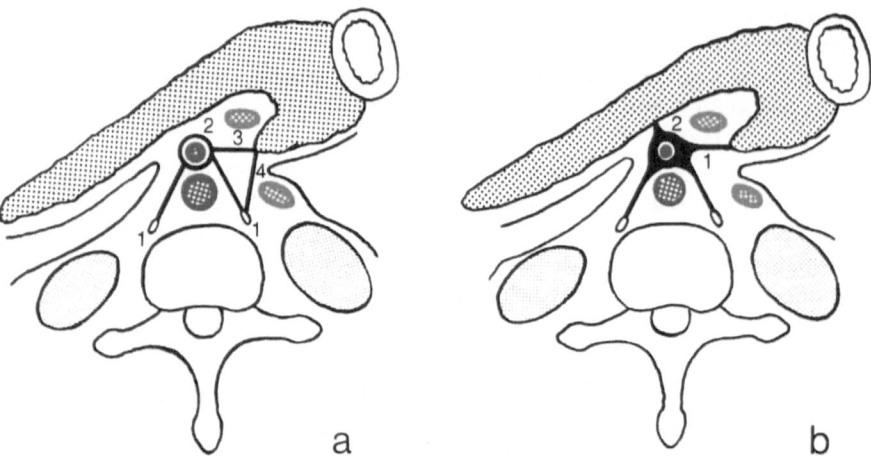

Fig. 7.2a, b. Posterior attachments of the pancreas. **a** (From Yoshioka and Wakabashi [87]) *1* celiac nerve nodes; *2* superior mesenteric artery; *3* uncomesenteric portion; *4* uncolunar portion. **b** (From Richelme et al. [65]) *1* right retroportal process; *2* left retroportal process

resented by the possible presence of a right hepatic artery [16, 70] (4% according to Rio Branco) [67]. When there, this hepatic artery emerges from the superior mesenteric artery, near its right edge of origin, and goes through the right retropancreatic process, making an oblique posterior crossing with the mesenteric portal axis, to finally exit on the right edge of the hepatic pedicle.

Besides these important arterial and venous relationships, we must stress the anatomical variations of the *posterior connections of the pancreas,* which are of great relevance in anatomical surgery, including cancer operations. Ideas on the distribution of these variations have recently been revised.

The pancreas is an organ with very little mobility, attached to the back by Treitz's fascia on the right, by the retropancreatic Toldt's fascia on the left, and by the hilum of the pancreas and the dorsal mesentery [13] to the isthmus. In 1959, Prioton and Laux [63] described the retroportal process as a thick wall stretched between the superior mesenteric artery and the median margin of the retrovenous pancreas. Earlier, Yoshioka (Fig. 7.2 a) [87] individualized the retrovenous postnodal extensions of the celiac plexus, with a right and left plexus termed "uncolunar" and "uncomesenteric lamina" by Couinaud and Huguet [14]. In 1982, Pissas gave a description of the left lateroportal process [60], and Richelme et al. [65] recently offered a synthesis of these connections and named these posterior formations the left and right retropancreatic processes (Figs. 7.2 b, 7.3). The right process corresponds to the final level of the mesoduodenum; the left one represents only an expansion of the latter, carried along by the dorsal pancreatic bud.

The right retropancreatic process is a fibroglandular element, 5–10 mm thick and reaching 6–8 cm in height. It is macroscopically difficult to see where the borderline between the fibrous and glandular tissues lies. It shares some important nerves with the postnodal semilunar fibers and includes some retrovenous pancreatic veins, some arterial elements for the uncinate process, the right hepatic artery

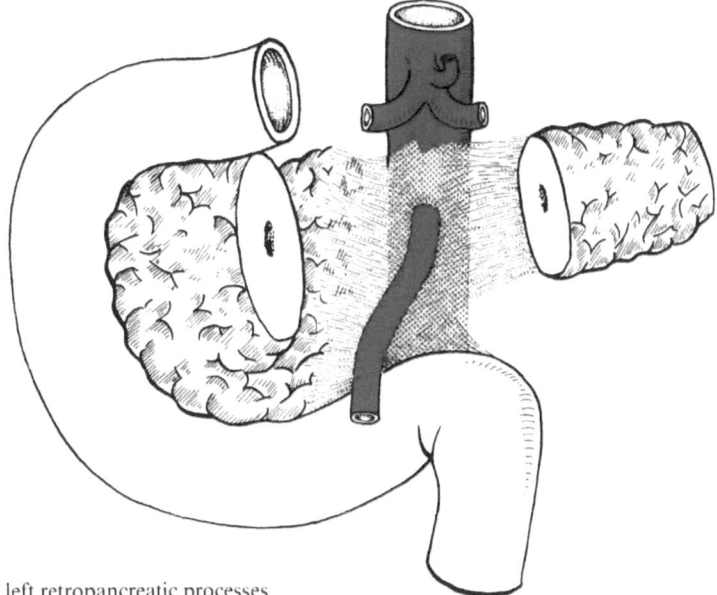

FFig. 7.3. Right and left retropancreatic processes

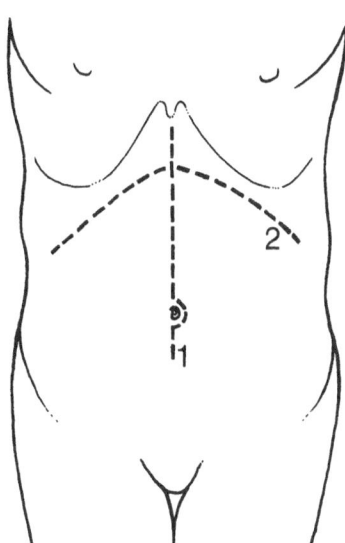

Fig. 7.4. Surgical approaches for pancreatectomy.
1 Median celiotomy; *2* transverse celiotomy (Ross)

when it originates from the superior mesenteric artery, and finally, some lymph-collecting vessels. The left retropancreatic process is thinner, never exceeding 1 mm in thickness; it is also not as high, stretched between the hilum of the pancreas, the superior mesenteric artery, and the back wall of the pancreatic body. Its fibrous tissue contains left postnodal semilunar fibers and some lymph-collecting vessels.

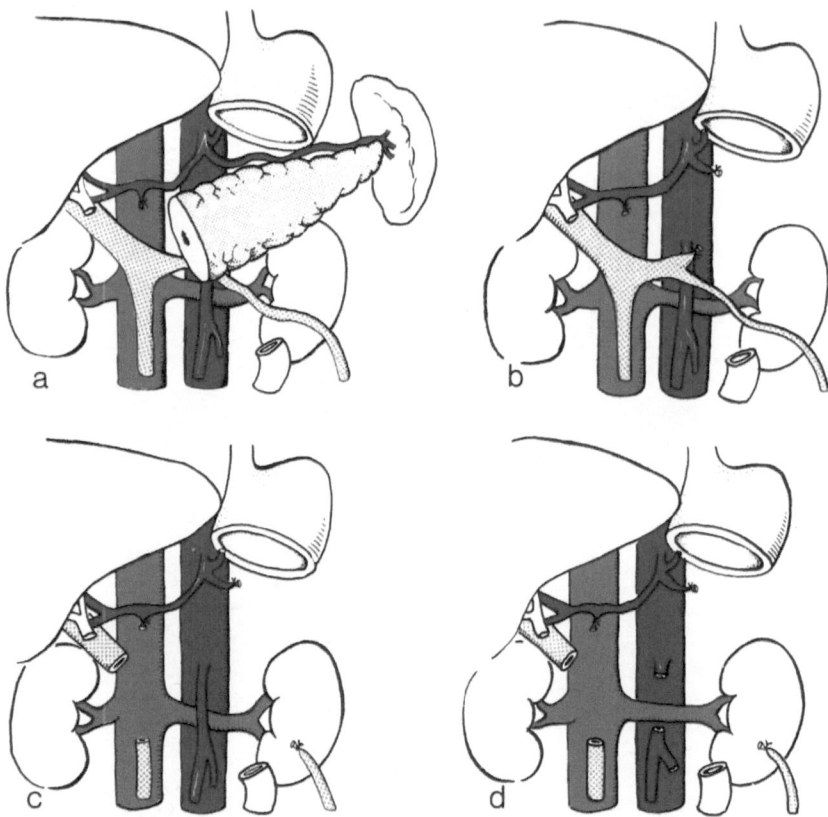

Fig. 7.5 a–d. Pancreatic resections. **a** Whipple's operation; **b** regional total pancreatectomy (RTP), Fortner type O; **c** RTP, Fortner type I; **d** RTP, Fortner type II a

We will not discuss again the lymphatic drainage of the pancreas since we have already dealt with the problem in the chapter on macroscopic pathological anatomy. We will have the opportunity to talk about it as well when studying the different techniques of pancreatectomies.

It seemed important to stress these notions, for some of them are recent and lead to more satisfactory surgery for carcinoma.

7.1.2 Surgical Approaches

The surgeon can choose between two different approaches, the supra- and periumbilical median approach and the Ross transversal approach, which is a bisubcostal incision (Fig. 7.4). One approach is not better than the other, but for a long time, surgeons preferred the median celiotomy, as it is easier to reconstruct and preserves the integrity of the muscles. Indeed, transection of the right and large abdominal muscles was reputed to damage the walls by the formation of fibrous muscular scars

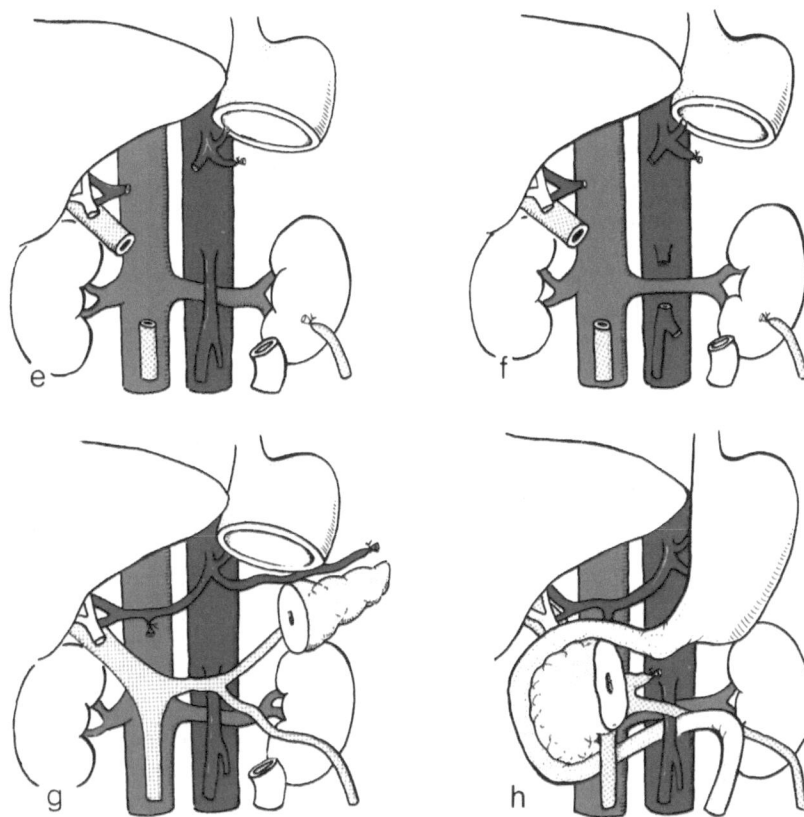

Fig. 7.5 e–h. e RTP, Fortner type II b; **f** RTP, Fortner type II c; **g** regional subtotal pancreatectomy; **h** distal pancreatectomy

and the section of certain nerves. Moreover, their reconstruction requires more time. In fact, curative surgery for cancer of the exocrine pancreas requires a large exposure of the upper abdomen, from the esophageal hiatus to the mesenteric root, and from the spleen to the right colic angle and the second duodenum. Only such an approach allows – under good conditions – total or subtotal resection with a regional lymphadenectomy. In our opinion, the ideal approach for this kind of surgery is the bisubcostal incision. If after the preoperative appraisal only palliative surgery by means of biliary or digestive bypass procedures can be considered, we start with a right subcostal incision which will be enlarged to the left if necessary. Another advantage is that this surgical approach allows for better exploration of the liver for secondary tumor localizations.

The parietal reconstruction does take longer than with a median celiotomy, but the walls are firm, and in our experience, there have not been any major parietal complications, in particular no evisceration. Besides, respiratory sequelae are less serious, the ventilatory parameter failure being lower than with the median approach. We therefore use this subcostal or bisubcostal approach and recommend it for pancreatic cancer surgery.

7.1.3 Techniques

Given the large number of right tumor localizations in exocrine pancreatic cancer, the principal technique has been the pancreatoduodenal resection. In the field of cancer surgery, the cephalic pancreatoduodenal resection was rapidly extended to the left, resulting in total pancreatoduodenectomy, and Fortner recently favored total and regional [21], then subtotal and regional pancreatectomy [23]. For left tumor localizations, the standard operation consists of a left pancreatosplenectomy with a pancreatic resection at the level of the isthmus. From that point, resection extended to the right can become a total or subtotal pancreatectomy.

We will now consider the various types of pancreatectomies (Fig. 7.5) and their major features.

7.1.3.1 Cephalic Pancreatoduodenectomy, or Whipple's Operation

Whipple's operation is a classical procedure, and need not be described in detail here. It consists of a right pancreatoduodenectomy with a resection at the level of the isthmus and a median gastric resection; the biliary duct is resected at the level of the common hepatic duct and the jejunum, below the angle of Treitz. Some surgeons follow this operation with a mechanical vagotomy. We will emphasize only a few points.

The most delicate step is the resection of the retrovenous pancreas and of the right retropancreatic process up to the superior mesenteric artery. To make it easier, Richelme proposed freeing the venous trunk and mobilizing it to the left mesentericoportal axis, beyond the superior mesenteric artery, for a good disengagement of the right retropancreatic process. The median border is liberated at the level of the mesenteric artery itself, by opening its wall and passing through a subadventicious plane, up to the anterior side of the aorta. The collateral vessels are then easily marked and ligated, especially if there is a right hepatic artery originating at this level and located in the median and upper part of the process. The only thing that remains to be done is the resection of the process from top to bottom, and the uncrossing of the duodenojejunum, which, as underlined by Richelme et al., becomes surprisingly easy (Fig. 7.6) [65].

Reconstruction of digestive continuity can be done in numerous ways. For a long time we have used the Child procedure involving the first or second jejunal loop. Pancreatojejunostomy is easy when an associated distal pancreatitis exists. On the other hand, considering the weakness of a normal pancreas, it appears to be much more difficult to perform. Two techniques are used here. The first is an end-to-side pancreatojejunostomy (Fig. 7.7a), and the second is an end-to-end pancreatojejunostomy with cuffing of the pancreatic stump (Fig. 7.7b). Obertop and Van Houten proposed closing the pancreatic plane of section with the GIA stapler and removing the centric staples to free the main pancreatic duct in order to perform an end-to-side wirsungojejunostomy, the remaining pancreatic slide being closed (Fig. 7.7c) [56]. Shiu ligates the duct of Wirsung with a slow-absorbing suture and performs an end-to-end pancreatojejunostomy by leaving a perforated tube in the

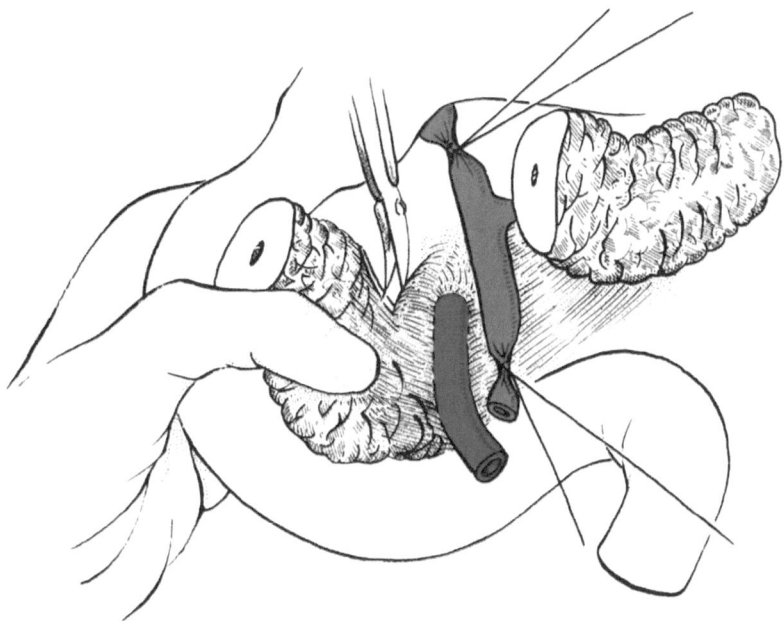

Fig. 7.6. Approach to right pancreatic process (from Richelme et al. [65])

jejunal loop. This is done in order to avoid exocrine pancreatic secretion during healing of the anastomosis (Fig. 7.7 d) [72]. Parc and Herbiere prefer to leave a jejunal length of 60 cm between the pancreatic and biliary anastomoses, changing a possible leakage of the pancreatic anastomosis into a pure pancreatic fistula, which is better accepted (Fig. 7.7 e) [58].

Contrary to the general way of thinking, Arendt et al. proved that pancreatojejunostomies do not evolve into fibrosis, becoming non-functional some years later; they were still efficient at least 7 years postoperatively [4].

Since Brunschwig's time, to avoid this possible leakage some surgeons are more likely to close the pancreatic stump after ligating Wirsung's duct. Mercadier et al. report an X-stitch suture of the pancreatic plane of section [48]. It is necessary to put a drain at the contact of the section to direct a possible pancreatic fistula. These appear in 25%–30% of cases and are pure pancreatic fistulas, generally reabsorbing themselves spontaneously [59]. We do not agree with this statement and think that this type of postoperative fistula remains a cause of high morbidity.

Other authors advocate the same procedure, stopping the leakage of pancreatic juice by an injection of biological glue into the main duct. Many such glues exist, and the laboratory studies are encouraging enough that this procedure could be applied in man [2, 31]. Within 10 days the residual pancreas becomes fibrotic. The occlusion would have no effect on the islets of Langerhans, and thus none on the endocrine function.

The following lymph nodes are resected in this operation: the pre- and retropancreatoduodenal node groups, part of the hepatic chain, the lymph-collecting vessels of the right retropancreatic process, and the first groups of the mesenteric root. As

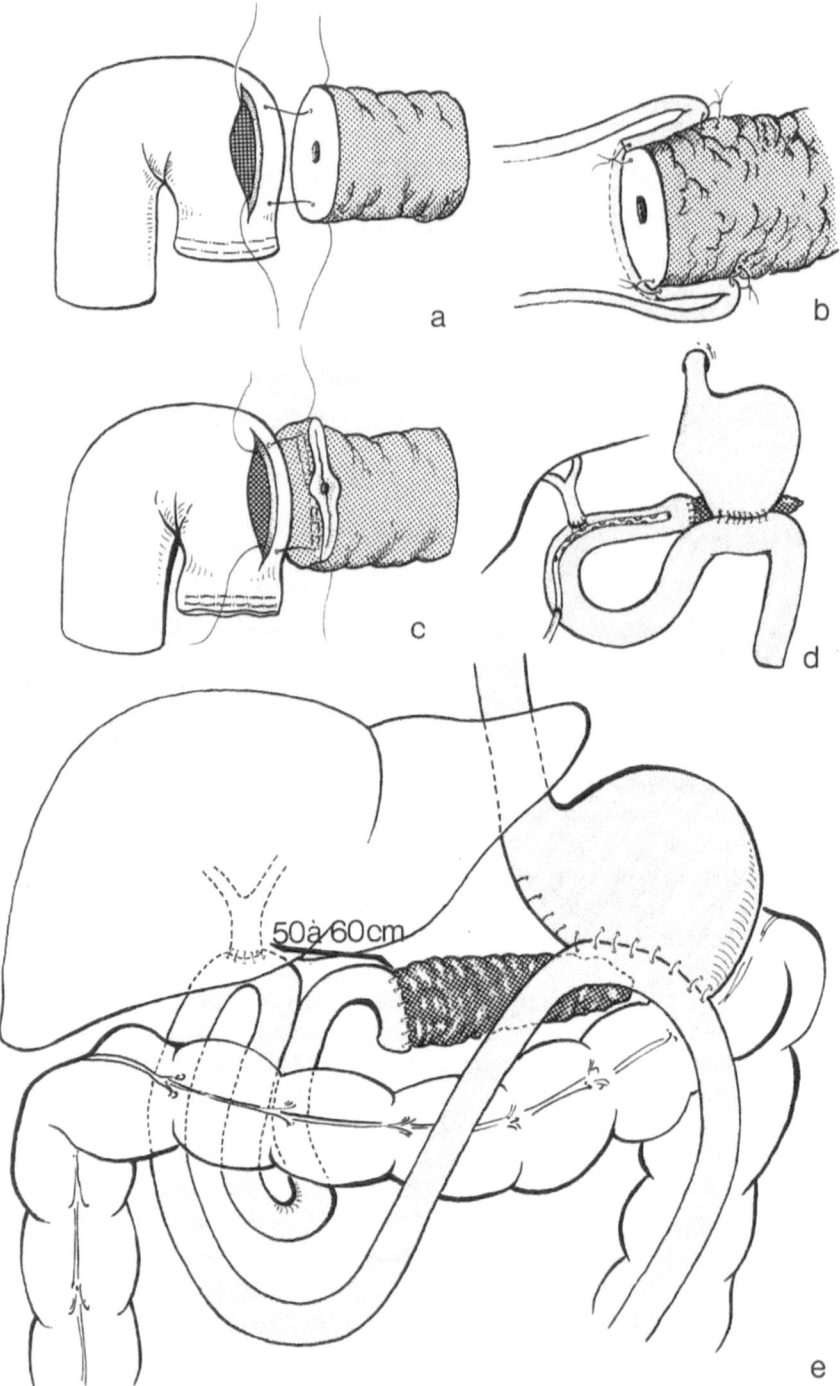

Fig. 7.7a–e. Pancreaticojejunal anastomoses. **a** End-to-side anastomosis; **b** end-to-end anastomosis, with cuffing of pancreatic stump; **c** Obertop's technique; **d** Shiu's technique; **e** Parc's technique

advised by Couinaud in 1967 [12], it appears useful to perform a complementary curage, removing the interaorticocaval-suprarenal groups, the gastric coronary chain, the celiac group nodes, and the hepatic pedicle nodes.

7.1.3.2 Total Pancreatectomy

This consists of the right pancreatoduodenectomy mentioned above completed by a left pancreatosplenectomy. It is a resection en bloc, without section of the isthmus. The dissection time is the same as for pancreatoduodenectomy, except that the isthmus is not separated from the portal vein and that after liberation of the main biliary duct, ligature of the gastroduodenal artery, and curage of the hepatic pedicle, we continue along the celiac trunk in order to link the splenic artery to its origin. To the left, the coloepiploic detachment proceeds straight down to the greater curvature of the stomach and is followed by resection of the splenogastric omentum and by the detachment and mobilization, when necessary, of the left colic angle. We then begin with the pancreatosplenic detachment, performed from left to right, with ligature and resection at the inferior margin of the pancreas, at the left of Treitz's angle of the inferior mesenteric vein. The splenic vein is ligated and resected at the level of the left retropancreatic process. Following the digestive sections, the whole of the pancreas is mobilized, sustained only by the posterior process, which in turn is centered by the superior mesenteric artery. We then arrive at the delicate part of the operation, with resection of the process and detachment of the retrovenous pancreas. This is done from left to right, starting with the resection of the left process and the superior mesenteric artery approach. We then divide the posterior side of the isthmus from the venous plane, and after applying one or two retractors around the portal vein in order to put it under slight tension, we can clip or ligate the small affluent veins of the retrovenous pancreas, as well as the posterosuperior pancreatoduodenal vein. The pancreas is, at this point, totally displaced to the right, and the only thing left to resect is the right process, as in the case of cephalic pancreatoduodenectomy.

To re-establish digestive continuity we use the second jejunal loop, placed through the mesocolon by means of end-to-side biliary and gastrojejunal bypasses (Fig. 7.8).

In addition to the nodes removed in a cephalic pancreatoduodenectomy, the lymph nodes of the hilum of the spleen, the splenic chain, and the inferior pancreatic chain are removed in a total pancreatectomy. This is not very different from the regional pancreatectomy – Fortner-type 0 – that we are going to examine. Moreover, in a total resection of the pancreas, we remove the intrapancreatic lymphatic anastomoses and also the secondary tumor foci of the multifocal types, present in 20%–25% of all cases.

7.1.3.3 Regional Pancreatectomy

In 1973, Fortner described and gave an organized basis for regional pancreatectomy [21]. It consists of a total pancreatoduodenectomy combined with a splenectomy, associated with a complete lymphatic dissection and a skeletonizing of the hepatic

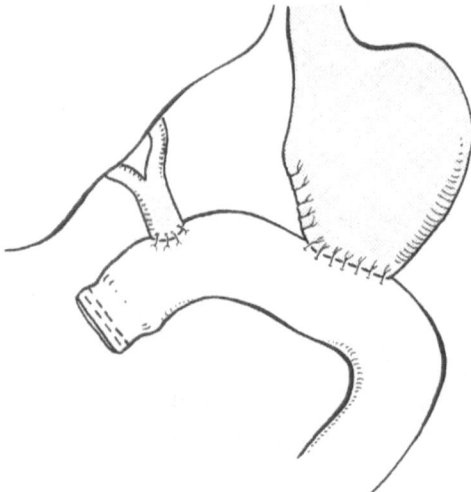

Fig. 7.8. Digestive continuity re-established after a total pancreatectomy

pedicle, the inferior vena cava, and the aorta from the diaphragm up to the origin of the inferior mesenteric artery; to this he added a subtotal gastrectomy and resection of the portal vein. The whole is resected en bloc. The idea was to treat this cancer by a resection at a distance from the neoplastic tissues, removing all the lymphatic relays with their regional lymphatic drainage. Concerning the pancreas, difficulties arise from the involvement of the retroisthmic vessels. On the other hand, the retroperitoneal nodes are rapidly metastasized. When all has been sectioned, the pancreas is removed en bloc, as are the invaded vessels and the nodal relays. This operation does present technical difficulties, and extensive experience with pancreatobiliary surgery is required, but Fortner's system gained widespread acceptance, as there is more than a theoretical justification for this radical surgery.

Looking back a little, to 1954, in a plea for total pancreatectomies, Ross [68] had already reported ten surgical cases, some of which were very closely related to regional resections. He had performed a portal resection with mesentericocaval anastomosis, described mutlifocal tumors, and, on a general level, advised good exposure, generous resections, an en bloc resection at the same time as a cholecystectomy with high resection of the main biliary duct, high gastric resection, entire removal of the duodenum, and finally, curage of all the peripancreatic lymphatic chains. In fact, some of his resections lack only aorticocaval lymphatic dissection to be Fortner's stage I. It should also be remembered that in 1965, Sigel et al. [73] reported a pancreatoduodenectomy with resection of the portal vein reconstructed by a venous autograft. In 1966, Prioton et al. were the first to succeed in a total pancreatectomy for cancer of the isthmus, with mesentericoportal and superior mesenteric arterial resection, followed by a mesentericocaval anastomosis and reimplantation of the superior mesenteric artery on the aorta [62]. In 1970, Remine et al. [64] proposed a regional total pancreatectomy procedure which would correspond to Fortner's type O. In 1971, Marchal et al. presented seven cases of pancreatoduodenectomies with vascular resections and reconstructions [47]. We will not give an exhaustive list of all the authors who have reported more or less extensive total pancreatectomies. They are very numerous, especially in Europe and in the United States, and one can perceive the trend to this regional operation developing along with the improvement of the technical environment and the reduction of the operative risk.

Based on publications and lectures since the codification of his technique in 1973, Fortner has listed the following three types of resection, to complete and modify his initial method:

1. Type 0 (see Fig. 7.5 b) refers to the transverse mesocolon, with the middle colic vessels and the regional and lymphatic nodes removed en bloc with the pancreas. This is combined with a subtotal gastrectomy, duodenectomy, splenectomy, cholecystectomy, and the largest possible resection of the main bile duct. The portal vein, hepatic artery, celiac trunk, and superior mesenteric artery are skeletonized. A retroperitoneal nodal dissection from the diaphragm to its superior mesenteric artery origin is then performed, associated with curage of the pararenal nodes, hilum, left renal vein, laterocaval, and interaorticocaval.

2. Type I (see Fig. 7.5 c) is the same operation as type 0, but adds resection of the retropancreatoduodenal mesenteric portal venous axis en bloc with the pancreas. The losses are compensated by an end-to-end mesenteric portal anastomosis, mobilizing the mesenteric root at the top in order to recover the 4 or 5 missing centimeters.

3. Type II consists of the type-I procedure complemented by some arterial resections, according to which Fortner distinguishes the three following subgroups:
   - Type II a (see Fig. 7.5 d) removes the retropancreatic portion of the superior mesenteric artery and the reconstruction is realized either by means of a end-to-end arterial anastomosis or by a reimplantation below the aorta, or occasionally by a substitution of the resected part by a venous autograft or an arterial prosthesis.
   - Type II b (see Fig. 7.5 e) removes a portion of the hepatic artery or the entire celiac trunk. The procedures of reconstruction are the same as for type II a.
   - Type II c (see Fig. 7.5 f) removes both the celiac trunk and the superior mesenteric artery. They are separately reconstructed or substituted with a bifurcated arterial prosthesis.

Some comments on these techniques are in order. First of all, the digestive continuity is reestablished by an end-to-side hepaticojejunal bypass, and then by a gastrojejunal bypass. Along with Fortner, we think that a T-tube for the biliary bypass is useless, as it can cause inflammatory diseases and secondary stenosis. The subtotal gastrectomy weakens the vascularization of the residual stomach. The only vascularizations left are diaphragmatic and cardial. With this in mind Fortner tends to perform frequent total gastrectomies. As far as the transverse colon is concerned, he removes the middle colic artery but keeps the vascular arcade of the transverse colon, which does not compromise colic vascularization. Finally, in Fortner's hands such an operation can last from 8 to 12 h, requiring a transfused blood volume of 5 liters, and the average postoperative hospitalization time is 53 days, 10 of which are spent in an intensive-care unit. These data are available for the first 18 regional pancreatectomies reported in 1977 [22]. The operative mortality at 30 days was only 16.6%, and the past decade has witnessed the adoption of Fortner's techniques with great interest by many teams, to improve the therapeutic results in exocrine pancreatic cancer. We understand that vascular sacrifices make one doubt in the oncological value of these regional resections, but we cannot agree with the idea which says that: "rather than mature thinking, this is effectively an imperative act of necessity as the communications are broken off and there is no way to go back" [32]. An aggressive attitude is better than a pessimistic point of view when the aim is to increase the number of cures.

7.1.3.4 Subtotal Pancreatoduodenectomy

Logically, based on tumor volume, this section should fall between "Cephalic Pancreatoduodenectomy" and "Total Pancreatectomy." But Fortner himself recently advocated subtotal pancreatectomy (see Fig. 7.5 g) with in the framwork of a regional resection [23]. How does he justify this when multicentric tumors are present and there are a large number of parenchymatous lymphatic anastomoses? According to him, the last 5 cm of the left pancreas are always free of secondary localizations and the splenic nodes are rarely metastasized. In studying 21 resected specimens of total pancreatectomies for right pancreatic cancer, Cubilla et al. [15] never found any metastasized nodes at the level of the hilum of the spleen group (Fig. 7.9). We and others favor the subtotal pancreatectomy with a regional lymphadenectomy. However,

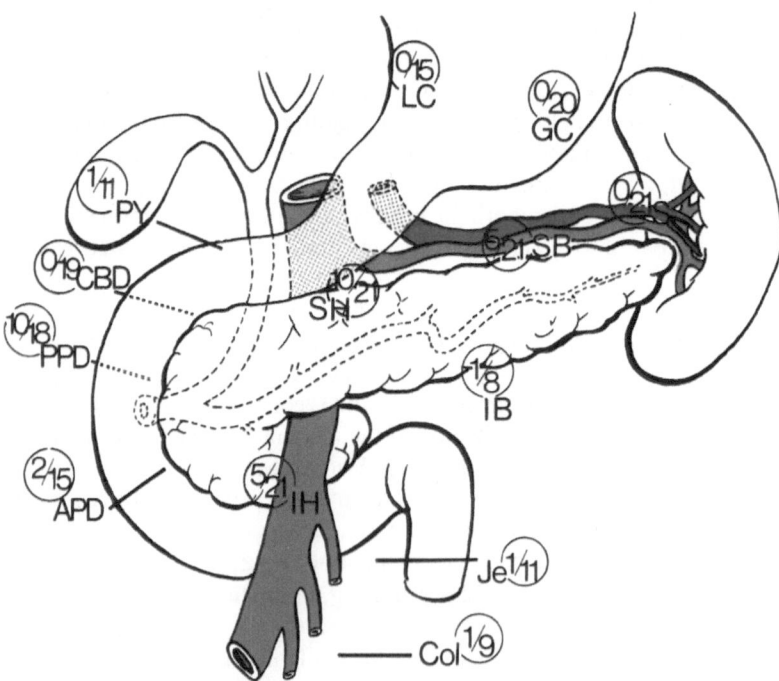

Fig. 7.9. Lymph node group involvement in 21 patients with duct cancer in the head of the pancreas (from Cubilla et al. [15]). *PY* pylorus; *CBD* common bile duct; *PPD* posterior pancreatic duct; *APD* anterior pancreatic duct. *Je* jejunum; *Col* colon; *LC* lesser curvature; *GC* greater curvature; *SH* superior head; *IH* inferior head; *SB* superior body; *IB* inferior body; *S* splenic

most surgeons do not reestablish the small pancreatic stump; we close it manually with separated X-stitches, after the ligature of the duct of Wirsung and the bevelling of the plane of section. We do not use autosuture staplers. But whether the suturing be done manually or by means of staplers, there is a high risk of exocrine pancreatic fistula, necessitating good drainage of the stump. However, these fistulas are not very serious and heal quite rapidly, in about 6 weeks in our experience. Another interesting solution to be considered is the obstruction of the ductal system by means of biological glue.

7.1.3.5 Left Pancreatectomy

Actually, there are two different types of left pancreatectomy: the true left pancreatosplenectomy with resection of the isthmus, and the left subtotal pancreatosplenectomy that leaves only one pancreatic rim surrounding the duodenum.

The *true left pancreatosplenectomy* (see Fig. 7.5h) stops at the plane of the portal axis with ligature of the splenic artery and vein, both at their origin and end. The inferior mesenteric vein is ligated unless it runs directly into the superior mesenteric vein. If after injection of contrast medium the pancreatic duct happens to be normal, with good passage through the duodenum, the pancreatic plane of section can be closed. If obstructed, it is advisable to perform a Roux-Y pancreatojejunal anastomosis. Concerning the lymphatics, only the groups of the hilum of the spleen, the splenic chain, and the inferior pancreatic chain are resected.

The *left subtotal pancreatectomy* involves a resection passing over the isthmus to remove the uncinate process. The incision is made 2 cm beyond the duodenum. One must be careful to avoid the main biliary duct by inserting a rigid tube as a landmark.

The criticisms are the same as those previously made of Fortner's subtotal pancreatectomy, because the nodal resection is limited and the existence of multifocal tumors is not taken into account. However, such operations are very seldom performed, as the left tumor distribution of cancer of the exocrine pancreas is diagnosed very late; the tumors are voluminous, and when surgery appears to be feasible, the operation of choice is not less than a total pancreatoduodenectomy.

7.1.4 Advantages and Disadvantages

We will evaluate these surgical procedures on a strictly technical level, but will also consider satisfactory oncological resection and the avoidance of postoperative complications.

We have reservations about the Whipple resection, which we consider unsatisfactory for the following reasons:
1. Malignant cells remain in the residual pancreas in about 20%–25% of cases, due to (a) direct spreading of the primary tumor (involvement of the slide of section), (b) tumor cell metastases along the main duct, (c) multifocal tumors, or (d) metastases through the intrapancreatic lymph network.

2. Nodal metastases exist in the groups which are not removed during this operation. We have already mentioned the findings of Cubilla et al. [15], which they summarized by giving a schematized representation of the nodal groups involved. Positive nodes were not found in only three groups: the lesser and greater curvature of the stomach, and the hilum of the spleen (see Fig. 7.9).

3. Anastomotic leak occurs after pancreatojejunostomy in 10%–50% of cases [58].

The third observation is only a relative contraindication, but the first and second represent some objective oncological disadvantages which should be taken into account. The anatomopathological examination of the plane of section, as is advised by many authors, does not preclude the presence of one or more distant foci in the left pancreas. Moreover, it is very difficult if not impossible, to perform a regional total lymphadenectomy and leave the left pancreas in place; this is easier to do with a total pancreatectomy.

Some questions remain: (a) In the case of a right pancreatic tumor, is a subtotal or a total pancreatectomy to be performed? (b) Is a total lymphadenectomy always required, including a large retroperitoneal one? (c) Can vascular resections be performed when the vessel walls are invaded by the tumor process? It seems very difficult to answer these questions here and now, as the results of important series reports have not yet been studied. For a left pancreatic tumor the size of the resection poses no problem; apart from exceptions, it will always consist of a total pancreatectomy, for we are unfortunately not able to diagnose small cancers of the left pancreas.

At the purely technological level, total pancreatoduodenectomies pose no more problems than subtotal ones – fewer perhaps – for we are not worried by the residual pancreatic stump. In this connection, let us mention the problem of postoperative *diabetes*, which for a long time was the main argument against total pancreatectomy. It is one reason why Fortner advocates subtotal resection of the gland for non-diabetic patients, for patients with small cancers of the head of the pancreas, and for patients who apparently would not tolerate diabetes associated with the digestive disorders consequent to a total resection [23]. According to Moossa [52], however, 34% of pancreatic cancers cause diabetes before the operation, and Schwartz et al. demonstrated that 47% of patients showed a pathological curve on the oral hyperglycemia test [71]. This rules out subtotal pancreatectomy for nearly one in two patients. On the other hand, one must remember that the tail end of the pancreas is rich in A cells providing glucagon, and it was noted that there were more significant residual secretions of glucagon than of insulin, which explains the occurrence of acido-ketosis more rapidly after subtotal pancreatectomies than after total pancreatectomies. We have often seen the onset of secondary diabetes within a few months after subtotal pancreatectomy; this rapidly becomes insulin dependent and is sometimes very difficult to balance. These difficulties seem to be less frequent after total resection. In Frey's series of 78 patients followed up after pancreatic resection, diabetes existed in 72% of the patients who had undergone a resection of 80%–95% of the gland, in 32% after resection of 40%–80% of the gland, and in 20% of the patients who had undergone Whipple's operation [24]. Consequently, we believe that the side effect of postoperative diabetes is no more of a risk in total than in subtotal pancreatectomies, perhaps even less.

As far as the lymphatics and nodal groups are concerned, in a total pancreatectomy, in addition to the splenic and digestive resection, we can easily remove the nodes of relays I and II en bloc with the gland. On the other hand, a lymphadenectomy of the retroperitoneal relays (relays III), resulting in a Fortner type-0 pancreatoduodenectomy, lengthens the operative time somewhat. Technically speaking, this poses no problem, since the upper abdomen is completely free of the gland, which can be bulky due to the large tumor volume. It is also no problem for a resection of the pancreatoduodenal segment of the portal vein, with the possible exception of the venous reconstruction. Paradoxically, the dissection is simplified and shortened, for it is only a question of the superior mesenteric artery approach with a resection of the retropancreatic process at this level. Thus, the occasionally delicate operation of unblocking the portal vein is avoided.

However, Fortner type II, especially type II c with its removal of the celiac and superior mesenteric arteries, lengthens the operative time; operations can last 12–14 h, and the surgeon's training and personal qualities play a very important role. It would seen at this point that the reasonable limits for such an operation are reached, in particular for a cancer whose curability is doubtful.

7.2 Symptomatic Treatment

Symptoms treated generally include jaundice, digestive stenosis, and pain. In this section we will deal only with surgical biliary bypass, internal and external nonsurgical biliary drainage, digestive bypass, and some analgesic treatments. Therapy for undernutrition (enteral and parenteral nutrition) and the antalgic treatments used by anesthetists and reanimation teams will be covered in Chap. 10.

7.2.1 Surgical Biliary Bypass

7.2.1.1 Biliary Anastomosis

Two biliary ducts are used: the gallbladder and the common bile duct, and two digestive ducts are possible: the first duodenum or a Roux-Y jejunal loop; the stomach is used only exceptionally. So far, four different types of diversion are commonly used: the cholecystoduodenostomies or jejunostomies and the choledocoduodenostomies or jejunostomies. The results of these four different techniques are superimposable and we perform any of them "on request." The environmental conditions and the indication for a diversion direct the technique. For instance, if there is a high cephalic tumor proximal to the portion of the cystic duct running into the common bile duct, it is better to avoid the gallbladder and duodenum because of the risk of invasion, and the anastomosis risks rapidly becoming nonfunctional.

Even if it is only meant as a temporary bypass before proceeding with a resection, it is of no use to perform a Roux-Y jejunal loop, and it is preferable not to compromise further the use of the common bile duct. On the other hand, when the

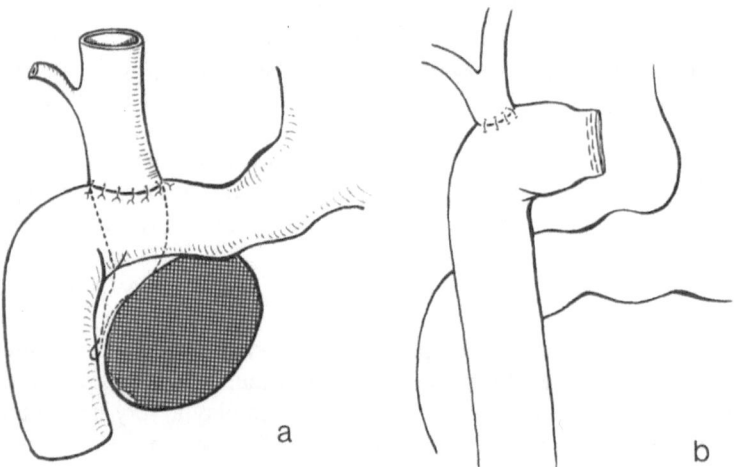

Fig. 7.10. a Side-to-side choledocoduodenal anastomosis. **b** End-to-side hepaticojejunal anastomosis

bypass is definitive, and the survival is estimated to be longer than a few months, it is important to create an efficient and durable bypass, such as a choledochojejunostomy.

We are likely to perform side-to-side choledochoduodenostomies as temporary bypasses and end-to-side choledochojejunostomies for the definitive cases. The former follow a transverse choledochotomy of the anterior hemicircumference of the common bile duct and a longitudinal incision at the upper anterior margin of the first duodenum (Fig. 7.10a). They are sutured by separated stitches with slow-absorbing thread. Various features have been described according to site and direction of the incision. We will refer only to Jurasz [38], who performs a posterior duodenotomy and then a choledochotomy as an extension of the first incision, and to Finsterer [19], who makes a vertical choledochotomy and a longitudinal duodenotomy on its upper margin. The latter are performed on a Y-jejunal loop set up through the mesocolon. The end of the jejunum is closed with an autosuture stapler; this forms an end-to-side anastomosis, high on the common bile duct, below the convergence, in order to prevent a rapid neoplastic invasion (Fig. 7.10b).

7.2.1.2 Surgical Biliary Drainage

Surgical biliary drainage is an interesting alternative when the tumor invasion of the common bile duct makes the bypass procedure too difficult. Three different types of drainage can be used:
1. Transtumor intubation of the common bile duct is done with a plain perforated polyethylene drain or with an endoprosthesis of the Lunderquist type. It is a tubular, rigid, arched, multiperforated drain, widening like a funnel, placed by means of a choledochotomy. The tube is easily placed when the lumen is not

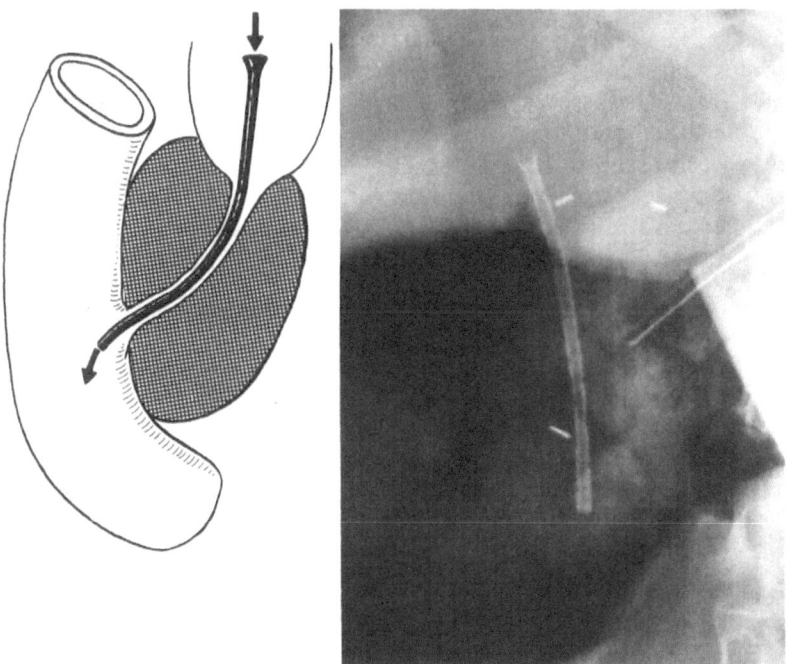

Fig. 7.11. Choledochal endoprosthesis of Lunderquist

completely obstructed (Fig. 7.11). Otherwise, the procedure is more delicate, for drilling of the tumor tissue carries with it the risk of false passage [37].

2. The U-tube palliative procedure proposed by Terblanche [78] and Praderi and Estefan [61] is a mixed internal and external drainage. The tumor is intubated by a drain, both ends exiting at the surface, allowing for daily cleaning. It is used mainly for tumors of the common bile duct and hepatic convergence, but sometimes it is applied for low tumor stenoses of pancreatic origin. This procedure is too demanding for the patient, however.

3. The bypass procedure by means of a Kron prosthesis consists of a silicon tube linked at one end to the common bile duct and at the other to the duodenum or the jejunum [40]. We have not yet tried this technique.

7.2.2 Nonsurgical Biliary Drainage (External and Internal)

The external techniques derive from direct biliary opacification via the transparietohepatic tract, developed by radiologists. Hoevels and the Swedish school [35], Mori et al. [53], Ferruci et al. [18], and Nakayama et al. [54], to name only a few, have described these techniques and analyzed their results. By the direct transparietal tract, most likely at the level of the median axillary line, approximately 10 cm above the angle of the tenth rib, a catheter is advanced into the right hepatic duct, pushed towards the convergence, and fixed to the skin. This drains the bile to the outside (Fig. 7.12). If internal biliary drainage is preferred, the catheter has to be pushed through the choledochal stenosis to enter the duodenum and receive the bile (Fig. 7.13). These techniques are derived from those of angiography, using supple metallized guide to pass the tumor stenoses. We, ourselves, use the techniques of the Swedish school of Lund [35]. They have been systematized and are quite reliable; drainage through this tract gives a 90% success rate with very few complications. In practice, they follow biliary opacification, which means that one can, at the same time, visualize the level, degree, and extent of the stenosis, rule out lithiasis, and perform a biliary drainage.

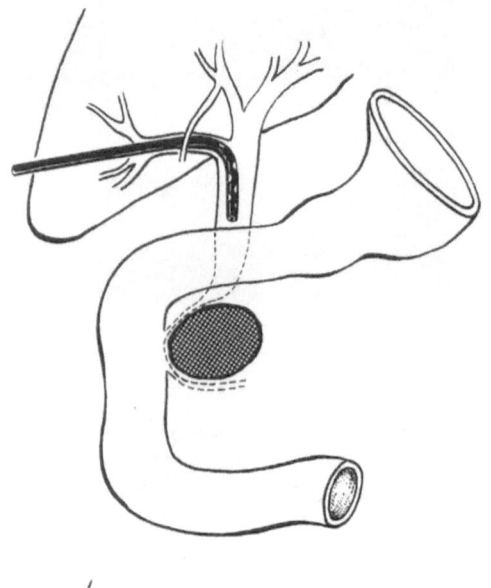

Fig. 7.12. External biliary drainage via the transparietohepatic route

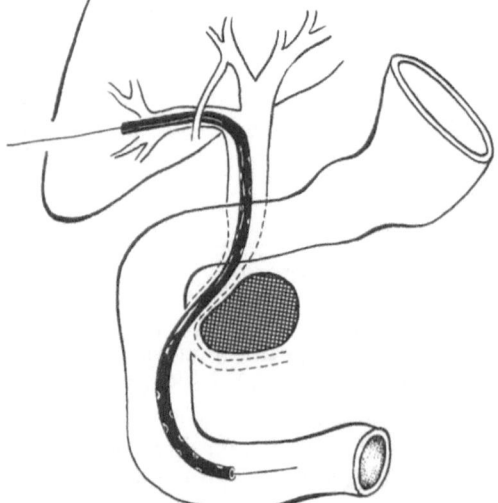

Fig. 7.13. Catheter for internal biliary drainage placed via the transparieto-hepatic route with wire guide

An internal biliary drainage can also be created through the endoscopic tract after a retrograde catheterization of the papilla. In this way it is possible to opacify both the common bile duct and the pancreatic duct, to do a biopsy if the tumor is adjacent to the papilla, and finally, to aspirate some pancreatic juice for cytology. When the tumor is not too advanced and has not completely stenosed the common bile duct, retrograde cholangiowirsungography - one of the most interesting examinations in the diagnostic pattern - allows the placement of an endoprosthesis into the common bile duct and avoids both parietal effraction and the risk of choleperitonitis or bleeding. However, it requires much experience and expertise on the part of the endoscopist.

7.2.3 Digestive Diversion

Gastrojejunostomy is done to shunt the duodenal or antral stenoses. When the anastomosis is done on the back of the gastric wall (Fig. 7.14a), by means of a transmesocolic isoperistaltic jejunal loop, it is said to yield the best functional result, but this is not always feasible because of the tumor volume itself or even the risk of invasion to the anastomosis. In the case of exocrine pancreatic cancer, surgeons often prefer to set up the jejunal loop on a precolic level and to perform a side-to-side anastomosis on the front wall of the stomach (Fig. 7.14b).

Digestive bypass is sometimes done concomitant with a biliary bypass in order to avoid the undesirable effects of a secondary stenosis. Prophylactic gastroenterostomy is controversial, and we will see in Chap. 8 whether this combination is significant for the increase in complications.

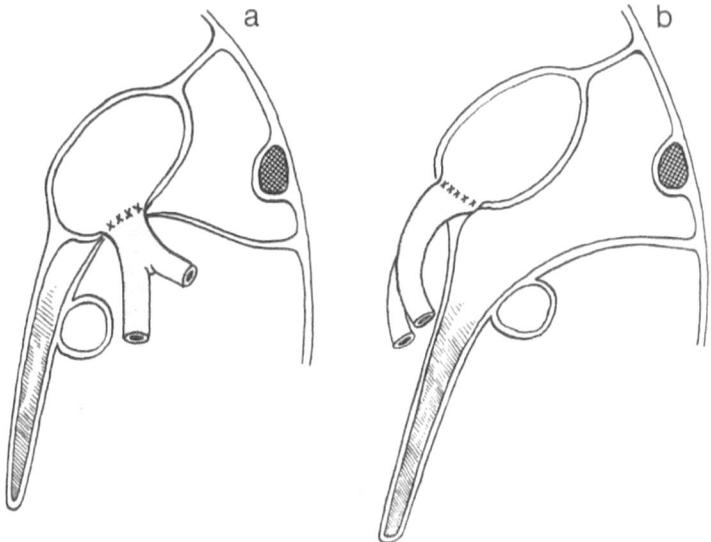

Fig. 7.14a, b. Gastroenterostomies. **a** Posterior transmesocolic gastrojejunostomy. **b** Anterior precolic transepiploic gastrojejunostomy

7.2.4 Analgesia

Pain, frequently debilitating, is often a presenting symptom. It increases during the course of the disease, associated with other symptoms.

Pain is treated by surgery, i. e., pancreatectomy. Unfortunately, due to the late diagnosis of pancreatic tumors, the number of such operations is limited. The only thing left to be treated is the symptom, and surgery is one of several therapeutic techniques for pain relief.

Neurotomies of the sensory tract are performed at different levels. Thoracic vagotomies and/or sympathectomies, which were once advocated [49, 66], appear to be very inefficient and therefore are very rarely done today. We just recall very seldom used operations such as rhizotomy, or section of the posterior nerve roots, anterolateral chordotomy, and lobotomy, in order to make a detailed study for *splanchnicectomy*, which is presently the operation of choice. In 1942, Mallet-Guy described the left splanchnicectomy for pain relief in chronic pancreatitis [44]. We perform a bilateral splanchnicectomy via the transhiatal tract according to the technique described by Dubois [17]. The greater splanchnic nerve, which originates from the 7th, 8th and, 9th node groups, is formed at the level of the 11th thoracic vertebra. It is 3 cm in front of the costal margin in the subpleural space. The lesser splanchnic nerve is variable and originates from the 10th and 11th node groups; it follows a posterior and external route compared with the greater splanchnic nerve. To free the pillars of the diaphragm, it is necessary to detach the pleura from the intravertebral body to the costal margin at the level of the two intravertebral bodies. The aorta does not hamper the operation very much, especially on the right. The greater splanchnic nerve has to be sectioned over many centimeters. The lesser splanchnic nerve, located posterior and lower, is more difficult to reach (Fig. 7.15).

Michotey [50] performed eleven splanchnicectomies through this tract for cancers of the body of the pancreas. He reported the antalgic effect to be striking for all

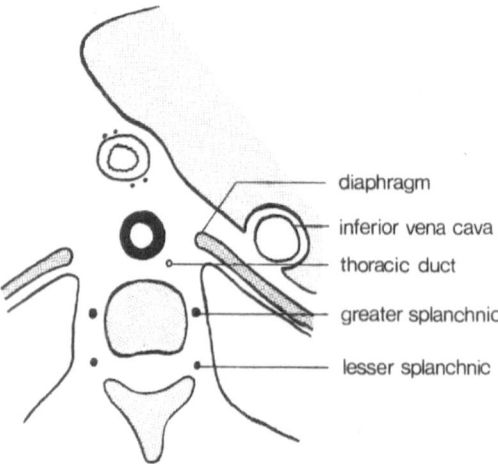

diaphragm

inferior vena cava

thoracic duct

greater splanchnic

lesser splanchnic

Fig. 7.15. Horizontal section of trunk at D-10 level, demonstrating laterovertebral location of greater splanchnic nerve

patients, as early as during recovery, and that this was a lasting effect. Five openings of the pleura proved not to have been essential, but one splenectomy was necessary. Among the various contraindications for this technique he noted invasion of the tumor process to the hiatus, a cardia already operated on for a hiatal hernia, and segmental portal hypertension.

In cases where a splanchnicectomy appears to be difficult because of large tumor volume, or is contraindicated, the surgeon can still perform a celiac block during exploratory laparotomy. It becomes a true chemical splanchnicectomy by bilateral infiltration of the celiac plexus with 25 cc of 50% ethanol [11, 82]. In the same way, 6% phenol can also be used. Flanigan and Kraft found relief from pain in 80% of 37 patients who had undergone chemical splanchnicectomy with or without biliary bypass as compared with 40% of patients who had undergone bypass alone; they reported no morbidity or mortality [20].

Besides neurotomies of the sensory tract, some authors propose decompression of the main pancreatic duct [3, 76]. In this case, of course, pain must be related to the distension of the excretory ducts, and the regional conditions must be favorable for this type of operation. Two techniques are reported: ductogastrotomy and the Puestow procedure.

In combination with these surgical procedures, radiation therapy has a significant value. The conventional external beam irradiation relieves pain in 33% of patients [80]. Goldson et al. reported remission in six of 19 patients (32%) treated by means of intraoperative electron beam therapy and bypass. He considers these remissions to be due only to the intraoperative electrotherapy [30]. In a comparative study of three different types of physiotherapy, Whittington et al. noted that the antalgic effect is more successful as the doses are increased (Table 7.1) [83].

7.3 Chemotherapy and Radiation Therapy

Chemotherapy and radiation are adjuvants to symptomatic treatments with a palliative intent, and they are just beginning to be used instead of pancreatectomy in treatments with a curative purpose.

7.3.1 Chemotherapy

A large number of drugs have been used to treat adenocarcinoma of the pancreas, but the objective positive reponses to monochemotherapy are few, so much so that this cancer was once regarded, with reason, as one of the most chemoresistant. Moreover, the therapeutic efficiency is difficult to estimate. Palliative chemotherapy is of interest for advanced tumors, in patients whose general health is often impaired and who are frequently jaundiced – factors which add to the difficulty of interpreting the results. In a synthetic study, O'Connel grouped the percentages of objective positive responses to the effectiveness of single agents, and only the re-

Table 7.1. Palliative effect of therapy on symptoms of patients with pancreatic cancer (from Whittington et al. [83])

	Palliative treatment	Precision high dose radiotherapy	^{125}I implant and external beam
Complete reponse	5/11	14/23	5/7
Partial reponse	1/11	7/23	1/7

Table 7.2. Objective reponses to monochemotherapy (from O'Connel [57])

Drug	No. of patients	Positive responses (%)
5-Fluorouracil	39	15
5-Fluorouracil	212	28
Mitomycin C	44	27
Streptozocin	27	11
CCNU	19	16
Methyl-CCNU	68	6
Adriamycin	25	8
Methotraxate	25	4
Actinomycin D	28	4
Phenylalanine mustard	43	2

sponses obtained with 5-FU and mitomycin C were encouraging (Table 7.2) [57]. Since then, chemotherapists have combined many drugs in the hope of increasing their activity, by analogy with the association of antitubercular or antibiotic agents. For instance, the Southwest Oncology Group Study (SOGS) included two trials, the first with M-F (mitomycin C + 5-fluorouracil), the second with SMF (streptozocin + mitomycin C + 5-fluorouracil); the objective response rates with the second were higher than with the first [8]. Nowadays, the association of various drugs produces positive and realistic response rates surpassing 40%. Among these various associations, the SMF and FAM (5-fluorouracil, adriamycin, and mitomycin C) regimens stand out. Brown et al. have obtained the same rate when 5-FU and streptozocin were combined with hexamethylmelamine [7]. We have grouped the main responses to the principal series in Table 7.3. It is clear that polychemotherapy, i. e., 5-FU associated with mitomycin, adriamycin, or streptozocin, represents an active and relatively nontoxic therapy. Waddel [79] noted a potentialization of the therapeutic effect when lactones, testolactone or spironolactone, were added to 5-FU. Lactones are administrated orally, and Waddel has demonstrated an improvement in survival with the combination of 5-FU and lactones as compared with 5-FU alone. There are more complications due to testolactone than due to spironolactone; they manifest mainly as gastroenterologic toxicity. At present we do not know what therapeutic effect the lactones have on tumors. However, Moertel et al. [51] are not yet ready to share Waddel's optimism, and more recent reports of the SOGS [43] and of the Eastern Cooperative Oncology Group [51] fail to confirm the initial results or even tend to contradict them.

These drugs are best administered systemically. A few trials of regional arterial chemotherapy, by means of a catheter intubated in the celiac trunk, were perform-

Table 7.3. Objective responses to polychemotherapy

Reference	Drugs	No. of patients	Objective responses (%)
Moertel [51]	5-FU + streptozocin	42	12
SOGS [77]	5-FU + mitomycin C	45	22
Horton [36]	5-FU + methyl-CCNU	41	10
Horton [36]	5-FU + methyl-CCNU + streptozocin	43	7
Brown [7]	5-FU + HMM[a] + streptozocin	15	40
Smith [74]	FAM	27	37
Bitran [6]	FAM	15	30
Wiggans [84]	SMF	23	43
Bukowski [8]	SMF	45	40

[a] HMM, hexamethylmelamine

ed, and some short series have been reported, especially by McCracken et al. [43] and Hafstrom et al. [33]. But this method of administration has no value. The results are not the same as those obtained with arterial or portal chemotherapy in the treatment of secondary hepatic cancer, and this must be due to the vascularization of the pancreas. The catheters are placed by a transbrachial or a transfemoral route and left for many days, during which the regimen is completed. Inherent difficulties in the technique have served to dampen the enthusiasm of clinical investigators.

In Chap. 8 we will report the effects of these treatments on the median survival, although today chemotherapy is not used as a single-modality treatment for pancreatic cancer.

7.3.2 External Beam Irradiation

Adenocarcinoma of the pancreas is not a radioresistant neoplasm, and radiation therapy has long been used in treating this type of cancer, in particuliar for large tumors estimated to be unresectable, for aged persons, or for high-risk patients for whom surgery is contraindicated. Photon beams delivered by a double-split course of cobalt teletherapy are the most frequently used, followed by linear accelerators. Improvements in the histological diagnosis and the careful delineation of tumor margins aid the use of high-energy transfer radiation, largely sparing the area surrounding the target. The precision high doses are related to the stage of development, the trial in which they are included, and the patient's state of health. External beam irradiation is thought to have only a palliative use. Photon-beam doses range from 3500 to 6500 rads. It is usually postulated that doses higher than 5000 rads are necessary to control the tumor but that, on the other hand, they increase the morbidity of the adjacent organs. Most of the time, irradiation follows an exploratory laparotomy, but it can also be administered prior to the operation, as was done by Whittington et al. in a physiotherapeutic protocol (Fig. 7.16). They consider that it minimizes the risk of parietal recurrence, but this must still be confirmed by other studies [83].

Histological confirmation of adenocarcinoma of the pancreas

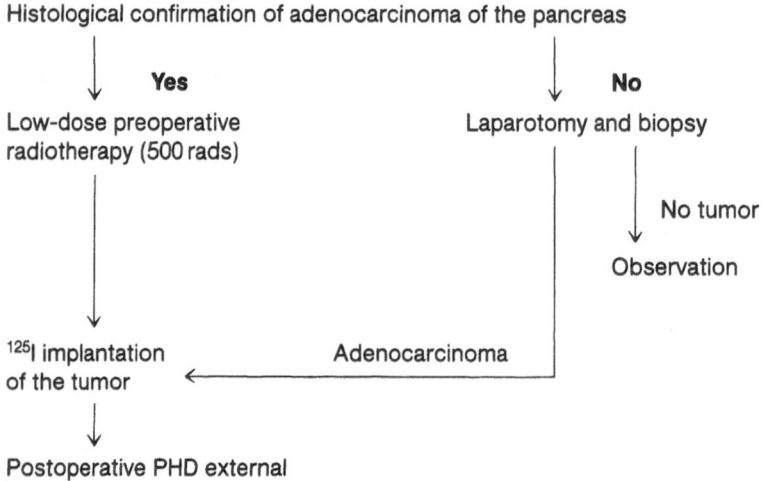

Fig. 7.16. Therapeutic protocol for localized, unresectable adenocarcinoma of the pancreas (from Whittington et al. [83])

Table 7.4. Toxicity of fast-neutron therapy in five patients (from Smith et al. [75])

Toxicity	Neutrons (1700 rads)
Median WBC nadir $\times 10^3$/cu mm	3.6
Median platelet nadir $\times 10^3$/cu mm	155
Skin erythema	5
Nausea/vomiting	3
Severe	
Mild to moderate	3
Diarrhea	1
Hemorrhagic gastritis	1
Hepatopathy	3
Esophagitis	0
Colitis	0
Myelopathy	0

For the past few years, several centers have been making trials with fast neutrons in addition to conventional photon-beam radiation therapy [39, 75]. Fast neutrons present a theoretical advantage, for they are more toxic than photon beams in hypoxic zones. Large, firm tumors, such as pancreatic adenocarcinomas, have a large number of malignant cells living in an environment of relative anoxia, and hypoxia could be a reason why some tumors in man are radioresistant [45]. The maximal doses are as high as 1700 neutrons rad, which represents the approximate equivalent of 5000 photon rad, over a 6-week period, four times a week. The disadvantages of such a method are no less than those of photon beams, at least in Smith's experience (Table 7.4) [75]. In a trial of fast neutrons compared with conventional photon beams at a maximum dose of 6000 equivalent rads, Bukowski [9] found moderate toxicity, due mainly to minor gastrointestinal reactions.

A study of patients treated by helium-ion therapy with a dose of 6000 co-equivalent rads in 7 weeks was recently reported [86], but here again, the undesirable side effects were more or less identical to those with other modalities of irradiation in the same doses.

7.3.3 Internal Radiation Therapy

The precise high doses of external beam irradiation must be higher than 5000 rads to control efficiently the development of pancreatic cancer; however, these doses are damaging to the adjacent tissues. For many years the enhancement of accurate dose delivery by direct intraoperative electron beam therapy has been proposed to avoid this damage. In 1941, Goin and Hoffman [28] attempted intravesical irradiation to treat cancer of the bladder. In Europe in 1944, Henschke [34] reported a study on intraoperative irradiation therapy. But owing to some technical problems, this method has been forgotten; it was only revived in Tokyo by Abe [1] in 1971, and by Goldson [29] in Washington D.C. in 1978.

Goldson et al. [30] use a linear accelerator placed in a normal sterile operating room. During laparotomy and following biopsies and staging, they deliver in one dose 1500–3000 rads with an electron beam through a special, sterilizable collimating lens. The doses rapidly decrease in depth, which spares normal tissues, especially those of the spina cord to the back. The target volume includes the pancreas, the adjacent lymph nodes, and a portion of the duodenum, from 30 to 180 cm^3. They then proceed to the biliary bypass with a gastroenterostomy. Between 1978 and 1981, in a phase-I study, they treated 19 advanced pancreatic unresectable cancers that had been proven on biopsy with internal beam irradiation and surgical bypass alone. They reported some slight side effects in 42% of cases, such as nausea, vomiting, or anorexia. Three patients presented major complications with pancreatic or peripancreatic necrosis leading to death; nevertheless, intraoperative electron-beam therapy is presently included in the therapeutic pattern of the Howard University Hospital in Washington D.C.

Warshaw and the investigators at Massachussets General Hospital in Boston [80] combine intraoperative irradiation at a dose of 1600 rads with external beam irradiation at a dose of 5000 rads. Eighteen patients suffering from localized but unresectable cancer underwent this protocol, and only three minor complications were reported (one pyloric stenosis and two duodenal ulcers).

Wood [85] treated 12 patients with intraoperative electron-beam therapy at a dose of 1652 rads for an average field diameter of 7 cm, combined with preoperative external photonradiotherapy at a dose of 2000 rads and postoperative photonradiotherapy at a dose of 2600 rads. In this study, Wood demonstrated that the precision high dose is slightly higher than 6000 rads and that it represents the biological equivalent of 8700 rads of a conventional fractional external beam irradiation.

Other investigators have tried surgical placement of radioactive isotopes – gold particles, and especially ^{125}I – into pancreatic neoplasms. Currently, the isotope of choice is ^{125}I, due to its physical qualities and its soft-emmitted X-ray. The technique is somewhat time-consuming, since the pancreas must be implanted with

Table 7.5. [125]I Implant complications in 18 patients treated for exocrine pancreatic cancer (from Whittington et al. [83])

Sudden death	2
Gastric ulcer →death	1
Pancreatic pseudocyst →death	1
Wound dehiscence	1
Bleeding	2
Superficial wound infection	2

14-gauge needles and injected with radioactive implants, and the needles must then be removed [55]. The precision high dose is 16000 rads, but over many weeks this represents the biological equivalent of 5000 rads delivered by conventional external beam radiotherapy. Warshaw et al. [80] do not report any complications with this technique and Nisar Syed et al. [55], reporting the results of 18 patients treated with [125]I (10000–15000 rads) and external beam irradiation (3000–5000 rads), regard the method as favorable, with few complications (one case of pancreatitis and one of pneumopathy).

Between 1978 and 1980, Whittington et al. [83] treated 18 patients presenting large but localized adenocarcinomas according to a program combining ^{125}I with external beam radiation therapy (see Fig. 7.16). The radioactive interstitial implantations were calculated to deliver 12000 rads. The postoperative irradiation began 5 weeks after implantation by means of photons in high-energy transfer in a field equal in size to the target volume. In this short series the complications appear to be significant (Table 7.5), since they include four deaths. Two of them were certainly the result of pulmonary embolism and dysrhythmia; the third was due to a complicated gastric ulcer and the fourth to a pseudocyst of the pancreas. In fact, only this last one can be directly related to the technique, and we think that this unfortunate series of Whittington must not lead to the dropping of this method.

Malt seems to prefer intraoperative irradiation to ^{125}I implantation, for the former treats more voluminous tumors with less damage for the adjacent tissues; the irradiation target is larger, and there is no risk of seeding a puncture tract with malignant cells [46].

In any case, whatever the technique, intraoperative irradiation therapy is a satisfying response to the problem of accurate dose delivery. Theoretically, it has many advantages and can lead to a great improvement in the physiotherapeutic treatment of cancer of the pancreas, for its complications are within reasonable margins. It now seems that these new techniques have a great deal to offer, but it is still too early to assess their palliative and curative values.

7.3.4 Combined Radiation Therapy and Chemotherapy

At the present time, radiation therapy and chemotherapy are very rarely used alone, as studies done in the past 10–20 years show a potentiation of effects from one method to the other. Prospective studies are now being done to determine the best drugs that can be associated with the best irradiation techniques.

Table 7.6. Toxicity of radiation therapy combined with 5-FU and methyl-CCNU in 62 patients (from Southwest Oncology Group Study [43])

Toxic reaction	No. of patients affected, according to severity					
	None	Mild	Moderate	Severe	Life-threatening	Fatal
Granulocytopenia	7	10	21	19	4	1
Thrombocytopenia	18	8	13	15	8	0
Nausea/vomiting	36	13	9	4	0	0
Anemia	55	2	3	2	0	0
Diarrhea	61	1	0	0	0	0
Allergy/rash	61	0	0	0	1	0
Alopecia	60	0	0	2	0	0
Hematuria	61	0	1	0	0	0
Mucositis/ulcers	60	1	0	0	0	0
Radiation enteritis	61	0	0	0	1	0

We will not summarize all the work being done in this field, but only the most recent, from the randomized trials of the Gastrointestinal Tumor Study Group (GITSG) reported in 1981 [25]. They compared high-dose radiation therapy alone (6000 rads) with high-dose radiation therapy plus concomitant and subsequent 5-FU and with moderate-dose radiation therapy (4000 rads) plus concomitant and subsequent 5-FU. Radiation therapy with adjuvant chemotherapy significantly increased the mean survival time; however, there was no difference in relation to the radiation doses.

In 1980, Mc Cracken et al. [43] reported the results of two series of SOGS; the first one combined radiation therapy (6000 rads), methyl-CCNU, and 5-FU, and the second consisted of a combination of radiation therapy (6000 rads), methyl-CNU, 5-FU, and testolactone. They did not find any difference between the two series, but did find a high toxicity rate (Table 7.6) related to the radiation dose (6000 rads) and to methyl-CCNU. This toxicity does not appear in the reports of the GITSG [25]. Since the beneficial value of methyl-CCNU is very small compared with its serious complications, it has been dropped from the study by SOGS. They then did a trial for localized but unresectable tumors, combining 5-FU by the celiac arterial tract with external beam radiation therapy (5000 rads), followed by systemic administration of mitomycin C and 5-FU. Nineteen patients underwent this program with moderate toxicity, but the troubles inherent to the arterial catheter and the lack of improvement in the results have caused the program to be dropped from the study as well [42].

On the other hand, some recent reports on the combination of 5-FU with fast neutrons [75] conclude that it is very highly toxic in comparison with 5-FU plus photonradiotherapy (Table 7.7).

Bukowski [9] combined a mixed radiation therapy (fast neutrons plus photons) with an SMF trial (streptozocin, mitomycin C, and 5-FU). Radiation therapy was given over 5 weeks at a maximum dose of 6000 rads, 720 rads of which were delivered by fast neutrons. When the blood constants were stabilized 3-4 weeks later, the SMF trial was started. The moderately undesirable effects of the irradiation consisted mainly of minor gastrointestinal disorders. As for the chemotherapy, there were

152   H. Baumel and B. Deixonne

Table 7.7. Toxicity of neutron therapy (1700 rads) combined with 5-FU
(from Smith [75])

	5-Fluorouracil	
	375 mg/m²	500 mg/m²
No. of patients	5	10
Median WBC nadir × 10³/cu mm	3.4	1.7
Median platelet nadir × 10³/cu mm	110	79
Skin erythema	5	10
Nausea/vomiting	3	9
Severe		3
Mild	3	6
Diarrhea	1	2
Hemorrhagic gastritis	1	3
Hepatopathy	2	5
Esophagitis	0	1
Colitis	0	2
Myelopathy	0	1

cases of nausea, vomiting, gastric ulcers, and gastric bleeding, as well as blood problems of leukopenia and thrombocytopenia.

Finally, in a curative strategy, radiation therapy and chemotherapy are also beginning to be combined with surgical resection. In particular, the GITSG did a prospective randomized study, the preliminary results of which are encouraging [5].

In summary, at present it appears that the combination of radiation therapy and chemotherapy is effective, that the most commonly used drug is 5-FU, that it is frequently combined in a SMF or FAM trial, and finally, that radiation therapy, whatever the particles, must be done with a minimum dose of 5000 rads.

References

1. Abe M, Fukada M, Yamono K (1971) Intra-operative irradiation in abdominal and cerebral tumors. Acta Radiol 10: 408–416
2. Alexiou D, et al. (1912) Occlusion des canaux pancréatiques par injection d' "éthibloc". Résultats d'une étude expérimentale chez le chien. J Chir 10: 597–602
3. Apalakis A, Dussault J, Knight M, Smith R (1977) Relief of pain from pancreatic carcinoma. Ann R Coll Surg Engl 59: 401–403
4. Arendt R, Reding R, Dummler W, Radker R (1982) Do pancreatico-digestive anastomoses remain open after duodeno-hemipancreatectomies? Digestion 25 (1): 15
5. American Society of Clinical Oncology (1985) Proceedings, 4 March, C-325
6. Bitran JD, Desser RK, Kozloff MF, Billing AA, Shapiro CM (1979) Treatment of metastatic pancreatic and gastric adenocarcinomas with 5-Fluoro-uracile, adriamycin and mitomycin C (FAM). Cancer Treat Rep 63: 2049–2051
7. Brown JC, Bruckner HW, Storch J, et al. (1980) Combination chemotherapy for pancreatic cancer. Proc Am Assoc Cancer Res 21: 420

8. Bukowski RM (1981) Randomized comparison of 5-FU and mitomycin C (MF) versus 5-FU, mitomycin C and streptozotocin (SMF) in pancreatic adenocarcinoma: A Southwest Oncology Group Study. Proc Am Soc Clin Oncol 22: 453

9. Bukowski RM, Gahbauer R, Rodriguez-Antunez A, Hermann R (1982) Mixed beam radiotherapy and combination chemotherapy in localized pancreatic adenocarcinoma, preliminary results. Int J Radiat Oncol Biol Phys 8 (7): 1231–1233

10. Cooper BH, Hawk JC, Rambo WM (1971) Long term incubation of the biliary tract with silastic catheters. Am Surg 37: 198–202

11. Copping J, Willix R, Kraft R (1969) Palliative chemical splanchnicectomy. Arch Surg 98: 418

12. Couinaud C (1967) Les pancréatectomies avec curage ganglionnaire. J Chir (Paris) 93: 397–410

13. Couinaud C (1970) Le méso-pancréatico-duodéno-ombilical. J Chir (Paris) 100: 249–266

14. Couinaud C, Huguet C (1966) Le temps d'exérèse dans la duodéno-pancréatectomie totale. J Chir (Paris) 91: 181–190

15. Cubilla AL, Fortner J, Fitzgerald PJ (1978) Lymph node involvement in carcinoma of the head of the pancreas area. Cancer 41 (3): 880–887

16. Doutre LP, Ducasse P, Kamuti J (1979) Artère hépatique droite et duodéno-pancréatectomie. Bordeaux Méd 12 (1): 9–11

17. Dubois F (1977) Splanchnicectomies par voie abdominale transhiatale. Nouv Presse Med 6: 2069–2070

18. Ferrucci JT, Mueller PR, Harbin WP (1980) Percutaneous transhepatic biliary drainage: technique results and application. Radiology 135: 1–13

19. Finsterer H (1952) Peut-on recommander la cholédoco-duodénostomie pour le traitement des maladies des voies biliaires? Mem Acad Chir 78: 499–502

20. Flanigan DP, Kraft RO (1978) Continuing experience with palliative chemical splanchnicectomy. Arch Surg 113: 509

21. Fortner JG (1973) Regional resection of cancer of the pancreas. A new surgical approach. Surgery 73 (2): 307–320

22. Fortner JG, Kim DK, Cubilla A (1977) Regional pancreatectomy: in bloc pancreatic, portal vein and lymph nodes resection. Ann Surg 186 (1): 42–50

23. Fortner JG (1981) Surgical principles for pancreatic cancer. Regional total or subtotal pancreatectomy. Cancer 47 (6): 1712–1718

24. Frey CF, Child GG III, Gry W (1976) Pancreatectomy for chronic pancreatitis. Ann Surg 184: 403–414

25. Gastro-Intestinal Tumor Study Group (1981) Therapy of locally unresectable pancreatic carcinoma: a randomized comparison of bright dose (6000 rads) radiation alone, moderate dose radiation (4000 rads + 5-Fluorouracil) and bright dose radiation + 5-Fluorouracil. Cancer 48 (8): 1705–1710

26. Gastro-Intestinal Tumor Study Group (unpublished) Essai n° 9173. Phase III. Study of combined 5-FU and supervoltage radiation therapy as an adjuvant to surgical treatement of pancreatic carcinoma.

27. Gilsdorf RB, Spanos P (1973) Factors influencing morbidity and mortality in pancreatico-duodenectomy. Ann Surg 177, 3, 332–337

28. Goin L, Hoffman E (1941) The use of intra-vesical low-voltage contact roentgen irradiation in cancer of the bladder. Radiology 37: 545–549

29. Goldson A (1978) Preliminary clinical experience with intra-operative radiotherapy. J Natl Med Assoc 70: 493–495

30. Goldson AL, Ashaveri E, Espinoza MC, et al. (1981) Single high dose intra-operative electrons for advanced stage pancreatic cancer: phase I pilot study. Int J Radiat Oncol Biol Phys 7: 869–874

31. Grosdidier D, Nesseler JP, Boissel P, Grosdidier J (1982) Le pancréas restant après duodéno-pancréatectomie céphalique. Son devenir et son traitement. J Chir (Paris) 119 (8–9): 485–490

32. Guillemin G, Berard P, Raymond DA Les pancréatectomies. Encycl Med Chir, Paris, Techniques Chirurgicales, Appareil Digestif, 4.3.03, 40880

33. Hafstrom L, Ihse I, Jonsson PE, et al. (1980) Intra-arterial 5-FU infusion with or without oral testolactone treatment in irresectable pancreatic cancer. Acta Chir Scand 146: 445–448

34. Henschke U, Henschke G (1944) Zur Technik der Operations-Bestrahlung. Strahlentherapie 74: 223–229

35. Hoevels J, Lunderquist A, Ihse I (1978) Percutanesous transhepatic intubation of bile ducts for combined internal-external drainage in pre-operative and palliative treatment of obstructive jaundice. Gastrintest Radiol 3: 23-31

36. Horton J, Gelber R, Engstrom P et al. (1981) Trials of single agent and combination chemotherapy for advanced cancer of the pancreas. Cancer Treat Rep 65: 65-68

37. Huguet C, Hakami R, Bloch P (1981) L'intubation transtumorale des obstructions néoplasiques du hile du foie. A propos de 36 observations. Ann Chir 35: 341-347

38. Jurasz (1923) Choledoco-duodenostomie als Methode der Wahl für die Drainage der tiefen Gallenwege. Zentralbl Chir 1000

39. Kaul R, Cohen L, Hendrickson F, et al. (1981) Pancreatic carcinoma: Results with fast neutron therapy. Int J Radiol Oncol Biol Phys 7: 173-178

40. Kron B, Sala F, Reynier J (1984) Dérivation par prothèses dans le traitement des ictères néoplasiques. Chirurgie 110 (8-9): 693-699

41. Leger L (1979) Sectorisation de la pathologie du pancréas. Nouv Presse Med 8 (3): 175-180

42. McCracken JD, Olson M, Cruz AB, et al. (1982) Radiation therapy combined with intra-arterial 5-FU chemotherapy for treatment of localized adenocarcinoma of the pancreas: a Southwest Oncology Group Study. Cancer Treat Rep 66 (3): 549-551

43. McCracken JD, et al. (Southwest Oncology Study Group) (1980) 5-Fluorouracil, methyl-CCNU and radiotherapy with or without testolactone for localized adenocarcinoma of the exocrine pancreas. Cancer 46 (7): 1518-1422

44. Mallet-Guy P (1942) La splanchicectomie gauche pour pancréatite chronique. Lyon Chir 38: 481-485

45. Malaise EP, Guichard M (1984) L'hypoxie est-elle une cause de radio-résistance des tumeurs humaines? In: Institut Gustave-Roussy (ed) Actualités carcinologiques. Masson, Paris

46. Malt RA (1983) Treatment of pancreatic cancer. JAMA 250 (11): 1433-1437

47. Marchal G, Balmes M, Vergue J, Grynfelt E, Selami (1971) Les problèmes vasculaires en rapport avec la chirurgie d'exérèse pancréatique. Montpellier Chir 17 (5): 407, 428

48. Mercadier M (1969) In: Patel J, Patel JC, Leger L (1969) Nouveau traité de technique Chirurgicale vol 12/2, p 552

49. Merendino KA (1964) Vagotomy for the relief of pain secondary to pancreatic carcinoma. Am J Surg 108: 1

50. Michotey G, Sastre B, Argeme M, et al. (1983) La splanchnicectomie par voie transhiatale de Dubois: technique, indications, résultats à propos de 25 sections nerveuses pour algies viscérales abdominales. J Chir (Paris) 120 (8-9): 487-491

51. Moertel CG, Engstrom P, Lavin PT, Gerber RD, Carbone PP (1979) Chemotherapy of gastric and pancreatic carcinoma. Surgery 85: 509-513

52. Moossa AR (1982) Pancreatic cancer. Approach to diagnosis, selection for surgery and choice of operation. Cancer 50 (11): 2689-2698

53. Mori K, Misumi A, Suguyama M, et al. (1977) Percutaneous transhepatic bile drainage. Ann Surg 185: 111-115

54. Nakayama T, Ikeda A, Okuda K (1978) Percutaneous transhepatic drainage of the biliary tract. Technique and results in 104 cases. Gastroenterology 74: 554-559

55. Nisar Syed AM, Puthawala AA, Neblett DL (1983) Interstitial iodine - 125 implants in the management of unresectable pancreatic carcinoma. Cancer 52 (5): 808-813

56. Obertop H, Van Houten H (1984) A new technic for pancreatectomy. Surg Gynecol Obstet 159 (1): 88-90

57. O'Connel MJ (1983) Oncologic treatment of pancreatic cancer. Mayo Clin Proc 58: 47-50

58. Parc R, Herbiere P (1983) Protection de l'anastomose pancréato-jéjunale après duodéno-pancréatectomie céphalique pour tumeur. Nouv Presse Med 12 (2): 99-101

59. Patel J, Patel JC, Leger L (1969) Nouveau traité de technique chirurgicale vol 12/2, p 552

60. Pissas A (1981) Essai d'anatomie clinique et chirurgicale sur la circulation lymphatique du pancréas. Thesis, University of Paris

61. Praderi R, Estefan A, Intubation canalaire pour cancer des voies biliaires. Encycl Med Chir Tech Chir Dig 4, 2, 40972

62. Prioton JB, Bernard JN, Olivier G (1966) Pancréatectomie totale pour cancer avec résection en bloc de l'axe mésentérico-portal et de l'artère mésenté rique supérieure. Réimplantation mésentérico-cave et mésentérico-aortique. Montpellier Chir 12 (3): 291-306

63. Prioton JB, Laux R (1960) La lame rétro-portale du pancréas céphalique. Incidence de sa topo-graphie en chirurgie pancréatique et portale. C R Assoc Anat 108: 667-673
64. Remine WH, Priestly JT, Judde S, King JN (1970) Total pancreatectomy. Ann Surg 172: 595-604
65. Richelme H, Birthwisle Y, Mitchetti C, Bourgeon A (1984) Les attaches postérieures du pan-créas. Incidence chirurgicale de la lame rétro-pancréatique droite. Chirurgie 110 (2): 150-157
66. Rienhoff WF, Baker BM (1947) Pancreo-lithiasis and chronic pancreatitis. JAMA 134: 20
67. Rio Branco (1912) Essai sur l'anatomie et la médecine opératoire du tronc coeliaque et de ses branches. Thesis, University of Paris
68. Ross DE (1954) Cancer of the pancreas. A plea for total pancreatectomy. Am J Surg 87: 20-33
69. Rouviere H (1948) Anatomie humaine, vol 1/2. Masson, Paris, p 932
70. Saubier EC, Lescoeur N, Patensky C, Barbe C (1978) Problèmes posés par une artère hépatique droite naissant de la mésentérique supérieure et duodéno-pancréatectomie céphalique. Lyon Chir 74: 223-226
71. Schwartz SS, Ziedler A, Moossa AR, et al. (1978) A prospective study of glucose tolerance, insu-lin, C-peptid and glucagon responses in patients with pancreatic carcinoma. Dig Dis Sci 23: 1107-1114
72. Shiu MH (1982) Resection of the pancreas without production of fistula. Surg Gynecol Obstet 154: 497-500
73. Sigel B, Basset JG, Cooper DR, Dunn MR (1965) Resection of the superior mesenteric vein and replacement with a venon autograft during pancreatico-duodenectomy. Ann Surg 162: 941-946
74. Smith FP, Hoth DF, Levin B et al. (1980) 5-Fluoro-uracile, adriamycin and mitomycin C (FAM) chemotherapy for advanced adenocarcinoma of the pancreas. Cancer 46: 2015-2018
75. Smith FP, Schein PS, McDonald JS, et al. (1981) Fast neutron irradiation for locally advanced pancreatic cancer. Int J Radiat Oncol Biol Phys 7: 1527-1531
76. Smith R (1973) Progress in the surgical treatment of pancreatic disease. Am J Surg 125: 143-153
77. Southwest Oncology Group Study (1979) 5-FU infusion with mitomycin C versus 5-FU infusion - methyl CCNU in the treatment of advanced upper gastro-intestinal cancer. Cancer 44: 1215-1221
78. Terblanche J (1976) Is the carcinoma of the main hepatic conduct junction an indication for liver transplantation or palliative surgery? A plea for the U-tube palliative procedure. Surgery 79: 127
79. Waddel WR (1973) Chemotherapy for carcinoma of the pancreas. Surgery 74: 420-429
80. Warshaw AL, Richter JM, Podolski DK, et al. (1982) A strategy against pancreatic cancer. J Clin Gastroenterol 4: 525-532
81. Whipple AO, Parsons WB, Mullins CR (1935) Treatment of carcinoma of the ampulla of Vater. Ann Surg 102: 763-779
82. White TT, Murat J, Morgan A (1968) The immediate surgical management of a mass in the head of the pancreas. Northwest Med 67: 731
83. Whittington R, Dobelbower RR, Mohuiddin M, Rosato FE, Weiss SM (1981) Radiotherapy of unresectable pancreatic carcinoma: a six-year experience with 104 patients. Int J Radiat Oncol Biol Phys 7: 1639-1644
84. Wiggans RG, Woolley PV, Mac Donald JS et al. (1978) Phase II trial of streptozotocin, mitomy-cin C and 5-Fluoro-uracile (SMF) in the treatment of advanced pancreatic cancer. Cancer 41: 387-391
85. Wood WC, Shipley WV, Gunderson LL, Cohen AM, Nardi GL (1982) Intra-operative irradia-tion for unresectable pancreatic carcinoma. Cancer 49 (6): 1272-1275
86. Woodruff KH, Castro JR, Quivey JM, et al. (1984) Post mortem examination of 22 pancreatic carcinoma patients treated with helium ion irradiation. Cancer 53 (3): 420-425
87. Yoshioka H, Wakabayashi T (1957) Traitement de la douleur des pancréatites chroniques par la neurotomie de la tête du pancréas. Lyon Chir 53: 836-835

8 Results of Therapy*

H. Baumel and B. Deixonne

Analyzing the results of various methods of treatment is difficult because the patient series providing these results are not homogeneous, and the stage of development of the tumor is not always determined using the same criteria from case to case. Nevertheless, we will try to point out, among the numerous therapeutic options, the advantages of each method as well as the path to be followed. To do this, we must answer three questions: 1. Do pancreatic resections improve the prognosis in comparison with palliative bypasses? 2. Which resections offer the best chance for a cure? 3. Which symptomatic and adjuvant therapies produce the maximum survival (length and comfort)?

8.1 Pancreatic Resection Versus Palliative Bypass

Actually, the question was first asked 20 years ago, when on comparison of the average survival rates following resection and bypass operations, the results were found to be identical. The first person to place any serious doubt on the resection procedure was Crile [10] in 1970; after comparing two series, he found that a bypass was better than a resection (Table 8.1).

In 1974, Hermreck et al. [21] criticized Crile's methods and demonstrated the superiority of resection, finding that the survival time was almost doubled for patients who underwent resection for a stage-I or -II pancreatic cancer (Table 8.2).

In 1975, Shapiro [37] found no difference in the median survival between two series of 24 patients. However, he pointed out that the cancer of 66% of patients with bypasses had not been histologically diagnosed during laparotomy. On the other hand, Brooks and Culebras [4] found that resections were genuinely advantageous, after they compared three series of patients treated with bypass, Whipple's operation, or a total pancreatectomy. The median survival during stages I, II, and III was 23 months following a total pancreatectomy and only 5.6 months following a bypass (Table 8.3). Why, then, do we find such contradictory results? Most likely this is

---

* *Author's Note.* This work does not relate our personal experience. Our patient series are limited and do not represent any scientific value and above all any statistical significance (81 surgical cases between 1977 and 1984, including only 15 partial or total resections and 51 by-passes). We deliberately chose to base this work on reviews of recent international studies. The large number of these studies did not allow us to quote them all.

Table 8.1. Comparison of bypass and radical procedure, 1953-1966 (from Crile [10])

Survival	Bypass ($n = 28$)	Radical duodenopancreatectomy ($n = 10$)
Average survival (months)	12	8.5
Median survival (months)	8	8
Died at 2 months (%)	7	10
Died at 4 months (%)	14	40
Lived 12 months + (%)	32	20
Longest survival (months)	41	22

Table 8.2. Survival in years according to stage of disease (Hermreck [21])

Surgical treatment	Stage			
	I	II	III	IV
Biopsy	0.20	0.21	0.08	0.14
Palliation	0.86	0.54	0.50	0.27
Resection	1.40	1.20	0.52	0.50

Table 8.3. Comparative survival (Brooks and Culebras [4])

Procedure	No. of patients	Mortality (%)	Mean survival (months)		
			Stages I, II, III	I, II	III
Bypass	35	14.2	5.6	5.8	5.4
DPC[a]	11	21	7.6	12.7	6
TP[b]	16	12.5	23	40	6

[a] DPC, Duodenopancreatectomy
[b] TP, total pancreatectomy

due to the fact that the results used in comparisons are usually overall results, which include all types of tumor as well as a jumbled assortment of tumor stages. Another point is that we cannot always be assured that a histological diagnosis has been performed.

When Hermreck et al. and later Brooks refined their results in relation to the stage of development of the tumor, they realized that only during an early stage could resection offer the patient the chance of being cured. It is understood that for well-advanced stages, today considered unresectable, the results with resections which were only palliative and those with bypasses are superimposable.

We cannot ignore the progress made in cancer resection during the period 1965-1975. Resections were extended, indications were more clearly defined, and cancer of the exocrine pancreas became better known. At the same time, the surgical environment offered better preparation for intervention and facilitated the fol-

Table 8.4. Comparison of bypass and radical procedure with regard to median survival (Mouiel [33])

Reference	No. of patients	Procedure	(%)	Median survival
Doutre [12]	172	Resection	23	12 months
		Bypass	69.5	5 months
Hollender et al. [25]	130	Resection	16	11.5 months
		Bypass	54.4	4.8 months
Grosdidier [19]	270	Resection	8.5	Four survivals at 4 and 5 years
		Bypass	88	7–9 months
Mouiel [33]	90	Resection	16.6	9 months
		Bypass	76.6	7.5 months

low-up. This led to the publication in 1975 of reports indicating the improvement of surgical resection results for cancers judged to be curable.

We are not able here to cite all the published results; however, all are concordant. We will restrict ourselves to French patient series. In 1984, Launois [27] reported 98 palliative bypasses, with a survival of 4% after 1 year and 0% after 2 years. He also reported on a series of 39 pancreatic resections with a survival of 45% after 1 year, 35% after 2 years, and 25% after 3 years. In 1983, Mouiel [33] published the results of several French series (Table 8.4) which again pointed out the advantages of resection over bypass.

At the present time, we can no longer reasonably contest the fact that the best chances for improving cancer prognosis is to perform a resection. The 5-year survivals are obtained only through resections. After a palliative bypass survival time is only slightly lengthened, and we cannot report any survivor after 5 years among patients presenting a histologically confirmed exocrine pancreatic cancer.

8.2 Results in Relation to Extent of Resection

The extent of resection is related to three parameters that cannot be dissociated: the possibility of resection, the percentage of cures, and the postoperative mortality and morbidity.

8.2.1 Rate of Resectability

In 1964, Mongé et al. [28] reported a resectability rate of 10%, based on the experience of the Mayo Clinic from 1941 to 1962 concerning 119 pancreatoduodenectomies of the head of the pancreas. Launois [27] found a resectability rate increasing from 15% to 35% when he compared two successive periods, and he increased the proportion of total pancreatectomies in relation to Whipple's operation.

Table 8.5. Resectability rate

Reference	Year	No. in series	Percent resectable
Nakase et al. [34]	1977	1819	18
Moossa et al. [31]	1979	157	33
Hollender et al. [25]	1980	130	16
Edis et al. [14]	1980	1272	13
Fortner [16]	1981	97	29
Solassol et al. [39]	1983	88	46.5
Launois [27]	1984	73	35

In 1977, Nakase et al. [34] gathered 1819 observations of cancer of the head of the pancreas originating from 57 Japanese hospitals, the majority of which had been treated by a Whipple procedure. The average rate of resectability was 18%. In 1980, Hollender et al. [25] reported 21 resections in 130 cases, in other words, a rate of 16%, whereas in a 1984 series Moreaux et al. reported 12 resections (11 Whipple procedures, one distal pancreatectomy) in 96 patients operated, giving a rate of 12.5% [32].

Total pancreatectomy, in relation to the Whipple procedure, increase the possibility for resection. Yet, in order to achieve perceptible progress we must undertake regional pancreatectomies and not hesitate to "go large" in including the required visceral and vascular removal.

In 1981, Fortner reported his experience with 151 patients operated on for periampullary pancreatic cancer. He was able to perform resections on 48 patients, resulting in a rate of 32%. Of the 48 resections, 36 were regional pancreatectomies, and 77% of these tumors had been previously explored and judged to be unresectable by other surgeons. In reality, only 97 of Fortner's patients had exocrine pancreatic cancer. For these he performed 22 resections, representing a rate of resectability of 29% [16]. Moossa et al. performed 52 resections in a total of 157 operations in 1979. Among the 33 total pancreatectomies done, some were Fortner's regional type 0 or I, resulting in a rate of resectability of 33% [31]. In 1983, Solassol et al. [39] reported the experience of the Cancer Institute in Montpellier with 88 treated patients, 41 of whom had been submitted to regional total or subtotal pancreatectomy, resulting in a rate of resectability of 46.5%.

We have presented these percentages of resectability in Table 8.5 and realize that they increase along with the extent of the resection. We must simply underline that these findings represent a bias toward regional resections.

8.2.2 Percentage of Cures

The interpretation and comparison of the results from a large series is awkward for the following reasons: (a) some series include pancreatectomies for cancer other than exocrine pancreatic; (b) some exclude survival figures and/or postoperative deaths; (c) percent survival is calculated according to different statistical criteria;

(d) the results do not take into account the stage of development, and when the stage is referred to, it is never with the same classification.

In reality, the simplest thing would be to determine the number of each type of resection done and then the number of patients surviving after a 5-year period for each type of resection. Very few published series allow this, and under these circumstances we cannot effectively compare the results of numerous series. Nevertheless, we will try to discuss the percentage of cures on the basis of several homogeneous series.

Between 1951 and 1975, a study was done at the Mayo Clinic of 124 Whipple procedures and 38 total pancreatectomies. Survival curves were calculated according to the method of Kaplan-Meier and reported using a logarithmic scale. The 5-year survival was 8% for the two techniques. Postoperative deaths were excluded, and the percentages were calculated for 32 total pancreatectomies and 101 pancreatoduodenectomies of the head of the pancreas (Fig. 8.1) [14].

Based on these results, Edis et al. recommended the Whipple procedure except in three circumstances: (a) where pancreaticojejunostomy is judged to be too risky, (b) in presence of an invasion of the pancreatic plane of section and (c) where there is preoperative insulin-dependent diabetes.

Van Heerden et al. later reanalyzed data from the Mayo Clinic dating from the period 1951–1978. Total pancreatectomy represented only 16% of all resections before 1970 but 41% after 1970. Between 1975 and 1978, 17 Whipple operations and 13 total pancreatectomies were performed. Van Heerden et al. are very qualified in their conclusions, but prefer total pancreatectomy. One of their arguments is to avoid performing a pancreaticojejunostomy [40].

Hicks and Brooks (Harvard Medical School) reported 91 surgical interventions for exocrine pancreatic cancer between 1956 and 1970, 11 pancreatoduodenectomies and 11 total pancreatectomies. The median survival rate after the total pancreatectomies was 15.4 months, versus 8.5 months after the pancreatoduodenectomies. When they presented these results in 1971, five patients who had had total pancreatectomies were still alive; one of them had undergone the surgery 4.5 years earlier. There was no survival of patients who had undergone a Whipple procedure. An anatomopathological examination of the pancreas following the 11 total pancreatectomies showed that four of 11 resected pancreas contained cancerous cells outside the normal limits for Whipple's procedure [23].

In 1976, Brooks and Culebras compared the median survival rates following Whipple procedures and total pancreatectomies in relation to the developmental stage of the cancer. Their findings ranged from 6 months for both techniques at stage III to 40 months following a total pancreatectomy and 12.7 months following a cephalic pancreatoduodenectomy at stages I and II. The advantage of the total pancreatectomy is unquestionable for the "curable" stages, but neither pancreatoduodenectomy nor total pancreatectomy can be considered other than palliative intervention for stage-III tumors (see Table 8.3) [4].

From 1970 to 1977, Moossa operated on 154 exocrine pancreatic cancers, performing 52 resections (19 Whipple procedures and 33 total pancreatectomies). He reports four survivals after a 5-year period following a total pancreatectomy and one following a cephalic pancreatoduodenectomy. The median survival was 27 months following total pancreatectomy and 18 months following Whipple's

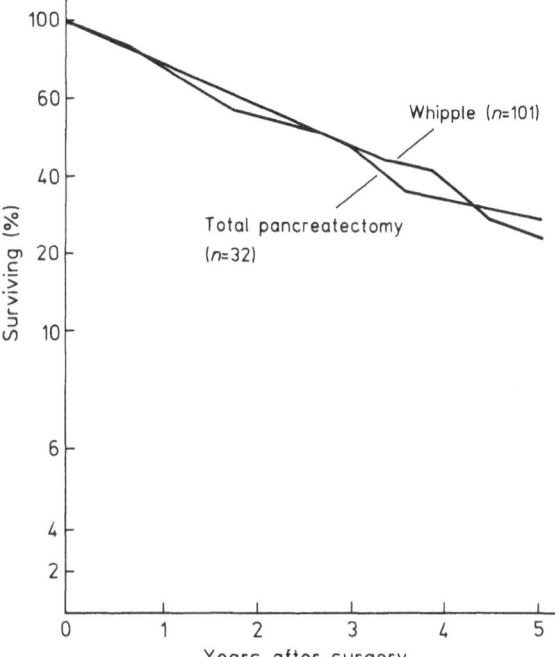

Fig. 8.1. Actuarial survival after Whipple's operation and total pancreatectomy for ductal carcinoma of the pancreas (26 operative deaths and three surviving reoperated patients are excluded; from Edis et al. [14])

procedure. Moossa believes that the best treatment is total pancreatectomy in combination with a regional lymphadenectomy [31]. This corresponds to a Fortner type-0 regional pancreatectomy. He presented five arguments in favor of this [30]:

1. In 30% of all cases cancer is potentially multifocal.
2. Histological invasion of the pancreatic section may follow a pancreatoduodenectomy.
3. Cancerous cells in the upper pancreatic duct can be a cause of recurrence.
4. The only way to correctly perform a regional lymphadenectomy is to totally remove the pancreas.
5. The risk of pancreaticojejunostomy is thus avoided.

Recently, Solassol et al. reported a series of 41 regional total or subtotal pancreatectomies performed at the Cancer Institute in Montpellier. Including postoperative deaths (six or 14.6%), there were two survivals after 5 years, representing 4.8%. According to Kaplan-Meier's method, the actuarial survival after 5 years is 28% (Fig. 8.2) [39].

The results of these five studies effectively show the progress that has been made in this field in the past 20 years, and it appears that extensive resection improves the median survival. We must also note, however, that other studies do not show this improvement after extended resection. In particular, Chigot et al. [9], Herter et al. [22], and Forrest and Longmire [15] did not find any improvement. We must repeat that it is very difficult to compare the results of these retrospective studies owing to the different treatments for cancers at different stages of development. It is possible, even likely, that we will not find improvement in 5 years survival rate, on a statistical level, if extended resections are reserved strictly for advanced tumors. In order to

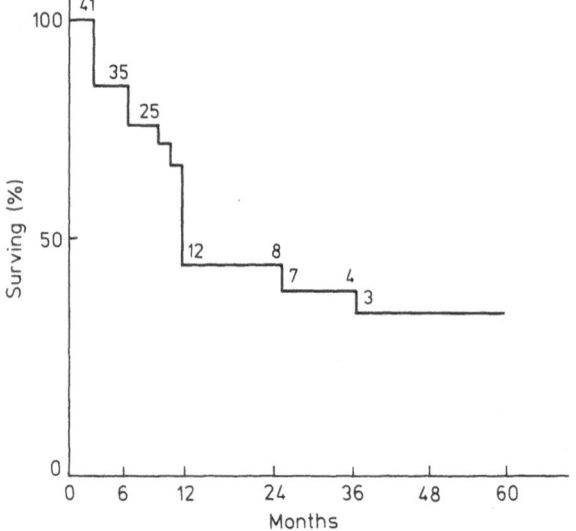

Fig. 8.2. Actuarial survival (Kaplan-Meier method) after regional pancreatectomy in 41 patients with pancreatic cancer (from Solassol et al. [39])

gain anything from this, a prospective study must be done comparing the results of each technique at a previously determined stage of development of the tumor. This requires adequate codification of the different techniques as well as of the stage of development. In the meantime, it seems logical to assume that, for a curative surgical strategy, wider resections must give the best results. This is a general oncological notion not always true, in particular when further treatments are used to control any residual cancer cells. This is not yet the case for pancreatic cancer, and the best chances for a cure remain with a wide resection.

Nonetheless, employing a treatment of radiation therapy associated with chemotherapy following pancreatectomy could improve the prognosis. Initial results of a randomized study of GITSG (protocol 9173) have just been published [1]. Two patient series are compared, the first treated with only a surgical resection and the second with a resection followed by 5-FU and external beam irradiation, at a dose of 4000 rads. In the former series, the survival after 2 years is 18%; in the latter it is 42%. Recurrence is more likely to follow the first option than when patients undergo supplemental radiation and chemotherapy (91% versus 67%). Kalser's and Ellenberger's study confirms the one of the GITSG. The median survival rate of the group treated by resection is only 11 months. The group treated by resection with adjuvant radiochemotherapy has a 20 months' survival rate [26]. These first results encouraging and will open new therapeutic perspectives.

To conclude on a positive note, we must remember the good results of cystoadenocarcinoma resections with a 5-year survival rate of 68% [24]. In 1984, Camprodon and Quintanilla found in the literature 28 childhood cases of pancreatic adenocarcinoma, usually very rare [7]. However, all of those that had been resected were subsequently cured.

Table 8.6. Primary causes of hospital mortality: Mayo Clinic experience (Edis et al. [14]

	Whipple operation		TP[a]	
	1951–1970 $n=95$	1971–1975 $n=29$	1951–1970 $n=18$	1971–1975 $n=20$
Intra-abdominal hemorrhage	5	0	2	0
Pancreatic leak	5	0	0	0
Intra-abdominal sepsis	4	0	1	1
Gastro-abdominal hemorrhage	2	0	0	0
Biliary leak	0	0	0	1
Gastric leak	1	0	0	0
Hepatic failure	2	0	0	0
Myocardial infarction	1	0	0	1
Total	20 (21%)	0 (0%)	3 (17%)	3 (15%)

[a] TP, Total pancreatectomy

8.2.3 Operative Mortality and Morbidity

As far as *operative mortality* is concerned, Launois found no significant difference between operative mortality with palliative bypasses, Whipple resections, and total pancreatectomies [27]. In a retrospective study of their experience at the Mayo Clinic from 1951 to 1975, Edis et al. [14] gathered the causes of operative mortality up to 30 days following a total pancreatectomy, during two successive periods, 1951–1970 and 1971–1975 (Table 8.6). In 1980, Doutre noticed an average mortality of 20% when he reviewed many international studies, with extremes ranging from 15% to 52% [12]. In 1983, De Battice et al. [11] reviewed operative mortality following cephalic pancreatoduodenectomy and total pancreatectomy, referring to the major series that had been published; they found an average rate of 17.1% for a total of 351 total pancreatectomies and the same rate of 17.1% for a total of 1554 Whipple procedures.

These figures seem high, but we should not lose sight of the fact that the series cover a long period of time. Today, some authors present more encouraging results. For example, Moossa et al. [31] report four deaths for 52 resections, or a mortality of under 8%. Unquestionably, progress in reanimation, better patient preparation, and enteral and parenteral nutritional support further lower the operative mortality figures.

We have too few references to judge the situation after regional pancreatectomies. Fortner [16] reports a 16% postoperative death rate, Solassol [39] 14.6%, but here again we see some improvement in the results. Actually, from 1973 to 1977, mortality was 21.7% for 23 regional pancreatectomies, whereas from 1978 to 1981 it was no more than 5.5% for 18 regional pancreatectomies.

Let us now look at *postoperative complications* from the experience of the Mayo Clinic following Whipple procedures and total pancreatectomies [14].

The attributable morbidity for these techniques is rather high (Table 8.7) – 52% following a cephalic pancreatoduodenectomy and 55% following a total pancreatectomy. The most frequent complication is a *disunited pancreatic anastomosis* fol-

Table 8.7. Postoperative complications: Mayo Clinic experience (Edis et al. [14])

	Whipple operation		TP[a]	
	1951–1970 $n=95$	1971–1975 $n=29$	1951–1970 $n=18$	1971–1975 $n=20$
Pancreatic anastomotic leak	10	4	0	0
Intra-abdominal hemorrhage	9	3	2	0
Intra-abdominal sepsis	6	1	1	3
Biliary anastomotic leak	5	1	0	1
Gastrointestinal hemorrhage	2	1	5	1
Gastric anastomotic leak	2	1	0	0
Wound dehiscence	0	1	1	2
Severe insulin reaction	2	0	3	0
Renal failure	3	0	1	0
Hepatic failure	2	0	0	0
Other	23	6	2	9

[a] TP, Total pancreatectomy

lowing the Whipple procedure, with a frequency on the order of 10%. Warren et al. [42] reported a 16% incidence of pancreatic fistulas with respect to the experience at the Lahey Clinic. Chigot et al. reported four pancreatic fistulas following 29 cephalic pancreatoduodenectomies; two of them followed a pancreaticojejunostomy and the other two were in the absence of anastomoses [9].

Postoperative *diabetes* presents a very unique problem. It is always present following a total and subtotal pancreatectomy and less consistent following the Whipple procedure. From 64 total pancreatectomies done between 1942 and 1973 at the Mayo Clinic, Pliam and Remine [35] summarized the problems of postoperative diabetic regulation (Table 8.8). They show that even in recent times (1969–1973) the average insulin doses required to regulate this diabetes were on the order of 21–24 U/day. Mongé et al. [28], also reporting on the experience of the Mayo Clinic from 1941 to 1962 regarding Whipple procedures, found that 22.3% of 119 patients who had undergone surgery for cancer developed diabetes. Daily doses of insulin varied from 10 to 45 U. It is normal to find less postoperative diabetes after a cephalic pancreatoduodenectomy than after a total pancreatectomy (where it is consistently found), but the average insulin doses are relatively identical. Generally, regulation difficulties are blurred when oral alimentation is resumed. Yet accidents such as hypoglycemia have been reported, notably by Van Heerden et al. [40] regarding two occurrences after 192 resections done at the Mayo Clinic. To reduce this accidental risk of hypoglycemia, the glucose levels of patients with pancreatectomies should be maintained above 1.5 g/l.

There do not appear to be any long-term vascular complications of insulin-dependent diabetes due to pancreatectomies, though a case of glomular sclerosis has been reported by Doyle et al. [13], a case of retinopathy by Burton et al. [6], and two cases of retinopathy by Pliam and Remine [35] in the literature from a series done at the Mayo Clinic before 1968.

As far as exocrine loss is concerned, it must be compensated for by pancreatic extracts, with the daily doses adapted to the extent of resection in order to avoid postoperative steatorrhea.

Table 8.8. Diabetic management after total pancreatectomy (Pliam and Remine [35])

Management	1942–1973	
	No.	%
Easy	25	50
Occasional hypoglycemic reaction treated orally with carbohydrates	9	18
Poor; persistent glyco-suria, brittle diabetes	2	4
Very difficult; ketoacidosis or hypoglycemia requiring hospital-ization	10	20
Difficult only with concomitant illness	4	8

8.3 Symptomatic and Adjuvant Therapies

We are no longer in the curative therapeutic pattern, and the question now is what to do with the patient who cannot undergo a curative resection, whatever the contraindications.

The goal of *symptomatic therapies* is to insure the passage of the bile and food and to relieve the patient of pain. This is mandatory for the comfort of the patient and gives a few months of respite before starting the adjuvant therapies. We will not review the bypass techniques again. Their results are comparable, even when considering over 8000 cases. Sarr and Cameron [36] showed that cholecystoenterostomies were not as burdened by postoperative mortality as were choledochoenterostomies, the rates being 16% versus 20%. Initially, the technique will depend upon the local conditions as well as the surgeon's habits. The most frequent condition is jaundice leading to an exploratory laparotomy. Must we associate a gastroenterostomy with a biliary bypass? Sarr and Cameron [36] found that 13% of all patients with bypassed bile must undergo a secondary gastroenterostomy. They compared the results of a group of patients who underwent only the biliary bypass with a second group who underwent a double bypass. The groups contained 107 patients each; in the first group, 26 patients had survived after a 1-year period, giving a median survival of 6.5 months, and in the second group, 21 patients had survived after 1 year, with a median survival of 5 months. Eight patients from the first group had to undergo a secondary gastroenterostomy 9 months after the first intervention. Blievernicht et al. [2] estimated identical mortality and morbidity as well, whether there were two bypasses or only one. Of 34 survivors after the biliary bypass alone, 13 had a secondary duodenal stenosis after an average delay of 4 months following the first intervention. They therefore advocated a prophylactic gastroenterostomy, as did Sarr. On the other hand, Warren [41] was not in favor of a prophylactic digestive bypass; for him, gastroenterostomy should be reserved only for duodenal stenoses, as it increases both mortality and morbidity. We do not have an absolute opinion on this problem and we react according to whatever the local conditions may be. However, it is true that a double bypass today does not modify postoperative morbidity and mortality to any great extent, and we perform more mechanical gastroenterostomies than we did a few years ago.

As far as the mortality figures following a palliative bypass are concerned, they are more or less identical to those following a resection. In France, Grosdidier [19] presented a figure of 25%, Hollender et al. [25] of 17%. Launois [27] reported 15.8% mortality following a bypass, 18.7% after a cephalic pancreatoduodenectomy, and 17.4% after a total pancreatectomy. In contrast, Van Heerden et al. [40], reporting on the experience of the Mayo Clinic from 1970 to 1975, found a relatively low mortality of 6% following a simple or a double bypass. These were cases of localized tumors. Moossa et al. [31] also reported 6% (two of 31) mortality for cephalic cancers treated with a bypass.

In the preceding chapter we spoke of antalgic treatments and gave some results, in particular for surgical or chemical splanchnicectomies. These now offering excellent analgesic possibilities; however, treatment for pain is not simply one therapy, and many true specialists working in pain centers are called into action where the problem is treated in its entirety. We can no longer calm the suffering of the cancer patient "on request" by empirical methods, always ending up with massive doses of morphine.

With respect to these analgesic therapies and bypasses, are radiation and chemotherapy beneficial? These *adjuvant therapies* bring a certain amount of progress which we will illustrate with several examples. In a series of 111 pancreatic cancers, Brooks et al. [3] reported 17% of cases with no intervention, 19% with laparotomy and biopsy, 16% with resections, and 48% with palliative bypasses. Among 51 patients with bypasses the average survival ranged from 6 months for a bypass alone to 8.5 months when the bypass was combined with radiation and chemotherapy.

The efficacy of these so-called adjuvant therapies depends upon whether or not there are distant metastases. For localized forms, after biliary bypass, or internal biliary drainage if the hepatic pedicle is invaded, one must identify the tumor with metallic clips and submit the patient to radiation and chemotherapy. In a double-blind study comparing external beam irradiation plus a placebo with radiation therapy plus 5-fluorouracil, Moertel et al. [29] showed that the average survival increased from 6.3 months to 10.4 months. The results of the GITSG are equally interesting: the 1-year average survival after 5-fluorouracil alone is 10%, but it increases to 40% when external beam irradiation is added. The dose can be either 4000 or 6000 rads [17]. Having treated 13 patients for localized nonmetastasized cancers with bypasses and clipping and by mixed-beam radiation (photons and neutrons) and an SMF chemotherapeutic protocol, Bukowski [5] found a median survival of 10 months.

We could improve greatly the results combining radiation therapy and chemotherapy. The median survival is generally 10 months without metastases and less than 6 months with them.

Does intraoperative radiation modify these figures? The results presently published are mainly of stage II attempts for voluminous unresectable tumors but without any extensive metastases. This way, combining intraoperative electrontherapy with external photontherapy and a FAM protocol, Wood et al. found a average survival rate of 15 months [43]. The number is more or less the same in the most recent series reported by Shipley et al. [38] and Gunderson et al. [20]. Goldson et al., on the contrary, treating 19 patients with internal radiation alone, reported an average survival rate of 5.5 months (ten patients presented however liver metastases). He was not able to make any judgment on the palliative or curative value of this technique [18]. It is too early to pass the least bit of judgement on the benefits of intraoperative irradiation. It has a theoretical justification as it augments the tumor dose without damaging the surrounding tissue. On the other hand, electrotherapy requires the installation of extremely costly equipment. Implantation radiation therapy appears to be easier to employ, not requiring this expensive equipment; only radioactive isotopes need be available.

We believe that it is useful to underline these facts regarding the different therapeutic methods. The figures are not very optimistic, as there are not many survivors after 5 years. In 1981, the American Cancer Society's figures for histologically proven cancer of the pancreas had an average survival rate after 1 year of 12% and after 5 years of 1%. The median survival was 3.3 months [8].

As far as pancreatectomies in particular are concerned, if we want to summarize the different results that we have just seen (objectively, this remains statistically impossible), it seems that about 25 of 100 diagnosed exocrine pancreatic cancers can be surgically resected. Of these 25 patients only one is likely to survive after 5 years (4%). Therefore, survival after 5 years for cancer of the pancreas, all stages taken together, is approximately 1%. These few figures clearly show that the majority of pancreatectomies with a curative intent are, in reality, only palliative interventions. Nonetheless, taking only the average survival as a reference criterion, pancreatectomy represents the best palliative intervention for theoretically curable stages.

In answer to the three questions that we asked at the beginning of the chapter we could say:
1. Do pancreatic resections improve the prognosis in comparison with palliative bypasses?
   Yes.
2. Which resections offer the best chance for a cure?
   The widest.
3. Which symptomatic and adjuvant therapies offer the longest and most comfortable survival?
   Bypasses, splanchnicectomies, and a combination of radiation and chemotherapy.

When all is said and done, extensive pancreatectomies increase the rate of resectability, and their morbidity and mortality is not greater than that of a Whipple procedure. Do they offer the best chances for a cure? This is rather likely, even if the results do not always demonstrate this. For this, it would be necessary to have at one's disposal all the results of regional pancreatectomies after 5 years for small cancers. All that we can say is that today there are some unquestionable theoretical arguments in favor of extended resections.

References

1. American Society of Clinical Oncology (1985) Educational symposium and educational workshops. May 19, p 13
2. Blievernicht SW, Neifeld JP, Terz JJ, Lawrence W (1980) The role of prophylactic gastro-jejunostomy for unresectable peri-ampullary carcinoma. Surg Gynecol Obstet 151 (6): 794-796
3. Brooks DL, Osteen RT, Gray EB, et al (1981) Evaluation of palliative procedures for pancreatic cancer. Am J Surg 141: 430-433
4. Brooks JR, Culebras JM (1976) Cancer of the pancreas: palliative operation, Whipple procedure or total pancreatectomy? Am J Surg 131: 516-520
5. Bukowski RM, Gahbauer R, Rodriguez-Antunez A, Hermann R (1982) Mixed beam radiotherapy and combination chemotherapy in localized pancreatic adenocarcinoma, preliminary results. Int J Radiat Oncol Biol Phys 8 (7): 1231-1233
6. Burton TY, Kearns TP, Rynearson EH (1957) Diabetic retinopathy following total pancreatectomy. Mayo Clin Proc 32: 735-739
7. Camprodon R, Quintanilla E (1984) Successful long-term results with resection of pancreatic carcinoma in children: favorable prognosis for an uncommon neoplasm. Surgery 95 (4): 420-426
8. Cancer Facts and Figures (1981) American Cancer Society, New York
9. Chigot JP, Riquet M, Ahualli C, Clot JP, Mercadier J (1982) Les résultats des exérèses dans les cancers de la tête du pancréas. J Chir (Paris) 119 (6-7): 411-414
10. Crile G (1970) The advantages of bypass operations over radical pancreatoduodenectomy in the treatment of pancreatic carcinoma. Surg Gynecol Obstet 130: 1049-1053
11. De Battice C, Fetelian D, Deltenre M (1983) Place de la pancréatectomie totale dans le cancer de la tête du pancréas. Acta Chir Belg 83: 89-94
12. Doutre LP (1980) Exérèse contre dérivation dans les cancers ictérigènes du pancréas. In: Chirurgie abdominale et digestive 2. Masson, Paris, p 56 (Actualités chirurgicales)
13. Doyle AP, Balcerzak SP, Jeffrey WL (1964) Fatal diabetic glomerulo-sclerosis after total pancreatectomy. N Engl J Med 270: 623-628
14. Edis AJ, Kiernan PA, Taylor WF (1980) Attempted curative resection of ductal carcinoma of the pancreas. Mayo Clin Proc 55: 531-536
15. Forrest JF, Longmire WP (1979) Carcinoma of the pancreas and peri-ampullary region. A study of 279 patients. Ann Surg 189: 129-138
16. Fortner JG (1981) Surgical principles for pancreatic cancer. Regional total or subtotal pancreatectomy. Cancer 47 (6): 1712-1718
17. Gastro-Intestinal Tumor Study Group (1981) Therapy of locally unresectable pancreatic carcinoma: a randomized comparison of bright dose (6000 rads) radiation alone, moderate dose radiation (4000 rads + 5 fluoro-uracile) and bright dose radiation + 5 fluoro-uracile. Cancer 48 (8): 1705-1710
18. Goldson AL, Ashaveri E, Espinoza MC, et al (1981) Single hight dose intra-operative electrons for advanced stage pancreatic cancer: phase I pilot study. Int J Radiat Oncol Biol Phys 7: 869-874
19. Grosdidier J (1981) Cancer du pancréas. Attitude chirurgicale: exérèse ou dérivation. In: Chirurgie abdominale et digestive 2. Masson, Paris, p 61 (Actualités chirurgicales)
20. Gunderson LL, Martin JK, Byer DE et al (1984) Intra-operative and external beam irradiation with or without resection: Mayo pilot experience. Mayon Clin Proc 59: 691-699
21. Hermreck AS, Thomas CY, Friesen SR (1974) Importance of pathologic staging in the surgical management of adeno-carcinoma of the exocrine pancreas. Am J Surg 127: 653-657
22. Herter FP, Copperman AM, Ahlborn TN, Antinori C (1982) Surgical experience with pancreatic and peri-ampullary cancer. Ann Surg 195: 274-281
23. Hicks RE, Brooks JR (1971) Total pancreatectomy for ductal carcinoma. Surg Gynecol Obstet 133: 16-20
24. Hodgkinson DJ, Remine WH, Weiland LH (1978) A clinico-pathologic study of 21 cases of pancreatic cystadeno-carcinoma. Ann Surg 188: 679-684
25. Hollender LF, Meyer C, Marrie A, Pierard T, Calderoli H (1980) Le cancer du pancréas. Réflexions à propos de 147 cas. Ann Chir 34: 775-777

26. Kalser MH, Ellenberger SS (1985) Pancreatic cancer. Adjuvant combined radiation and chemo-therapy following curative resection. Arch Surg 120: 899-903
27. Launois B (1984) La chirurgie du pancréas pour cancer. Bordeaux Med 17: 115-118
28. Mongé JJ, Judd ES, Gage RP (1964) Radical pancreatectomy. A 22-year experience with the complications, mortality rate and survival rate. Ann Surg 160 (4): 711-719
29. Moertel CG, Childs DS, Reitemeier RJ, et al (1969) Combined 5-fluoro-uracil and supervoltage radiation therapy of locally unresectable gastro-intestinal cancer. Lancet 2: 865-867
30. Moossa AR (1982) Pancreatic cancer. Approach to diagnosis, selection for surgery and choice of operation. Cancer 50 (11): 2689-2698
31. Moossa AR, Lewis MH, Mackie CR (1979) Surgical treatment of pancreatic cancer. Mayo Clin Proc 54: 468-474
32. Moreaux J, Catala M, Marzano L (1984) Les résultats du traitement chirurgical du cancer du pancréas. Etude d'une série de 96 opérés. Gastroenterol Clin Biol 8: 11-16
33. Mouiel J (1983) Dérivation ou exérèse dans le cancer pancréatique? Med Chir Dig 12: 475-478
34. Nakase A, Matsumoto Y, Uchida K, Honjo I (1977) Surgical treatment of cancer of the pan-creas and the peri-ampullary region: cumulative results in 57 institutions in Japan. Ann Surg 185: 52-57
35. Pliam MB, Remine WH (1975) Further evaluation of total pancreatectomy. Arch Surg 110: 506-512
36. Sarr MG, Cameron JL (1982) Surgical management of unresectable carcinoma of the pancreas. Surgery 91 (2): 123-133
37. Shapiro TM (1975) Adenocarcinoma of the pancreas: a statistical analysis of biliary bypass vs Whipple resection in good risk patients. Ann Surg 6: 715-721
38. Shipley WU, Wood WC, Tepper JE et al (1984) Intra-operative electron beam irradiation for patients with unresectable pancreatic carcinoma. Ann Surg 200: 289-294
39. Solassol C, Joyeux H, Yakoun M, Blanc F, Bories P (1984) La pancréatectomie régionale dans le traitement de l'adénocarcinome du pancréas. A propos de 41 cas. Gastroenterol Clin Biol 8: 17-21
40. Van Heerden JA, Remine WH, Weiland LH, et al (1981) Total pancreatectomy for ductal ade-nocarcinoma of the pancreas. Am J Surg 142: 308-311
41. Warren KW, Braasch JW, Thum CW (1968) Carcinoma of the pancreas. Surg Clin North Am 48: 601-605
42. Warren KW, Braasch JW, Thum CW (1968) Diagnosis and surgical treatment of carcinoma of the pancreas. Curr Probl Surg 70: 3-10
43. Wood WC, Shipley WV, Gunderson LL, Cohen AM, Nardi GL (1982) Intra-operative irradia-tion for unresectable pancreatic carcinoma. Cancer 49 (6): 1272-1275

9 Present Treatment Strategies

H. Baumel and B. Deixonne

The poor quality of therapeutic results in pancreatic cancer incites us to bring together along with an earlier diagnosis all our knowledge and means in order to determine the best treatment strategies available today. Since a long time, surgery had proven its superiority, to such an extent that it was essentially the only therapy being used at the expense of the other techniques, initially radiation therapy and later on chemotherapy.

Surgical resection must take first place today in therapeutic management. It represents the only hope for a cure, all the more so as modern techniques allow for more extensive and audacious, and hence apparently more effective operations. We can no longer ignore, however, the usefulness of adjuvant treatments, as a great deal of work has demonstrated their beneficial action. Moreover, recent progress in symptomatic treatments has had a not inconsiderable effect on the comfort and pain relief of patients.

An analysis of these diverse treatments can for the most part only be done retrospectively, using a very limited number of homogeneous patient series. Many studies have no statistical value, as they are biased from the start. Some do not show a positive histological proof of cancer [40], others include tumors involving the pancreas but with diverse origins (duodenum, ampulla, biliary ducts). It is therefore important to define relatively homogeneous patient groups with the aim of performing exploitable clinical trials and establishing the most effective protocols. It is in function with these groups that the different treatment strategies should be proposed.

9.1 The Various Patient Groups

The anatomical features of the tumor (volume, right or left localization, staging, histological type), or its clinical symptoms (jaundice, malnutrition) can mean many variables in a prospective study. They must be taken into account as prognostic factors, but it is also necessary to define three important notions in the approach to therapeutic strategies: operability, resectability, and curability. A certain confusion reigns on this subject. The three notions depend on the general pretherapeutic workup of the patient and also on the extent of the tumor. The picture is completed by a precise inventory obtained during laparotomy.

9.1.1 Operability

Surgery performed for pancreatic cancer is usually major. Even if it is simply palliative, this surgery entails not inconsiderable risks of mortality and morbidity, in spite
of recent progress in this field [24, 28, 32, 40, 41, 55]. It is therefore important to
assess the risk factors before taking the decision for anesthesia and surgery.

Concerning the *general fitness* of the patient, of greater importance than age are
nutritional status and the presence of organic insufficiencies (cardiorespiratory, renal, or hepatic) in the determination of whether or not surgery can be performed.
Jaundice and malnutrition, often improved by appropriate treatments, can be temporary criteria of inoperability.

The *stage of development* of the tumor in itself can be a definite contraindication
for surgical intervention. This is the case for cancers which have progressed to systemic invasion associated with hepatic and peritoneal metastases, ascites, or other
secondary localizations (e.g., lung, brain). Systemic invasion is not always recognized during a pretherapeutic workup. Peritoneal metastases are not easily demonstrated, except by - a little practiced exploration - laparoscopy. If hepatic metastases do not frequently escape discovery during examination, other localizations are
not as consistently discovered. This explains a certain number of useless laparotomies. However, they are fewer now (10% as opposed to 27%) [53] due to progress in
preoperative appraisal.

There is no point in operating on pancreatic cancers which are at an inoperable
stage of development as the survival is little influenced by palliative surgery. Moreover, symptomatic, nonsurgical treatments can be just as effective in giving the patient relief.

It is occasionally the association of local and general factors that indicate inoperability (a large palpable tumor in an aged patient with poor general health). The
group of inoperable patients remains small (10%) relating above all, based on the
criteria chosen by most of the teams, to their general state of health.

9.1.2 Resectability

This notion is derived from a locoregional evaluation of whether or not the pancreatic tumor mass can be surgically removed, whatever the importance of the resection.

Subjectivity, therefore, plays a large role in the assessment of resectability. With
the exception of a tumor invading the posterior aortocaval plane, tumors are almost
always resectable, on condition that the resection is extended into the neighboring
invaded tissues (stomach, colon, juxtapancreatic vessels). Therefore, the decision is
a function of the audacity, training, and philosophy of the surgeon. This decision is
extremely variable: some believe that if a tumor is removable, everything must be
done to carry out the resection. Others are more reserved on the utility of some resections that are in reality palliative. This explains the large number of discrepancies between series regarding this point.

Resectability is independent of the stage of development of the tumor and does not take into account an invasion into the lymphatic nodes. A stage-IV tumor can be resectable, whereas one of stage III might not be. In principal, stages I and II are always resectable. It is during the pretherapeutic appraisal that one must begin to look into this possibility. At the present time, different morphological examinations, especially CT scanning and arteriography [52], can provide interesting information. Unfortunately this information is rarely definitive. Laparotomy allows a better assessment of resectability, by giving a complete inventory of the tumor and its extensions.

Resectability is sometimes superimposable on curability, giving it a curative value and occasionally leading to a cure. On the other hand, resectability is considered palliative if there is any tumor tissue remaining. This is the case for incomplete tumor resections, for partial pancreatectomies of multiple foci cancers, and for resections which ignore nodal invasion, or those that are performed in spite of metastases. This can be either deliberate or unintentional on the part of the surgeon.

The differentiation between curative and palliative resectability is important. Resections performed for a curative purpose, and which at the time are the only possibility for a cure, should be done at every opportunity. Those which are only palliative in aim are less justifiable and will be discussed later on.

In reality, the resectability rate varies, according to the patient series, from 10% [37] to 46.5% [50]. We have explained the reasons for such variations. The rate is higher for right head localizations than it is for left body and tail of the pancreas localizations, which are diagnosed at a later stage. By calculating an average rate of most series, the obtained result is on the order of 25%.

9.1.3 Curability

This notion is complementary to the preceding one. In effect, some resectable cancers are curable and others are not. Those cancers considered to be curable are those in which resection allows a total removal of all intraglandular, lymphatic, and surrounding tumor tissue. Only this can give the patient a chance of long-term survival.

Yet "curability" is a theoretical notion which is not synonymous with "cure". Indeed, only a small percentage (5%–10%) of patients said to be curable are, in fact, cured after 5 years. Real curability, that is to say leading to a cure after the appropriate treatment is undertaken, is a progressive notion which can never be defined in advance.

It is therefore very difficult to evaluate curability in practice, as it is more of a presumption than a certainty. Assessment can be made with a certain degree of objectivity, on condition that the surgeon submits himself to a rigorous discipline in his research; unfortunately this happens all too rarely. Numerous surgeons content themselves with a subjective evaluation of the tumor's resectability.

It is much easier to speak with certainty on the incurability of cancer of the pancreas; for example, the presence of distant hepatic and/or peritoneal metastases are definitive indications of incurability. Lymphatic involvement – at least invasion of the lymph nodes of the first and second relay – is not a definitive indication of incurability in our eyes since the nodes are theoretically removable, and this has led to some effective cures. This was also the opinion previously expressed by Child [12]. Others are not in agreement, and consider that nodal invasion at all levels signifies an incurable case [27, 54]. An invasion of the lymph nodes at the level of the third relay (stage IV) is more debatable, as it is situated at the limit of regional and systemic dissemination, and hence at the limit of curability. We, ourselves, consider this a criterion of incurability.

The degree of curability is therefore, on the whole, dependent on the stage of the tumor, stages I and II being by definition the most curable. Whatever the stage, it is never possible to affirm with certainty that all of the tumor tissue has been removed. The high relapse rate (90%-95%) after surgery which was previously considered to be curative attests to this fact.

A very rigorous, methodological and difficult appraisal, in particular of lymph node involvement, is necessary during a laparotomy in order to arrive at a presumption of curability for the lesion. In the case of Whipple's procedure, it is necessary to ascertain by an extemporaneous examination the integrity of the section [9, 34, 36, 40]. This is not always a proof of the integrity of the remaining pancreatic tissue as would be the case for multicentric tumors. All these procedures lengthen the duration of surgery, occasionally to a considerable extent. For this reason, only highly trained surgeons are qualified to perform such a workup. It is also necessary to have a real work team, which includes the pathologist charged with the carrying out of all these extemporaneous tests. We will further analyze the means to be used in such an appraisal.

In spite of its theoretical aspect, the notion of curability is very important. When all is said and done, the surgeon's classification of his operation as a palliative or curative strategy is based upon his assessment of curability. In the first case (curability) all can be envisaged (regional pancreatectomy) to give the patient the maximum chance of achieving a cure. In the second case (incurability) it is useless to perform a resection of the lesion at all costs, even if the tumor is resectable, when one considers the futility of this action. Such surgery has too many grave consequences. When a resection with a curative aim in mind has been decided upon, the degree of curability must permit the surgeon to adapt the degree of resection to the requirements of the tumor invasion. This is particularly true in the case of partial pancreatectomies, where the risk of residual lymphatic or glandular tumor tissue is higher than in total pancreatectomies.

Does the notion of curability modify the resectability rate? In principal it does, if all resectable but incurable tumors are not subjected to resection. Tryka and Brooks, considering all cancers with invaded lymph nodes to be incurable, report a resectability rate of less than 10% for total pancreatectomy [54]. In fact, for a curative strategy, the presumption of curability - being in itself a favorable factor towards an extended resection - should in relation slightly increase the rate. These two factors have a tendency to cancel each other out. We agree with the presumption of curability up to and including stage III, and we think that regional pancreatectomy is a legitimate therapy. At stage IV, however, it is better to abandon all curative procedures.

Without being able to give a precise figure, we estimate that the presumption of curability is on the order of 15% of all cases. This rather low figure results from diagnoses which are made too late in the course of the disease. In fact, few surgeons consider curability, confusing it with resectability; the average number of resections performed – being on the order of 25% of all cases – indicates that many palliative resections are still performed unintentionally.

Let us then review the three patient groups, according to the notions of:
1. *Operability* – a notion that permits one to know:
   a) If the patient's general state of health permits consideration of anesthesia and surgery
   b) If the extent of the tumor permits surgery (curative or palliative) rather than a simple laparotomy
2. *Resectability* – a local notion that is often subjective, permitting to judge whether the tumor mass can be the object of a complete resection, whatever the necessary vascular sacrifices (vessels, adjacent organs). Resectability is not necessarily dependent upon the stage of the tumor or its curability.
3. *Curability* – a theoretical notion, more presumptive than definitive in nature, which attempts to establish whether or not all the tumor tissue (pancreatic and extrapancreatic) can be removed by the appropriate surgical procedure. It is not synonymous with a cure and is related to the stage of development of the cancer. In case of incurability, it is futile to consider resection of the tumor.

9.2 Exploratory Laparotomy

We recognize the importance of laparotomy, and feel that all operable patients should undergo this procedure. It is, at the same time, the final diagnostic step (see Chap. 6) and the first treatment step, because the final decision as to whether or not a resection should be done is made during this surgical exploration.

The macroscopic estimates resulting from palpation by the examiner are not sufficient, even after direct access to the bursa omentalis, after a large pancreato-duodenal detachment, and after an exploration of the celiac region and the principal vascular pedicles. The exact tumor volume itself can be difficult to determine due to perineoplastic pancreatitis.

Four surgical approaches are mandatory during an exploratory laparotomy to complete the manual study performed by the surgeon. These are: pancreatic biopsy, the search for hepatic and peritoneal metastases, the study of the vascular connections to the tumor, and the search for lymph node involvement. The surgeon is helped in this evaluation by intraoperative ultrasound and extemporaneous microscopic examinations.

9.2.1 Pancreatic Biopsy

Pancreatic biopsy specimens must be taken each time, especially if there is not a biopsy-proven malignancy before surgery. The tissue biopsy poses no problem in the case of a superficial invasion or of accessible metastases. It can be difficult and dangerous in the case of a small intraglandular tumor surrounded by pancreatitis. This explains the disadvantages of this procedure as mentioned by different authors [6, 26]. Among these are the false negatives (15%), the mortality, which is low but still important (1%), and the morbidity (5%: pancreatic fistula, hematoma, pancreatitis).

It is for this reason that some prefer a needle biopsy permitting the removal of a tissue core (Tru-Cut system). This method, which is more precise for deeply located tumors, seems to have a greater sensitivity and to present a lesser danger than the biopsy. In reality, it is not exempt from complications. These are even more frequent in certain patient series [31, 33, 48], because this procedure is used for deeply located, extremely inaccessible tumors, whereas a classical biopsy is of more interest for superficially located tumors.

Today the thin, inframillimetric (0.6 mm) needle cytopuncture proposed by Swedish authors [13, 21] seems to be preferred. This technique appears to be the most reliable and least dangerous [2]. The majority of series show no accidents and give this procedure reliability of 87%-100%. With 38 intraoperative cytopunctures of the pancreas, Boutelier [6] obtained 28 true positives and 4 false negatives in 32 cancers. The tumor can be punctured directly approached via a transduodenal route. Multiple punctures (10-12 slides) are necessary in order to increase the sensitivity of the test and to diminish the false negatives due to pancreatitis. We have indicated that ultrasound is not of interest in the guidance of this intraoperative puncture. The slides must be prepared (cf. Sect. 2.2.2) and subjected to an extemporaneous cytological examination. The cytologist must be highly trained for the delicate interpretation that is required in this test. For small tumors, therapeutically speaking the most interesting, a needle biopsy at surgery must supplant the much more difficult percutaneous cytopuncture.

Some people emphasize the importance of looking for tumor extensions that involve the prepancreatic peritoneum and are of grave significance. They recommend that an extemporaneous histological verification be carried out [50].

9.2.2 Abdominal Metastases

The search for abdominal metastases is a matter of attentively exploring the liver as well as the peritoneal cavity, particularly at the level of the upper abdomen for small metastases either proximal or distant to the primary tumor. Here, again, any doubt should be removed by an extemporaneous histological examination.

The liver should be manually searched for palpable metastases. When a small superficial and suspicious node is found, it should become the object of an extemporaneous examination. The absence of any hepatic anomaly should be confirmed by intraoperative ultrasound, which is sensitive to the detection of occult metastases [4, 5].

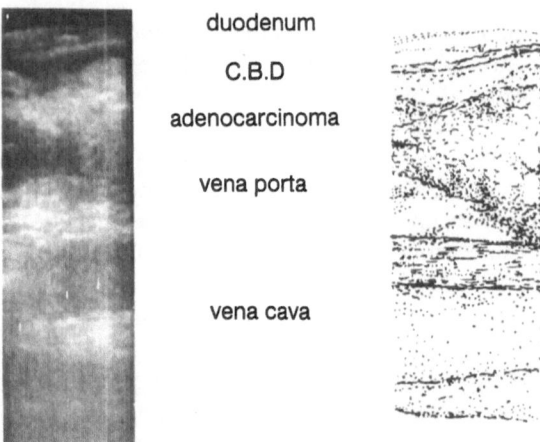

duodenum

C.B.D

adenocarcinoma

vena porta

vena cava

Fig. 9.1. Intraoperative echograph showing stenosis of portal vein

9.2.3 Invasion of Adjacent Vessels

Peritumoral vascular invasion can be uncovered through a manual exploration. This is sometimes the case for the mesenteric portal venous axis. An invasion of the arterial pedicles can be indicated during the preoperative period by the CT and angiography results. The degree of vascular invasion is difficult to define, and vascular resection is determined in accordance with this degree. Intraoperative ultrasound is capable of giving this type of information (Fig. 9.1). We believe that it should be systematically employed in this fashion during a laparotomy. Vascular invasion is not always neoplastic and can be caused by an associated pancreatitis. Only an examination of the tissue biopsies can differentiate between the two, and the prognostic value of this test has been indicated by Moossa et al. [40].

9.2.4 Lymph Node Involvement

The state of the lymph nodes must be methodically verified. Any therapeutic decision is largely dependent upon whether or not they have been invaded. It is therefore necessary to take repeated biopsies and give them to the pathologist for an extemporaneous evaluation. Nodal biopsies are guided by the location of the tumor and by a good knowledge of its lymphatic drainage; care should be taken, if possible, to examine the juxtapancreatic nodes of the first relay as well as those of the second and third. Access to the retroperitoneal nodes can be difficult in the early stages of intervention due to the pancreatic mass. It is sometimes only after eight, ten, or twelve successive extemporaneous examinations that the surgeon will ask the pathologist for information concerning the evolutive stage of the tumor.

We realize how much time is required to carry out this exploration precisely and thoroughly. It is nevertheless useful to submit a patient to this procedure in order to direct selectively the therapeutic indications. It is actually during an exploratory laparotomy that a decision is made on whether to perform a surgical curative resection or simply a palliative procedure. This decision is based on the degree of resectability and curability of the lesion.

9.3 Curative Strategies

These must be reserved for those tumors deemed curable, and must be applied according to the patient's general state of health. Treatments with a curative aim are largely dominated by pancreatectomies. We will see that the occurrence of jaundice can pose a problem for a preliminary biliary drainage, that the evolutive stage of the tumor has little influence on resection technique, and that adjuvant treatments have an equal place in curative protocols.

9.3.1 Pancreatectomies

Knowing that no pancreatic cancer can be cured without resection, what type of pancreatectomy should be proposed in a curative strategy? Along the same vein, is there, at present, a place for partial pancreatectomies? Although the Whipple procedure is strongly defended by Longmire et al. [34], we do not concur, owing to the frequency of tumors that extend outside of the limits of the slice, to multicentric tumors, and to the particularities of the lymphatic drainage of the pancreas. As early as 1952, Orr considered the Whipple procedure a simply palliative measure [45]. In 1954, Ross pleaded in favor of the total pancreatectomy [49]. In 1967, Couinaud recommended en bloc lymphatic curage. In 1983, Malt [35] counted only 65 cures resulting from 15000 Whipple resections.

    At present, it is therefore the total pancreatectomy with extended lymphadenectomy to the upper abdomen which represents the curative intervention of choice, as has been proposed for several years by numerous authors [9, 15, 20, 32, 37, 39, 49, 51]. This holds even if the tumor is small and localized within the gland. In effect, it is the combination of small tumor and large resection that leads to the best chances for a cure in a young patient.

    A subtotal pancreatectomy, acceptable at the oncological level, poses the problem of what to do with the residual stump and of postoperative diabetes that can be difficult to equilibrate. However, Whipple's procedure cannot be totally removed from curative resections. It is of value when a regional total pancreatectomy is inadvisable owing to the age and/or general well-being of the patient presenting a small tumor in the head of the pancreas (stage I or II).

9.3.2 The Problem of Jaundice

Jaundice merits discussion as it is the most frequent (80%) presenting symptom of right-side localizations, which in themselves are the most frequent. In practice, the question is the following: must jaundice and its cause be treated simultaneously or should jaundice be treated first and then its cause? Numerous studies have dealt with this subject and we will now summarize them.

Denning et al. [17] studied the influence of jaundice on the mortality and the complications of resection from two patient groups operated with or without preliminary biliary decompression by transparietal external biliary drainage (Table 9.1). There was a significant difference in morbidity but not in mortality. The biliary drainage was maintained for an average of 13 days and the fall into the mean bilirubin level was 55.8% ± 18%. Recently, in France, Chapuis et al. [11] conducted a retrospective study on the influence of biliary retention on the operative mortality of pancreatic cancer. They concluded that the duration of jaundice had no influence on the mortality, whereas the degree of intensity was significant. Regarding 279 Whipple resections, 224 of which were for cancer of the head of the pancreas and 55 for chronic pancreatitis, Braasch and Gray [7] reported a relationship between the intensity of preoperative jaundice, the frequency of complications, and postoperative mortality, in particular for patients having a bilirubinemia higher than 200 mg/l. These observations were not surprising, as we know that cholostasis has an effect on the blood crasis, renal functions, immune response, and the healing process. The hepatic functions of synthesis are diminished leading to such associated consequences as proteinemia, albuminemia, coagulation factors.

In addition, it appears that a jaundiced kidney, like the liver, is more sensitive to ischemia, further exposing itself to postoperative weakness through a hepatorenal syndrome. Fourtanier [22] has also shown, in regards to 56 jaundice-associated cancers of the head of the pancreas, a higher operative risk in patients whose bilirubin titers were higher than 200 mg/l. Fortner et al. [20] although they have not demonstrated this, declared that a biliary decompression is indispensible on account of the higher morbidity and mortality in jaundiced patients. In a retrospective study of 88 pancreatectomies for cancer, Gilsdorf and Spanos [23] found a significant difference in morbidity and mortality when the bilirubin titer was higher or lower than 100 mg/l. This same significant difference is found when the lumen of the principal

Table 9.1. Operative morbidity and mortality in patients with and without preoperative biliary decompression (from Denning et al. [17])

Tumor	Drainage			No drainage		
	Number	Morbidity	Death	Number	Morbidity	Death
Benign	3	0	0	6	4	1
Malignant	22	7	4	26	14	7
Resection	3	1	1	6	4	3
Palliation	14	6	3	15	7	3
Biopsy	5	0	0	5	3	1
Total	25	7	4	32	18	8

biliary tract is more or less than 1 cm. Using external percutaneous drainage, Naka-yama et al. [43] noticed a reduction in operative mortality when the drainage is per-formed before surgery (8.2% as opposed to 28.3%). Taking up the work of Hatfield et al. [25], Belghiti et al. [3] thought that preliminary biliary drainage is not justified in principal, as the expected pathophysiological benefits are not always confirmed. Moreover, the improvements in mortality and morbidity are counterbalanced by the real complications of this drainage: 24.2% for Ferrucci et al. [19], 27% for Pollock et al. [46]; the most frequent of these are cholangitis, hemoperitonitis, and choleperi-tonitis. The procedure in itself is not exempt from a certain mortality [44]. Neverthe-less, Belghiti et al. remain advocates of the diversion whenever there is a cholangitis which cannot be controlled by antibiotic therapy.

Actually, the interpretation of results is difficult due to the multiple variables that exist, in particular, the age of the patients. In the patient series reported by Hu-guet et al. [29], it was shown that jaundice has no specific incidence in patients un-der the age of 55. On the other hand, in older patients with a bilirubin titer above 200 mg/l it appeared to be preferable to carry out a biliary decompression.

External biliary drainage, or better still, internal biliary drainage achieved by en-doscopy or the transparietal tract, represents the best solution in this case, although the absence of a laparotomy does not permit a precise workup of the lesion to be done. It is for this reason, and also so as not to delay treatment, that some surgeons prefer a surgical exploration. If the tumor appears to be resectable and curable, they perform a resection either immediately or in two steps, preferably after the biliary diversion (biliary bypass, transtumoral intubation in favorable cases, and some-times a simple cholecystostomy in the meantime). In order to make this choice, it is essential to take into consideration the severity of the jaundice, the patient's general state of health, the extent of the proposed resection, the surgeon's skill in perform-ing the resection [35, 40], and the skill of his personnel (recovery team). The interval between these two interventions is approximately 3 weeks, during which time it can be beneficial to carry out an external radiation program (2500 rads) and/or renutri-tion.

9.3.3 Localization and Stage of Development

The localization of the tumor and its staging has only a small influence upon cura-tive resection techniques. Whether it is situated on the right or left side of the pan-creas, a resectable cancer judged to be curable must be the object of a regional pan-createctomy. This is more frequently possible for a cephalic cancer than for a cancer of the body and tail of the pancreas because the latter are more extensive at the time of intervention. The following pancreatectomies can be performed for all stages ex-cept stage IV and in the absence of general contraindications; a preliminary biliary drainage is also possible:
1. For stage I and II a regional total (or subtotal) pancreatectomy, Fortner's type 0 is appropriate.
2. For stage III a the resection will be distant to the invaded tissues and can entail a subtotal, or better yet, a total gastrectomy and/or partial colectomy.

3. For stage III b vascular resections must be carried out according to the degree of invasion of the vessels (pancreatectomies types I and II a, b, or c).
4. For stage IV the incurability is certain when there are distant metastases (i.e., liver, peritoneum, etc.). Yet, for some authors [10, 36] the presence of an unique hepatic or peritoneal metastasis would not be an absolute contraindication to a curative resection under exceptional conditions (small pancreatic tumor that is easily resectable with only one small and removable metastasis). This attitude is similar to that proposed in certain curable Dukes'-D colorectal cancers. We are more reserved as to the value of resection for stage-IV cancer of the pancreas, and we consider it as a palliative strategy.

In the absence of distant metastases, but in the presence of an invasion of the nodes of the third relay, the problem becomes more delicate, as we are at the borderline between regional and systemic extensions. This stage appears to represent a reasonable barrier to curative resections, which can only be envisaged with prudence and are reserved for young healthy subjects who also present favorable local factors, notably vascular, and who undergo postoperative adjuvant treatments.

Our present knowledge is not sufficient to say if such an undertaking is justified or not. Only prospective studies defining this nodal invasion can permit a well-founded judgement.

9.3.4 Adjuvant Treatments

Do adjuvant treatments now have a place beside surgery within the context of a curative strategy? This is difficult to affirm, even though the efficacity of chemotherapy and radiation therapy is well known today.

In our experience, the only case of survival after 5 years among a total of 81 exocrine pancreatic cancers treated between 1977 and 1984 consisted of a stage III a (two nodes of the second relay were positive and there was duodenal invasion) and was treated as follows: biliary bypass procedure for jaundice, clipping of the tumor, external photoradiation therapy (2000 rads), regional subtotal pancreatoduodenectomy.

Many trials are now underway associating radiation therapy and/or chemotherapy with surgical resection. The initial results are favorable [1]. However, we must wait before judging, as numerous randomized prospective studies linking these techniques are necessary. It is likely that progress will be possible due to their association in curative strategies.

9.4 Palliative Strategies

Palliative strategies must be considered whenever the pretherapeutic workup or the laparotomy shows that the tumor is not resectable, or that it is resectable but not curable. This is usually the case for stage-IV cancers but can also be true for tumors at an earlier stage, theoretically resectable and even curable, but for which an extensive resection is not feasible because of the age or the general state of health of the patient.

9.4.1 Palliative Surgery

A simple laparotomy, followed by the closing of the abdominal wall when the tumor is not removable, must be avoided at all costs, as the postoperative persistence of a major symptom (pain, jaundice, digestive stenosis) is always poorly received on the part of the patient, the family, and the doctor! In our opinion, it is better to abstain from surgery than to do an isolated laparotomy; the importance of a pretherapeutic workup and a search for the criteria of inoperability must be emphasized in order to reduce the number of useless laparotomies [53] still being performed in 3.5%–10% of all cases. It can be of interest to perform palliative surgery in order to relieve the patient once the laparotomy has been done.

We have mentioned what we think of deliberately palliative pancreatectomies which knowingly leave glandular or extraglandular pathological tissue in place. Although their aim is immediate improvement of the symptoms, notably pain, they must be avoided in our opinion. The mortality of these resections is high [24]. The consequences of these interventions are too heavy, as they have virtually no beneficial value in regards to increasing the mean survival time. Actually, we do not have the means today of effectively controlling residual tumor tissue. There is a possibility that in the future the practice of internal intraoperative irradiation or the discovery of new chemotherapeutic techniques will modify this point of view and justify these tumor-reducing operations, as is the case for the cancers of other organs.

When during the course of a laparotomy the surgeon decides not to perform a resection, palliative surgery must be done with the aim of improving the patient's comfort and survival. When a biliary diversion must be performed, our preference is the biliary bypass (choledochoduodenostomy or choledochojejunostomy) with gastroenterostomy. This is especially true when the projected survival time is long. Transtumor intubation does not appear to be a good solution, as there is a risk of obstruction. It should be used only as a last resort and should be reserved for short-term palliation. This technique is not exempt from complications (mortality, cholangitis, pancreatic fistulas, choleperitonitis). It is more appropriate for neoplastic hiliary or pedicular jaundice than for pancreatic cancers [16, 30]. In the case of an isolated digestive diversion or one which is associated with the preceding case, a precolic gastrojejunostomy must be done. More rarely, a pancreaticojejunostomy is decided upon, and occasionally a section or phenolization of the splanchnic nerves. Marking the tumor target with metallic clips is good preparation for possible postoperative radiation therapy [40]. We must remember that the operative mortality of these interventions is not negligible (6% [40, 55] to 30% [18]).

9.4.2 Adjuvant Therapies

Are adjuvant therapies useful in a palliative strategy? This question is difficult to answer with absolute certainty. Yet, as the median survival is influenced by the association of radiation and chemotherapy [8, 37], this must be proposed to the patient and the family. It is not, however, always psychologically acceptable, owing to its palliative character.

Practically speaking, radiation therapy must have a minimal dose of 5000 equivalent rads. It can be external, internal, or a mixture of the two, all at one time or in sequential treatments. As far as chemotherapy is concerned, the most effective protocol (PA102), used at the Institut Gustave Roussy (Paris) in the context of a phase-II trial, combines radiation therapy delivered by a linear accelerator in three series of 2000 rads per series with an alternating treatment of 5-fluorouracil, adriamycin, and mitomycin C (FAM) (Fig. 9.2).

The effects of the treatment must be closely monitored by ultrasound and/or CT scans. Tumor markers can be very useful in this case, as their levels are elevated at the time of diagnosis.

9.5 Inoperable Patients

Inoperability is not very frequent, as it is always difficult to make a decision that will deprive a patient invaded by cancer of the pancreas of his only chance of a cure. The treatment can therefore be palliative only, knowing that the survival rate will not be more than a few weeks, or at best a few months. Only very serious reasons such as age, general state of health, tumor extension (distant metastases), or the refusal of intervention can contraindicate a laparotomy. Without surgical intervention, it is nevertheless possible to treat the principal symptoms (jaundice, malnutrition, pain) in order to relieve the patient and improve his comfort.

9.5.1 Jaundice

Internal biliary drainage is the best solution to the problem of jaundice, whether it is put into place via a transparietal tract or endoscopically. The success rate for placement of the endoprothesis by the above methods (always beginning with endoscopy) is on the order of 90% [16]. Only a complete stenosis of the principal biliary duct prevents it; in this case one must be satisfied with an external transparietal biliary drainage. This is not always a good solution, considering that we must compensate for the losses and deal with the problems brought about by this type of drainage, mainly infection or displacement of the catheter due to body movements. We have already discussed these techniques, which were perfected by the Chiba University School of Medicine and at Lund. It should be kept in mind that transparietal biliary drainage is possible in 94% of cases for the Department of Radiology team at the

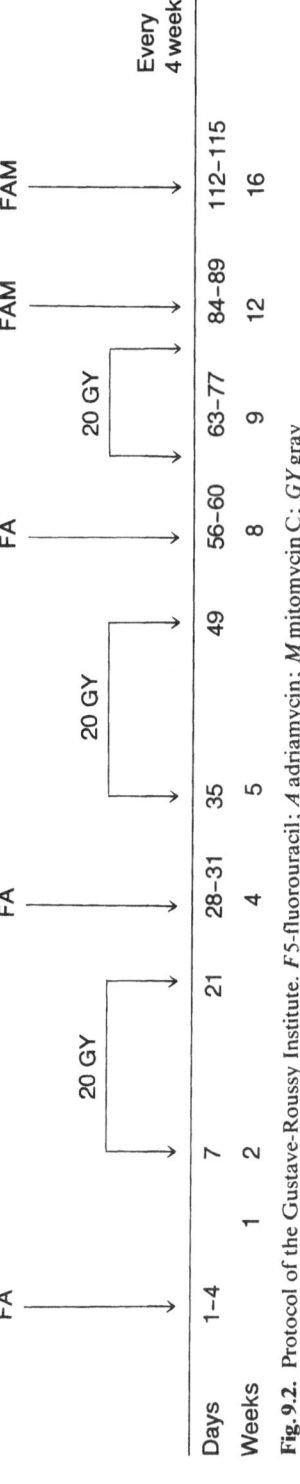

Fig. 9.2. Protocol of the Gustave-Roussy Institute. *F* 5-fluorouracil; *A* adriamycin; *M* mitomycin C; *GY* gray

Harvard School of Medicine (72% internal drainage and 22% external drainage) [19, 42]. The complications of these techniques are not negligible (about 30%) and their mortality is about 6% [41].

9.5.2 Nutrition

Nutrition is of particular importance when a duodenal stenosis is aggravated by anorexia. Two possibilities can serve as nutritional supports in a palliative treatment: parenteral nutrition or feeding by jejunostomy. The inconveniences and limitations of prolonged catheterization usually lead to the second option. The jejunal feeding tube can be put into place *à minima* with the patient under a local anesthetic and allows enteral feeding by means of a constantly outflowing pump (see Chap. 10).

9.5.3 Pain

All analgesic therapeutic resources must be employed in relation to the intensity of the pain (see Chap. 10).

9.5.4 Radiation Therapy and Chemotherapy

Radiation therapy and chemotherapy have no great value for patients judged to be inoperable. These treatments are not very compatible with the general factors of inoperability (age, poor general state of health) and are very inefficient in the case of extensive tumor spread (metastases).

If, as an exception, radiation therapy can be envisaged in some cases after family approval, the protocol used should be similar to that previously described (see Sect. 9.4.2). Tolerance is judged according to digestive and hematological levels. Remember, in the lack of a better treatment, that radiation therapy has an analgesic effect.

In the majority of cases, we must take into account the realistic hope of survival for these patients; whatever the tumor stage, it is useless to submit these patients to the therapeutic constraints of radiation and chemotherapy. Generally, in these cases only jaundice and pain are treated, where possible.

9.6 Conclusion

The principal therapeutic strategies are summarized in Fig. 9.3.

The definition of homogeneous groups of patients is indispensible in the undertaking of prospective studies and controlled therapeutic trials. Useless operations

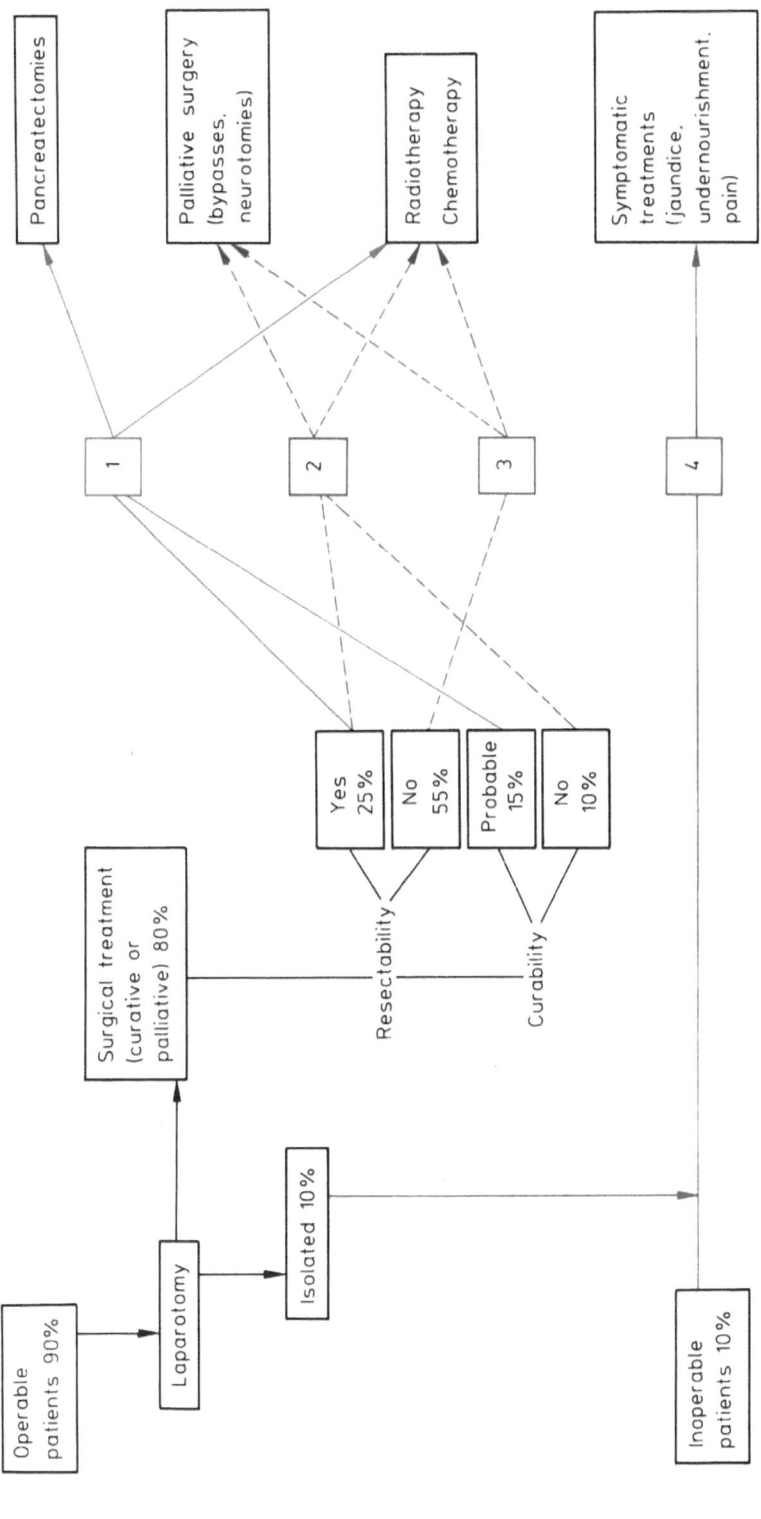

Fig. 9.3. Summary of therapeutic strategies; averages estimated in percent. *1* Curative; *2, 3* palliative; *4* inoperable

(isolated laparotomies, palliative resections) must be avoided through a better appreciation of operability, resectability, and curability.

Exploratory laparotomy, essential and lengthy, must be done with patience, rigor, and discipline in order that the surgeon can choose a well-founded curative or palliative strategy. Curative strategies must, in all cases, consist of extended surgical resections (total pancreatomies with lymph node dissections). Partial pancreatomies should not be emphasized in these strategies. Radiation and chemotherapy play an increasingly important role in both curative and palliative strategies.

The improvement of results in treating cancer of the pancreas depends among other elements, on a very particular methodology. Only very specialized teams and well-trained surgeons are presently capable of meeting these demands.

References

1. American Society of Clinical Oncology (1985) Educational symposium and educational workshop, May 19, p 13
2. Beazley RM (1981) Needle biopsy diagnosis of pancreatic cancer. Cancer 47 (6): 1685–1687
3. Belghiti J (1983) Le drainage biliaire pré-opératoire est-il utile? Gastroenterol Clin Biol 7: 732–734
4. Belghiti J, Menu Y, Nahum H, Fekete F (1984) Apport de l'échotomographie per-opératoire dans la chirurgie des tumeurs du foie. Presse Med 13 (30): 1839–1841
5. Bismuth H, Castaing D, Kunstlinger F (1984) L'échographie per-opératoire en chirurgie hépato-biliaire. Presse Med 13 (30): 1819–1822
6. Boutelier P, Callard P, Champeault G (1984) La cytoponction per-opératoire dans les tumeurs solides du pancréas. In: Chirurgie abdominale et digestive 2. Masson, Paris, p 84 (Actualités Chirurgicales)
7. Braasch JW, Gray BN (1977) Considerations that lower pancreatoduodenectomy mortality. Am J Surg 133: 480–485
8. Brooks DL, Osteen RT, Gray EB, et al (1981) Evaluation of palliative procedures for pancreatic cancer. Am J Surg 141: 430–433
9. Brooks JR, Culebras JM (1976) Cancer of the pancreas: palliative operation, Whipple procedure or total pancreatectomy? Am J Surg 131: 516–520
10. Brunschwig A (1954) cited by Patel J, Patel JC, Leger L (1969) Nouveau traité de technique chirurgicale, vol 12/2. Masson, Paris, p 511
11. Chapuis Y, Place S, Bonnette P (1983) Influence de la rétention biliaire sur la mortalité opératoire dans les cancers ictérigènes du pancréas: étude rétrospective de 111 cas. Med Chir Dig 12 (5): 327–331
12. Child CG, Frey CF (1966) Pancreatico-duodenectomy. Surg Clin North Am 46: 1201
13. Christoffersen P, Poll P (1970) Per-operative pancreas aspiration biopsies. Acta Pathol Microbiol Scand [Suppl] 212: 28
14. Couinaud C (1967) Les pancréatectomies avec curage ganglionnaire. J Chir (Paris) 93: 397–410
15. Collins JJ, Craighead JE, Brooks JR (1966) Rationale for total pancreatectomy for carcinoma of the pancreatic head. N Engl J Med 274 (11): 599–602
16. Cremer M, Adler M, Dunham F, et al (1982) Intubation non opératoire des sténoses néoplasiques des voies biliaires. In: Actualités digestives médico-chirurgicales, 3e series. Masson, Paris, pp 103–111
17. Denning DA, Ellison EC, Carey LC (1981) Pre-operative percutaneous transhepatic biliary decompression lowers operative morbidity in patients with obstructive jaundice. Am J Surg 141: 61–65
18. Doutre LP, Perissat J, Bobois JP, Grenet J (1975) La survie post-opératoire des cancers ictérigènes du pancréas. Chirurgie 101 (11): 836–843

19. Ferrucci JT, Mueller PR, Harbin WP (1980) Percutaneous transhepatic biliary drainage: technique results and application. Radiology 135: 1-13

20. Fortner JG, Kim DK, Cubilla A (1977) Regional pancreatectomy: in bloc pancreatic, portal vein and lymph nodes resection. Ann Surg 186 (1): 42-50

21. Forsgren L, Orel S (1973) Aspiration cytology in carcinoma of the pancreas. Surgery 73: 38

22. Fourtanier G (1984) L'ictère est-il un facteur de gravité? In: Chirurgie abdominale et digestive 2. Masson, Paris, p 3 (Actualités chirurgicales)

23. Gilsdorf RB, Spanos P (1973) Factors influencing morbidity and mortality in pancreatico-duodenectomy. Ann Surg 177 (3): 332-337

24. Grosdidier J (1980) Exérèse contre dérivation dans les cancers ictérigènes du pancréas. In: Chirurgie abdominale et digestive 2. Masson, Paris, p 61 (Actualités chirurgicales)

25. Hatfield ARW, Tobjas R, Terblanche J, et al (1982) Pre-operative external biliary drainage in obstruction jaundice. A prospective controlled clinical tiral. Lancet 2: 896

26. Hermann RE (1979) Manual of surgery of the gallbladder, bile ducts and exocrine pancreas. Springer, Berlin Heidelberg New York

27. Hoffman (cited in [51])

28. Hollender LF, Meyer C, Marrie A, Pierard T, Calderoli H (1980) Le cancer du pancréas. Réflexions à propos de 147 cas. Ann Chir 34: 775-777

29. Huguet C, Tussiot J, Parc R, Loygue J (1981) Faut-il décomprimer les voies biliaires avant d'opérer les ictères par obstruction? Gastroenterol Clin Biol 5 (1): 219 A

30. Huguet C, Hakami R, Bloch P (1981) L'intubation transtumorale des obstructions néoplasiques du hile du foie. Ann Chir 35: 341

31. Issacson R, Weiland LH, McIllrath DC (1974) Biopsy of the pancreas. Arch Surg 109: 227-230

32. Launois B (1984) La chirurgie du pancréas pour cancer. Bordeaux Med 17: 115-118

33. Lightwood R, Reber HA, Way LW (1976) The risk and accuracy of pancreatic biopsy. Am J Surg 132: 189-194

34. Longmire WP, Traverso LW (1981) The Whipple procedure and other standard operative approaches to pancreatic cancer. Cancer 47 (6): 1706-1711

35. Malt RA (1983) Treatment of pancreatic cancer. JAMA 250 (11): 1433-1437

36. Mercadier M, Clot JP, Melliere D, Camplez P (1967) Technique des duodéno-pancréatectomies céphaliques. Ann Chir 21: 11-12, 672-680

37. Monge JJ, Judd ES, Gage RP (1964) Radical pancreatectomy. A 22-year experience with the complications, mortality rate and survival rate. Ann Surg 160 (4): 711-719

38. Moertel CG, Childs DS, Reitemeier RJ, et al (1969) Combined 5-fluoro-uracil and supervoltage radiation therapy of locally unresectable gastro-intestinal cancer. Lancet 2: 865-867

39. Moossa AR (1982) Pancreatic cancer. Approach to diagnosis, selection for surgery and choice of operation. Cancer 50 (11): 2689-2698

40. Moossa AR, Lewis MH, Mackie CR (1979) Surgical treatment of pancreatic cancer. Mayo Clin Proc 54: 468-474

41. Mouiel J (1983) Dérivation ou exérèse dans le cancer pancréatique. Med Chir Dig 12: 475-478

42. Mueller PR, van Sonnenberg E, Ferrucci JT (1982) Percutaneous biliary drainage: technical and catheter related problems in 200 procedures. AJR 138: 17-23

43. Nakayama T, Ikeda A, Okuda K (1978) Percutaneous transhepatic drainage of the biliary tract. Technique and results in 104 cases. Gastroenterology 74: 554-559

44. Norlander A, Kalin B, Sundblad R (1982) Effect of percutaneous transhepatic drainage upon liver function and postoperative mortality. Surg Gynecol Obstet 155: 161

45. Orr TG (1952) cited by Leger et Brehant J (1956) Chirurgie du pancréas. Masson, Paris, p 411

46. Pollock TW, Ring ER, Oleaga JA, et al (1979) Percutaneous decompression of benign and malignant biliary obstruction. Arch Surg 114: 148-151

47. Remine WH, Priestly JT, Judde S, King JN (1970) Total pancreatectomy. Ann Surg 172: 595-604

48. Reuben A, Cotton PB (1978) Operative pancreatic biopsy: a survey of current practice. Ann R Coll Surg Engl 60: 53-57

49. Ross DE (1954) Cancer of the pancreas. A plea for total pancreatectomy. Am J Surg 87: 20-33

50. Solassol C, Joyeux H, Yakoun M, Blanc F, Bories P (1984) La pancréatectomie régionale dans le traitement de l'adénocarcinome du pancréas. A propos de 41 cas. Gastroenterol Clin Biol 8: 17-21

51. Spay G (1981) Problèmes et modalités techniques de l'exérèse pancréatique totale pour adéno-carcinome. Incidences du curage. J Chir (Paris) 118 (3): 161–168
52. Susuki T, Imamuram M, Tamura K, et al (1979) Correlative evaluation of angiography and pan-créato-ductography in relation to surgery for cancer of the pancreas. Surgery 85 (6): 644–651
53. Trede M (1985) The surgical treatment of pancreatic carcinoma. Surgery 97 (1): 28–35
54. Tryka AF, Brooks JR (1979) Histopathology in the evaluation of total pancreatectomy for ductal carcinoma. Ann Surg 190 (3): 373–381
55. Van Heerden JA, Remine WH, Weiland LH, et al (1981) Total pancreatectomy for ductal ade-nocarcinoma of the pancreas. Ann J Surg 142: 308–311
56. Warshaw AL, Richter JM, Podolski DK, et al (1982) A strategy against pancreatic cancer. J Clin Gastroenterol 4: 525–532

10 Intensive Care

F. d'Athis and J. J. Eledjam

Three problems are posed in particular by intensive care in pancreatic cancer:

Immunonutritional deficiency is generally rapid in onset and severe, and is responsible for morbidity and/or mortality. Estimates of its severity must be made, and it must be adjusted efficiently and rapidly by means of pre- and postoperative nutritional support.

Pain is often a presenting symptom of pancreatic cancer. It is congruent with the invasion of the tumor, and is also frequently associated with palliative surgery. When performed immediately following surgery, efficient analgesic treatment can comfort the patient while minimizing the risk of respiratory complications normally associated with upper abdominal surgery.

Organic predisposition is difficult to define. The perioperative risks are likely to be related either to age or to associated cardiovascular, respiratory, or metabolic dysfunction. Surely, when age plays a role, the major risk factor is respiratory insufficiency, which requires attentive preparation *prior to* surgery.

10.1 Nutritional Deficiency and Support

As do other cancers of the digestive tract, cancer of the pancreas leads to a more or less significant malabsorption caused by several factors [16]. They are related to the elevated energy expenditure due to the tumor's energy consumption and/or to metabolic disorders [23]. This malabsorption is responsible for a high complication rate: poor wound healing resulting in the opening of stitches, fistulas [34], and wound infections [1]. The risk of infection is closely related to the cellular immunity always observed with serious malnutrition.

10.1.1 Nutritional Deficiency

The energy reserves split into compartments within the organism. The major source of available energy is in adipose tissue, but other sources may be mobilized in the case of a poor supply or in response to an increase in protein synthesis. In establishing a nutritional profile one must include not only a systemic evaluation, but also an investigation of the adipose tissue and protein compartments.

Body weight gives preliminary information on the nutritional status of the patient. Weight loss can be estimated from the ideal weight worked out from Lorentz's formulas referring to the size in centimeters, or from the patient's usual weight compared with his or her present weight. Whatever the method chosen, the percentage of weight loss or variation will be reckoned. Weight loss of about 10% must be regarded as malabsorption, between 10% and 20% as severe, and more than 20% as serious. The duration of weight loss may be damaging even when the weight variation is 10%.

Total lipids: the adipose tissue compartment must be investigated during the clinical examination by measuring the triceps skin fold. This method allows accurate estimates of the subcutaneous fatty mass, as reported by Simon et al. [45], who performed some ultrasonographic measurements. Any variation of 10% or more must be related to a decrease in the lipid energy reserves. However, errors can be made owing to the increase of proteins in obese patients and the presence of edemas of decubitus.

Total proteins: a modification of the total proteins changes the muscular and visceral proteins. Muscular proteins are estimated either from anthropometric (arm muscle circumference and triceps skin fold), from dynamometric (muscular strength), or from biochemical (creatinine/size index expressed in mg/cm and 3-methyl histidinuria) measurements. This last index is advocated by Forber and Bruining [20] as the most easily used clinically. The only contraindication is renal insufficiency. However, given the daily variation of the urinary volume, a cumulative appraisal over 3 days is required. According to Nixon et al. [36], a titer of less than 8.4 mg/cm/day in men or 4.5 mg/cm/day in women assesses a real loss. The 3-methyl histidine urinary assay over 24 h is more reliable for muscular proteolysis [51]. It consists of a fibrous protein marker giving a good evaluation of protein catabolism, whatever its origin may be [40]. Unfortunately, such a standard assay appears to be difficult.

Visceral proteins fall into two groups. Short half-life proteins such as transferrin, pre-albumin-binding thyroxine, and retinol-binding protein are very sensitive to both malnutrition and nutrition. Their diagnostic value is very dependent upon large individual variations. On the contrary, plasmatic albumin is a protein with a long half-life, less sensitive to malnutrition, whose loss always indicates severe malabsorption [36]. Moreover, some of the variations are due to intravascular transfer factors as well as to the hydration condition.

Inherent immunity: immunologically competent cells can be used as nutritional indicators. The most important immunological impairment refers to the cell-mediated immunological responses. The loss of energy reported during severe malnutrition seems to be linked to an impairment in antibody production due to a reduction of thymus-dependent cells. Chandra [12] showed that in the case of protein-caloric deficiency, the number of T4 helper cells decreases, with only a slight effect on the suppressive cytotoxic T8 cells; the ratio T4/T8 would then be greatly diminished.

The clinical examination consists of multiple cutaneous tests of retarded hypersensitivity which are becoming increasingly simple, standardized, and quantitated. A response is said to be positive when there is induration of more than 10 mm in men or 5 mm in women. The patient is normal when at least two of these tests are positive, hypoergic when only one test is positive, and anergic when all of the tests are negative. Their negativity depends upon the erosion of muscular mass, and especially on the onset of complications due to infection [8]. Along with Belghiti et al. [7] and Rao et al. [39], we think that it is somewhat difficult to establish a relationship between the immune deficiency volume and tumor resectability. In addition to cell-mediated immunological impairment, the complement system, the opsonic function of the plasma, and the "killing" capacity of the segmented neutrophils are all minimized in a state of severe malnutrition.

Nutritional indexes would be of great value in helping to screen high-risk patients. The prognostic nutritional index proposed by Bubzy et al. [11] on the basis of the triceps skin fold, albuminemia, transferrin, and delayed hypersensitivity skin tests, seems to be quite sensitive but also requires calculation of the algebraic sum of variation coefficients and comparison of the results with the threshold values. This complexity limits its clinical application. In a more recent study of patients who had undergone major visceral surgery, Di Constanzo et al. [17] tried to define a simpler multifactorial nutritional index. Unfortunately, this index only includes three discriminative variables and thus results in a 50% predictive value. This is not enough, due partly to other factors that make up the preoperative risk and that are not taken into account. Baker et al. [3] conclude that only simple parameters such as percentage of weight loss (greater than 30 g/l) and clinical examination are to be considered in the screening for high-risk patients. In any case, preoperative malnutrition does not necessarily contraindicate surgery, but requires administration of nutriments to correct the postoperative risk for these patients to the level of others.

10.1.2 Nutritional Support

Nutritional support must be continued after surgery to avoid protein catabolism and, in patients presenting malabsorption, to restore the muscular mass and the energy reserves. There are three important factors: the duration of preoperative nutrition, the level of nitrogen-caloric intake, and the intake components.

10.1.2.1 Duration of Preoperative Nutrition

In order to be effective, preoperative nutrition must last 7–10 days. Mullen et al. [33] showed that a 7-day duration would statistically minimize complications in high-risk patients. On the other hand, a 3-day duration appears to be inefficient. It permits only repair of the electrolytic and albumin blood deficits, and avoids the hemodynamic risk at the induction of anesthesia. Jaundiced patients present quite a different pattern. In their case, the preoperative delay must be as short as possible, aiming to correct a hemostasis deficiency as well as a renal function insufficiency. The ideal response would be to perform a biliary drainage (whatever the method), and then to adjust the nutritional deficit before proceeding with surgery (see Chap. 9).

10.1.2.2 Level of Nitrogen-Caloric Intake

The nitrogen-caloric intake level has to be a function of the energy deficits. This level can be calculated from Harris and Benedict's formula. A more rational approach is given by calorimetry. Though direct calorimetry is the method of reference, indirect calorimetry is more adapted to clinical practice [29]. It is of great value for three reasons: to measure the energy deficit, to determine the optimal intake, and to study the metabolic usage of the substrates during nutritional assistance. For a long time now, the level of the energy deficit has been overestimated, leading to hyperalimentation which causes major metabolic complications. Through direct calorimetry on 200 cancer patients, Knox et al. [28] determined three groups according to the metabolic level. Half of the patients were normometabolic and the other half fell into the hypo- and hypermetabolic categories. Neither age, nor tumor extent, nor nutritional status was correlated to the energy level, but rather to the clinical duration of the disease. Under these conditions, it seems difficult, if not impossible, to determine this metabolic level. These failures have led to many discussions about the dubious necessity of preoperative nutritional support [6]. With these means, it has been demonstrated that the energy deficit of undernourished patients was 1.25–1.50 times the energy metabolism at rest. At the optimal intake, reserves are restored and maintained without inducing any metabolic complication. Any additional intake tends to increase the deficits and diminish the output.

10.1.2.3 Intake Components

Regimens consisting exclusively of glucides must be avoided in undernourished patients. When used as the essential energy source, glucides can induce respiratory complications by increasing the respiratory quotient with no remarkable effect on malnutrition. Nitrogen regimens, proposed by Blackburn et al. [9], with or without lipids, are of value only in patients with no malabsorption syndrome who have oral alimentation. Other undernourished patients must be given total parenteral alimentation before undergoing surgery. Lipids must represent at least 30% of the energy intake [2] in order to allow direct oxidation of the carbohydrates and avoid any fat storage [24]. The most common lipid emulsion in use contains soya oil and egg-yolk lecithin. When this is well tolerated, it provides a sufficient supply of essential fatty acids. Management should be directed towards medium-chain fatty acids, which seem to have more effective results [15]. The nitrogen intake is obtained from amino acids. The mean need ranges between 0.20 and 0.30 g nitrogen/kg/day. Augmentation with branched-chain or essential amino acids does not seem to increase the nitrogen reserve. Thus, a protocol suggested for this kind of patient is 30–40 glycolipid Kcal/kg/day. This level is reached progressively in the case of serious malnutrition and is increased in the case of complications. The intake must be correlated to an optimal 150–200 Kcal/g nitrogen ratio. The fluid and electrolyte intakes are estimated daily, taking the metabolic fitness, adjuvant treatments, and biochemical data into account. Additional potassium and phosphate intakes are frequently necessary at the onset of renutrition. The vitamin and trace element needs are significant for patients presenting malabsorption, since any loss can lead to complications or be responsible for the lack of modulation of the immune response [13].

10.1.2.4 Appraisal of Nutritional Support

Efficacy can be estimated from the weight gain; this can appear to be rapid at the beginning, and is linked to the water- and salt-adjusted deficit. In any case it must be correlated to the anthropomorphic data and the biochemical markers as well. The nitrogen workup gives a good estimation of therapeutic efficiency, but due to the daily variation, a cumulative appraisal is necessary. Since a complete preoperative correction of the immunonutritional failure cannot even be contemplated, surgery can be performed only on patients in whom the best balance has been reached.

10.1.2.5 Route of Administration

Nutritional support is usually administered parenterally through a deep vein, but this exposes the patient to mechanical complications and infections [44]. Thus, it is often replaced with continuous enteral nutrition postoperatively, via a nasojejunal probe or a jejunostomy placed during surgery. The nitrogen reserve is equal to the caloric protein intake obtained by parenteral administration. However, it is preferable to use monomeric or polymeric regimens which are better tolerated by the digestive tract [19]. Enteral supply can start as early as 24 or 48 h after the operation. At first it is administered along with parenteral nutrition, which is progressively reduced. In addition to careful monitoring for complications, enteral supply requires constant control just as parenteral supply does.

10.1.2.6 Glucide Balance

In case of pre-existing diabetes, insulin supply is required. After surgery, glycemic imbalance depends upon the extent of the resection. In the case of total pancreatectomies, the balance is usually attained with low doses of insulin. The main risk is an insulin overdose leading to hypoglycemia, increased by the lack of glucagon-like proteins. Partial pancreatectomies can affect the glycoregulation, can be followed by a simple glucidic intolerance, or can even induce a real diabetes free of insulin-dependence characteristics, as happens after total pancreatectomies. Immediately after surgery, administration of insulin with the glucidic supply avoids the uncontrolled glycemic fits. As soon as the process of alimentation is in order, diet alone or associated with oral medication (sulfonamides, biguanides) is sometimes sufficient.

But the increased glycocaloric requirement frequently results in glycemic imbalance, and the lack of weight gain requires a substitutive insulin therapy after a longer period of time.

10.2 Pain

Pain is found in two different situations. The immediate need of patients suffering from prolonged or chronic pain, secondary to an invasive cancer which is beyond all forms of surgical intervention, is analgesia. Postoperative pain requires short-term relief to insure patients' comfort, rapid mobilization, and early respiratory physiotherapy.

10.2.1 Chronic Pain

Chronic pain is linked to an invasion or to the compression of the celiac plexus or its neighboring structures; it consists of deep pain with frequent crises requiring immediate attention. Such pains very quickly influence the patient's language and affect physical activity, general well-being, and sleep. The possible therapeutic responses can be either surgical (see Chap. 7) or medicinal. Whatever the method used, the only goal is to ensure the patient's comfort with respect to his foreseeable survival.

10.2.1.1 Peripheral Analgesics

Peripheral analgesics inhibit prostaglandin synthesis. They are often ineffective, which means the dosage must be increased or they must be combined with other therapies such as steroids or psychotropic drugs. Steroids are of interest not only for their anti-inflammatory and antiedemic properties, but also for their effect upon the psyche and energy. The use of delta nonfluorinated derivatives is recommended, except for cortisone and hydrocortisone. This is to avoid a mineral-corticoid effect, muscular atrophy, and hypophyseal and adrenal slowdown.

10.2.1.2 Narcotic Drugs

The failure of peripheral analgesics has caused therapists to turn to narcotics. The chief aims are analgesia which translates itself into a higher pain threshold, inhibition of the pain message, and an overall reduction in the degree of pain. Morphine is chosen because of its powerful and long-lasting effect. Powerful but short-acting narcotics are reserved for intraoperative use. They can also be used at the terminal stage of the disease but require frequent injections or infusions. For ambulatory patients morphine is preferred, as it remains the best narcotic for controlling intractable pain.

The way of administering the drug is an important consideration. Direct administration by contact with medullary and encephalic receptors permits smaller doses, increases the duration of the effect, and limits the number of injections. The peridural route, very useful for postoperative analgesia, is rarely used. A tunneled catheter must be placed surgically to avoid any risk of infection. Morphine is given either in repeated doses or by a continuous pump, external or implanted, depending upon the estimated survival, as proposed by Stoyanov et al. [46]. The average dose of morphine used by these authors for effective analgesia is 6-9 mg/24 h. Ventricular administration, described by Roquefeuil et al. [41], was first proposed for a late-stage cancer of the pancreas. It required a ventricular cannula put into place in a neurosurgical environment, with the patient under premedication and local anesthesia. The morphine is either injected into a reservoir implanted under the skin or autoadministered from a bag. This is a very effective technique but is reserved for terminal neoplastic pain.

10.2.1.3 The Lytic Celiac-Plexus Block

This technique was described by Kappis in 1919 [26]. It accurately interrupts the pain originating in the pancreas. This has been confirmed by Bridenbaugh et al. [10] and Gorbitz and Leavens [21]. The percutaneous posterior approach blocks the afferent nerves of the solar plexus, with no direct effect, and therefore it can only be done surgically. This is the technique described by Moore et al. [31]. With the patient in a prone position and slightly sedated, the puncture is made with a 20-gauge needle, 7 cm, from one side of the processus spinalis L1 to the other. The needle, at a 45° angle and with a brightness amplifier, searches for the bony contact. When it touches the bone, the needle is advanced 1.5-2 cm in order to bypass the vertebral body. The position of the needle can be controlled with a radiopaque index. Usually, the solution injected is 45% alcohol (50 ml). The quality of analgesia is unequal, indicating either an increased dose (but high doses must be avoided because of the risk of toxicity) or the use of opiates. In a series of 20 celiac blocks, Moore et al. [31] obtained a level of 95% effectiveness within 72 h. For 33 patients, 58% of whom had cancer of the pancreas, Batier et al. [5] had 75% good results, but in 25% of the cases deep pain persisted to the extent that it was necessary to return the patient to morphine therapy. The complications linked to this technique are varied. Postural hypotension by an extended sympathetic block required the supine position for a 24-h period. Puncture of the major vessels has no serious repercussions. The presence of lumbar pain and myalgia for 48 h involves the use of heavy doses of analgesics for the first few hours. Therefore, the celiac block is an effective approach to severe pain originating in the pancreas. Even considering the difficulty of performing this technique, it should be done without delay if other methods have failed.

10.2.2 Postoperative Pain

Pancreatic surgery induces nociceptive stimulations originating in neuroendocrine reactions that are responsible for metabolic and clinical changes. The changes that have been shown in ventilatory dynamics [22] are linked to different causes (diaphragmatic dysfunction, suppression of physiological sighs) and are increased by pain. In effect, this limits the cough mechanism and causes respiratory difficulties. Though it has been shown [27] that neuroendocrine reactions are reduced by heavy doses of intraoperative narcotics and/or by locoregional anesthesia, stress-free anesthesia is restricted to the operation time and does not cover the postoperative period. Pain following major visceral surgery is constant and noxious. It is recognized during the patient interview from both clinical and behavioral signs. Its evaluation is difficult, however, owing to the lack of objective methods and the existence of possible modulating factors: ethnic, cultural, age, and sex. Postoperative analgesia can be given parenterally, peridurally, or by a staged intercostal nerve block.

10.2.2.1 Parenteral Analgesia

Morphine hydrochlorate is the reference product due to its powerful and long-lasting effect. A dose of 0.1 mg/kg produces effective analgesia for 4–6 h. The minimum required dose can be calculated by fractional intravenous injections, under clinical supervision, until relief is obtained. This appears to be the safest method while responding to the needs of the patient [38]. Other morphine-like drugs can also be used. The most interesting are fentanyl citrate, alfentanil, and lofentanil; they are powerful but of short duration, requiring continuous administration [35]. Buprenorphine and nalbuphine hydrochlorate have actions similar to morphine; their antagonistic properties diminish the risk of respiratory depression inherent in narcotic drug usage. Different parenteral techniques are possible: analgesia on request implies recurring pain, but this can be underestimated by the prescriber or overestimated by the patient. Systematic prescriptions, taking into account the pharmacokinetics of the narcotic used, must be adapted to the pain level. This can lead to insufficient treatment or to excessive therapy. Autoadministration is the ideal method [47]; it does not bring about overuse and appears to be well adapted to the level of pain. However, the patient must be well informed and cooperative and must enjoy the confidence of the referring surgeon, and sophisticated equipment should be used.

10.2.2.2 Peridural Analgesia

At present, peridural analgesia is the most popular. It can be achieved either with local anesthetics or with morphinic drugs. The placing of the catheter, possible in patients taking anticoagulants, must be done in a surgical environment. The catheter is isolated by an occlusive dressing and the injections are given aseptically by the medical staff.

Long-lasting local anesthetics can be used. Administration is either by repeated injections every 4–6 h or by infusion. A sympathetic block requires hemodynamic supervision and can aggravate a pre-existing hypovolemia.

Peridural administration of a narcotic drug – more frequent than the subarachnoid approach, which requires repeated punctures – produces a more effective analgesia than that obtained with local anesthetics. For about 18 h of analgesia the dose of morphine must be 0.05 mg/kg. Nevertheless, an installation delay of 60 min requires that analgesia be started in the recovery room after surgery. Other opiates can be used, but only lofentanyl and buprenorphine have a duration comparable to that of morphine. The risk of late respiratory depression necessitates a prolonged period of supervision, even when minimal doses are used and no concomitant parenteral morphine injections are given. However, a weak and continuous parenteral dose of naloxone in association does not change the analgesic quality and does reduce the risk of a respiratory depression. This analgesia is carried out for 48–72 h.

10.2.2.3 Intercostal Nerve Block

Intercostal nerve blocks must be bilateral and layered. They require long-lasting local anesthetics, often in large quantities, carrying the risk of an overdose. The average duration of analgesia is 12 h, and therefore repeated injections are required. The effect it can have on ventilation contraindicates this technique for patients suffering from chronic respiratory insufficiency.

10.3 Organic Predisposition

10.3.1 Age

Age increases the intraoperative mortality risk in that it reduces the body's capacity to adapt to different organic functions. According to Cogbill [14], in major abdominal surgery – other than in all associated pathologies – the mortality changes from 1% for subjects under 65 years to 14% for patients over 65. The intraoperative cardiovascular risk increases with age; it is very slight for patients under 70 but becomes very significant thereafter. Age also brings about a progressive reduction of the expiratory capacity and flow [32], and a reduction in the cough reactivity [37]. All of these factors tend, even more than an already existing respiratory pathology, to increase the perioperative risk of complications.

10.3.2 Respiratory Function

Abdominal surgery brings about quasi-inevitable failures in respiratory function, even in otherwise healthy patients. These failures, bearing on time capacity and forced expiratory volume appear as important as the height of the resection. The nature of the incision, median, vertical, or transverse, is blamed for the reduction of the ventilatory parameters and for the occurrence of postoperative complications. Overall, the results are in favor of transverse incisions [48], though this is contested [49, 50]. The effect on the respiratory system of upper abdominal surgery requires a systematic and rigorous preoperative attempt to detect high-risk patients. The practice, at the patient's bedside, of apnea duration and simple spirometry (total volume and forced expiratory volume) permits selection of patients who must undergo a complete functional respiratory exploration and blood gas measurements. High-risk patients must undergo an average of 7 days' preoperative preparation, preferably using the incitive spirometric technique described by Bartlett et al. [4]. The ideal is a respiratory apprenticeship for all patients, which would allow immediate and active postoperative physiotherapy. Besides patient preparation, can the technical choice of anesthesia influence postoperative respiratory function? This type of surgery requires good muscular relaxation and neurovegetative protection. General anesthesia is most frequently chosen to achieve the above requirements, because a T-4 level is necessary with regional anesthesia. This can be done by placing a thoracic catheter in T-10 and using a mixture of 0.5% bupivacaine and 1% etidocaine with epinephrine. This technique produces good relaxation with no noticeable hemodynamic effect and with neurovegetative protection superior to that obtained with neuroleptanalgesia [18]. However, it is necessary to use tracheal intubation with artificial ventilation under light anesthesia in order to minimize the risks of intraoperative alveolar hypoventilation. If the superiority of this technique is not evident for patients suffering from chronic respiratory insufficiency, it nevertheless permits – without the use of opiates and muscle relaxants – long-term intervention with rapid recovery, early extubation, and immediate postoperative peridural analgesia.

References

1. Apelgren KN, Rombeau JC, Miller RA, Waters LN, Carson SN, Twomey P (1981) Malnutrition in veterans administration surgical patients. Arch Surg 116: 1059-1061
2. Askanazi J, Carpentier YA, Elwyn DH (1980) Influence of total parenteral nutrition on fuel utilization in injury and sepsis. Ann Surg 191: 40-46
3. Baker JP, Detsky AS, Wesson DE (1982) Nutritional assessment, a comparison of clinical judgement and objective measurement. N Engl J Med 306: 969-972
4. Bartlett RH, Brennan M, Gazzanniga AB, Hanson EL (1973) Studies of the pathogenesis and prevention of postoperative pulmonary complications. Surg Gynecol Obstet 137: 925-933
5. Batier C, Roquefeuil B, Blanchet P (1985) Le bloc solaire (coeliaque) dans les algies néoplasiques rebelles de l'étage digestif sous diaphragmatique. Cah Anesthesiol 33: 31-34
6. Belghiti J, Langonnet F, Wessely JY, Fekete F (1981) Faut-il corriger la dénutrition des malades ayant un cancer de l'oesophage ou du cardia en période pré-opératoire? Nouv Presse Med 10: 2273-2279
7. Belghiti J, Langonnet F, Bourtyn E, Fekete F (1983) Surgical implications of malnutrition and immunodeficiency in patients with carcinoma of the oesophagus. Br J Surg 70: 334-341
8. Bistrian BR, Sherman M, Blackburn GL, Marshall R, Shaw C (1977) Cellular immunity in adult marasmus. Arch Intern Med 137: 1408-1411
9. Blackburn GL, Flatt JP, Clowes GH, O'Donnel TE (1973) Peripheral intravenous feeding with isotonic amino acid solutions. Am J Surg 125: 447-454

10. Bridenbaugh LD, Moore DC, Campbell DD (1964) Management of upper abdominal cancer pain. JAMA 190: 877-882
11. Bubzy GP, Mullen JL, Mattews DC (1980) Prognostic nutritional index in gastrointestinal surgery. Am J Surg 139: 160-167
12. Chandra RK (1983) Numerical and functional deficiency in T helper cells in protein energy malnutrition. Clin Exp Immunol 51: 126-131
13. Chandra RK (1985) Nutrition et immunité: bases théoriques et applications pratiques. Immun Med 8: 13-17
14. Cogbill CL (1967) Operation in the aged. Mortality to concurrent disease, duration of anesthesia and elective emergency operation. Arch Surg 94: 202-205
15. Denisson A, Ball M, Crowe P, Watkins R, Hands L, White K, Grant A, Kettlewell (1984) A comparative trial of medium- and long-chain triglycerides during parenteral nutrition. 6th Congress of the European Society of Parenteral and Enteral Nutrition, Milan
16. Dewis WD (1977) Anorexia in cancer patients. Cancer Res 37: 2354-2358
17. Di Costanzo J, Martin J, Cano N, Cros RC, Sastre B, Noirclerc M, Pelissier G (1983) Prognostic nutritional index in gastrointestinal surgery. Gastroenterol Clin Biol 7: 851-856
18. Eledjam JJ, Bonnafoux J, Pougnon I, Poupard P, Deslandes JC, Vidal J, D'Athis F (1985) Metabolic and endocrine response during abdominal surgery performed under general anesthesia or extradural analgesia. 4th International Meeting of the European Society of Regional Anaesthesia, Rome
19. Fairfull-Smith RJ, Freeman JB (1980) Immediate postoperative enteral nutrition with a nonelemental diet. J Surg Res 29: 236-239
20. Forber GR, Bruining GJ (1976) Urinary creatinine excretion and lean body mass. Am J Clin Nutr 29: 1359-1366
21. Gorbitz C, Leavens ME (1971) Alcohol block of the coeliac plexus for contral of upper abdominal pain caused by cancer and pancreatitis. J Neurosurg 34: 575-581
22. Graig DB (1981) Postoperative recovery of pulmonary function. Anesth Analg 60: 46, 57
23. Harvey KB, Bothe A, Blackburn GL (1979) Nutritional assessment and patient outcome during oncological therapy. Cancer 43: 2063-2069
24. Horton ES (1983) An overview of the assessment and regulation of energy balance in humans. Am J Clin Nutr 38: 972-977
25. Howat DDC (1971) Cardiac disease, anaesthesia and operation of the cardiac patient. Br J Anaesth 43: 488-490
26. Kappis M (1919) Sensibilität und lokale Anästhesie im chirurgischen Gebiet der Bauchhöhle mit besonderer Berücksichtigung der Splanchnicusanästhesie. Beitr Klin Chir 115: 161-175
27. Kehlet H (1979) Stress-free anesthesia and surgery. Acta Anaesthesiol Scand 23: 503-506
28. Knox LS, Crosby LO, Fleurer ID, Bubzy GP, Miller CL, Mullen JL (1983) Energy expenditure in malnourished cancer patients. Ann Surg 197: 152-162
29. Lerebours E, Denis P (1984) La calorimétrie indirecte: application à l'assistance nutritionnelle en pathologie digestive. Gastroenterol Clin Biol 8: 595-598
30. MacFie J, Holmfield JHM, King RFG, Hill GL (1983) Effect of the energy source on changes in energy expenditure and respiratory quotient during total parenteral nutrition. J Parenter Enterol Nutr 7: 1-5
31. Moore DC, Bush WH, Burnett LL (1960) Celiac plexus block: a roentgenographic, anatomic study of technique and spread of solution in patients and corpses. Anesth Analg 160: 369-379
32. Morris JF, Koski A, Johnson LC (1971) Spirometric standards for healthy nonsmoking adults. Am Rev Respir Dis 103: 57
33. Mullen JL, Bubzy GP, Mattews DC, Smale BF, Rosato EF (1980) Reduction of operative morbidity and mortality by combined preoperative and postoperative nutritional support. Ann Surg 192: 604-613
34. Mullen JL (1981) Consequence of malnutrition in the surgical patients. Surg Clin North Am 61: 465-487
35. Nimmo WS, Todd JG (1985) Fentanyl by constant-rate i. v. infusion for postoperative analgesia. Br J Anaesth 57: 250-254
36. Nixon DW, Heymsfield JB, Cohen AE, Kutner MH, Ansley J, Cawson DH, Rudman D (1980) Protein-calorie undernutrition in hospitalized cancer patients. Am J Med 68: 683-690
37. Petterson DD, Pack AI, Silage DA, Fishman AP (1981) Effect of aging on ventilatory and occlusion pressure responses to hypoxia and hypercapnia. Am Rev Respir Dis 124: 387-391

38. Pflug AE, Bonica JJ (1977) Physiopathology and control of postoperative pain. Arch Surg 112: 773-781
39. Rao B, Wanebo HJ, Pinsky C, Stearn M, Dettgen MF (1977) Delayed hypersensitivity reactions in patients with carcinoma of the colon and rectum. Surg Gynecol Obstet 144: 677-681
40. Rodier M, Richard JL, Bringer J, Cavalier G, Mirouze J (1984) Thyroid status and muscle-protein breakdown as assessed by urinary 3-methylhistidine excretion. Metabolism 33: 97-100
41. Roquefeuil B, Benezech J, Batier C (1985) Intérêt de l'analgésie morphinique par voie ventriculaire dans les algies rebelles néoplasiques. In: Simon L, Roquefeuil B, Pelissier J (eds) La douleur chronique, vol 1. Masson, Paris, pp 212-219
42. Rowlands BJ, Giddings AEB, Johnston AOB (1977) Nitrogen sparing effect of different feeding regimes in patients after operation. Br J Anaesth 49: 781-787
43. Rutten P, Blackburn GL, Flatt JP (1975) Determination of optimal hyperalimentation infusion rate. J Surg Res 18: 447-483
44. Ryan JA, Abel RM, Abott WM (1976) Catheter complications in total parenteral nutrition. A prospective study of 200 consecutive patients. N Engl J Med 290: 1037-1040
45. Simon C, Durckel J, Vignon F, Schlienger JL, Walter J (1985) Evaluation du tissu sous cutané par la mesure de l'épaisseur des plis cutanés et par la mesure échographique. Presse Med 14: 696
46. Stoyanov M, Muller H, Hempelmann G (1985) Application morphinique péridurale continue au moyen d'une pompe. In: La douleur chronique, vol 1. Masson, Paris, pp 201-206
47. Tamsen A, Sakuoara T, Walhstrom A, Terenius L, Harivig P (1982) Postoperative demand for analgesics in relation to individual levels of endorphine and substance P in cerebrospinal fluid. Pain 13: 171-183
48. Vaughan RW, Wise L (1975) Choice of abdominal operative incision in the obese patient: a study using blood gas measurements. Ann Surg 181: 829-835
49. Wightman JA (1968) A prospective survey of the incidence of postoperative pulmonary complications. Br J Surg 55: 85-91
50. William CD, Brenowitz JB (1975) Ventilatory patterns after vertical and transverse upper abdominal incisions. Am J Surg 130: 725-728
51. Young VR, Munro HN (1978) 3-MH and muscle-protein turnover: an overview. Fed Proc 37: 2291-2300

11 Treated Patients

B.Deixonne

11.1 Prognostic Factors

As for all other cancers, but especially in the case of adenocarcinoma of the pancreas, it is necessary to determine the prognostic factors, given the poor therapeutic results. The factors which play a role in the patient's survival fall into three categories: general, oncological, and therapeutic. As far as we know, the epidemiological factors have not been clearly determined, except perhaps for the sex ratio - the median survival rate for unresectable pancreatic cancer appears to be higher for men than for women (4.5 versus 3.5 months) [8].

11.1.1 General Factors

11.1.1.1 Age

Cancer of the pancreas occurs more frequently in people over 60 years of age, with a mean age of 67.6 ± 1.8 for men and 71.5 ± 2.5 for women, yet age does not seem to represent a real factor in the prognosis. In two series of patients (younger than 65 in the first and older than 65 in the second) who had undergone surgical resection, we find somewhat identical percentages of complications and postoperative mortality; at least there is no statistically significant difference [10]. The results from an adjusted survival curve are in the same range, at least for patients younger than 55, between 55 and 74, and older than 74 years, based on findings reported in the tumor register for the Cote d'Or region of France (Fig. 11.1) [8].

11.1.1.2 Nutritional Status

Malnutrition is frequently a presenting symptom in digestive diseases, but has no univocal cause and is partly responsible for a depression of the immune system. To Belghitti [3], malabsorption and immunodeficiency are simply symptoms linked to the evolution of a pathological process which in itself is the chief factor in the prognostic pattern.

Nutritional status can be estimated from various signs. Weight loss compared with the ideal or previous weight helps to rapidly and easily determine the percent-

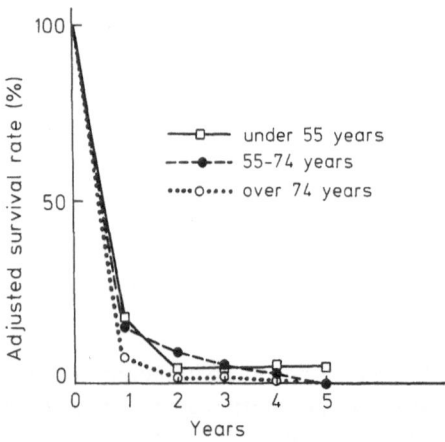

Fig. 11.1. Age-adjusted survival curve for pancreatic cancer (from Faivre et al. [8])

age of variation. Time must be taken into account, for the rapidity of the loss is a significant element, and for us, an assessment of bad prognosis. Total protein in the muscular mass, the state of the visceral proteins, and the immunological assays must be considered, since their value is significant.

On the basis of these various nutritional parameters, a large number of authors have proposed a nutritional prognostic index which would divide patients into high-, mean-, or low-risk groups [4, 6, 17]. They believe that mortality and morbidity are more significant for high-risk patients. Yet such a determination is quite difficult, and hence not very commonly used. Baker et al. [1] have suggested that only simple parameters be considered, such as the degree of weight loss (greater than 10%), the serum albumin rate (less than 30 g/l), and the clinical examination, which are helpful in screening high-risk patients.

Preoperative renutrition seems to benefit these patients. According to Mullen et al., it should be continued for more than 7 days, as a 3-day trial is ineffective [16]. Di Constanzo et al. believe it is necessary to add a treatment for a possible woundinfection, as the standardization of each of these factors is not theoretically feasible on a separate basis [6].

11.1.1.3 Jaundice

Jaundice represents an operative risk factor, as its severity can affect diverse functions (renal, immunological, wound healing). This factor is related to age and the bilirubin titer (see above). In a study on the factors of operative risk, Gilsdorf and Spanos report a significant difference in mortality and morbidity for patients with or without clinical presentation of jaundice, with a main bile duct caliber greater or smaller than 1 cm, and with a prothrombin time of more or less than 15 s [10].

11.1.1.4 Patient Fitness

Reviewing the study of Gilsdorf and Spanos, we note that they report alcoholism and associated cardiopathy as factors of operative prognosis [10]. The cardiovascular risk can be estimated according to the multifactorial protocol defined by Goldmann et al., the accuracy of which is greater than that of the ASA classification [11]. The operative prognosis is also linked to the onset of respiratory complications whose frequency increases relative to the pre-existing pathology. A diaphragmatic dysfunction is usually the cause [9], the type of the incision having little effect in the end.

The question could be raised of whether diabetes and endocrine pancreatic dysfunction are factors of prognosis. We could not find any relationship in our experience.

11.1.2 Oncological Factors

11.1.2.1 Histological Features

Exocrine pancreatic cancers are ductal and acinous carcinomas, cancers of uncertain histogenesis, and sarcomas. The first represent 90%-95% of the whole, and, whatever the histological feature might be within each group, the prognosis is equally poor. However, there are two exceptions: the first is the mucinous cystadenocarcinoma, with a 5-year survival rate of 68% reported by Hodgkinson et al. [13]. This is striking compared with other pancreatic cancers. However, this type occurs very rarely, having a frequency of about 1%. The second is the cystic papillary carcinoma, belonging to the group of cancers of uncertain histogenesis. Its evolution appears to be nonmalignant, since only two metastatic disseminations have been found among the 60 or so cases reported (cf. chap. 2.2.1.3).

11.1.2.2 Site and Size of Tumor

Cephalic localizations are the most frequent and have the best prognoses. According to Cubilla et al., the actuarial 1-year survival, whatever the treatment, is 17% for cancers of the head of the pancreas and only 1% for the cancers of the body and tail of the pancreas [5]. In the Cote d'Or region of France the findings are more or less the same; the adjusted survival rate at 3 years is 3% for cancers of the head and 0% for cancers of the body of the pancreas. There is no specification concerning cancers of the tail of the pancreas [8] and invasion of the uncinate process has never been reported. This localization should theoretically have the worse prognostic value, however, because of the contiguous mesentericoportal axis and the absence of nodal relays I and II.

Tumor size also represents a factor of prognosis for Cubilla et al. In their series, tumors smaller than 3 cm mean a median survival of 12 months, tumors ranging from 3 to 5 cm of 5 months, and tumors larger than 5 cm only 1 month [5]. On the other hand, Gilsdorf and Spanos found no significant difference in the operative risk for tumors larger or smaller than 4 cm [10].

Finally, if we compare the median survival as a function of both tumor size and localization, as Cubilla et al. did, the best prognosis would be for small tumors of the head of the pancreas. They consider that, even when small, tumors of the tail of the pancreas have a very bad prognosis [5].

11.1.2.3 Staging

In this pattern, the prognostic factors are the same as those for tumor size and localization. The larger a tumor is, the greater the risk of invasion to the adjacent organs and lymph nodes. It is normal in oncology to say that the prognosis worsens with the stage of development. This is demonstrated by the adjusted survival curve in the register of the Cote d'Or regarding localized tumors with regional involvement or distant metastases (Fig. 11.2) [8].

While in the case of metastases we can assess the prognosis as a function of the regional invasion, this is more difficult regarding nodal involvement or invasion to the mesenteric vessels. Present classifications do not distinguish between invasion to the various lymph node groups; not one statistical study compares the survival curves as a function of the nodal groups invaded. The prognosis is indeed damaged by a nodal involvement, but one can give different prognostic values to an invasion of nodal relays I and II, to that of retroperitoneal relay III located on the main lymph collecting vessels proximal to the thoracic duct. Only a prospective study taking into account the lymph drainage of the pancreas will reveal whether this distinction is an ancillary help in prognosis.

Invasion to the mesenteric vessels is also serious. The venous axis can rapidly become invaded by the malignant process and some buds can be seen in the vascular lumen, even causing an obstruction. The arterial wall is more resistant; however, when there is an invasion of a lymph network in the adventitis the prognosis is worsened. As far as we know, only one 5-year survival has been reported after regional pancreatectomy with vascular resection [19].

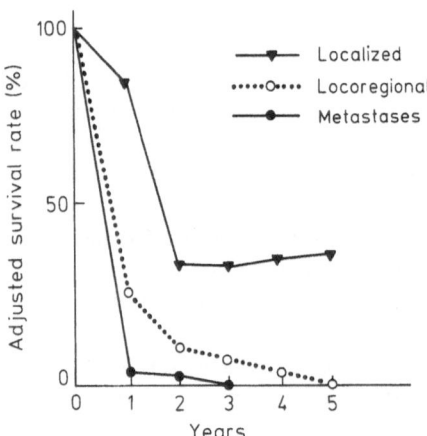

Fig. 11.2. Adjusted survival according to stage of pancreatic cancer (from Faivre et al. [8])

11.1.2.4 Tumor Markers

There are no reports of a formal correlation between the CEA or CA-19-9 rates and the prognosis of pancreatic cancer, especially when the serum rate is low. After performing a surgical resection, Barkin et al. did not find any relationship between the CEA rate and survival [2]. However, the marker rates are elevated when there is a voluminous tumor mass or a cancer with hepatic metastases. Under these conditions, it is probable that a correlation will be established in the future.

11.1.3 Therapeutic Factors

11.1.3.1 Therapeutic Management

We will not review everything covered in the chapter on treatment. We would just like to stress that only resections lead to 5-year survivals, and that without any treatment, except symptomatic, the survival rate is less than 5 months.

11.1.3.2 Therapeutic Possibilities

By this concept we mean human as well as material resources which may modify a prognosis. Exocrine pancreatic cancer is a complex digestive pathology requiring sophisticated methods and very well trained and motivated teams. Some results reported by Gilsdorf and Spanos hold great promise for the operative prognosis at the Veterans Hospitals of Minneapolis. Three skillful surgeons performed 16 pancreatectomies with no subsequent mortality or postoperative complications. At the same time, 72 resections were performed by other surgeons on the staff, with 22% complications and 28% postoperative mortality [10].

Diagnostic and therapeutic difficulties, the present poor results, and the need for randomized prospective studies on a large number of patients demonstrate the necessity of specialized centers; numerous investigators before us have emphasized the positive effect of such centers on the prognosis [7, 12, 14, 15].

11.2 Quality of Survival

Given the therapeutic strategies used for pancreatic cancer and their poor results (1% cure over 5 years, median survival less than 6 months), we will consider the aspect of survival rather than of cure, and for only a limited number of patients.

Survival, whatever its duration, is generally disappointing, either short (a few months) resulting from palliative treatment and from the growth of the tumor process, or longer owing to surgery, extensive resections performed with a curative intent. Actually, the parameters of survival quality are numerous and must be studied in relation to the therapy chosen by the referring surgeon.

11.2.1 After Resection

Cephalic pancreatoduodenectomy, or Whipple's resection, is functionally well tolerated by the patient. In contrast, total or subtotal pancreatectomies cause digestive disorders such as steatorrhea or dietary deficiency syndrome, which must be compensated for by the administration of pancreatic extracts. Weight loss frequently occurs in such cases. The onset of postoperative diabetes (after total or subtotal pancreatectomies) creates an insulin dependence damaging to the quality of the patient's survival. When chemotherapy is an adjuvant treatment to surgical resection, it also diminishes the quality of the survival. This aspect is prominent in descriptions of survival. And finally, long-term survival requires numerous follow-up medical examinations.

11.2.2 After Palliative Treatment

Patients who cannot undergo pancreatic resection generally receive palliative treatment. Their survival is relatively short and is disturbed by the symptoms associated with the evolution of the disease and by the adjuvant therapies such as radiation or chemotherapy. Before proceeding to such therapies, it is necessary to determine both the advantages and the disadvantages. Only in the case of jaundiced patients does a palliative bypass or drainage improve the quality of their survival by overcoming their jaundice. We have already seen that one can also relieve pain.

11.2.3 Inoperable Patients

Patients who have not been operated can only hope for a very short survival. It is always of very poor quality because of the prominence of debilitating symptoms (pain, jaundice, digestive disorders) as well as the effects of the drugs administered in such cases.

With few exceptions, patients harboring a cancer of the pancreas do not face the problem of rehabilitation into daily life. They cannot go back to their jobs and the only possible reinsertion is familial, owing to the poor conditions imposed by the survival. In order to accurately estimate the quality of the survival with pancreatic cancer, we refer to the classification reported by the World Health Organization; (1) normal activity with no symptom; (2) nearly normal activity, symptom-related; (3) decubitus for less than 50% of the day; (4) decubitus for more than 50% of the day; (5) no possibility of standing up.

11.3 Follow-up

For the pancreatic cancers no follow-up protocol exists, such as one for cancer of the colon. The seriousness of the former, its quasi-incurable recurrences or metachronous metastases and the reduced number of curative resections easily explain the present pattern in the field of follow-up - empirical control by the referring surgeon.

Recurrences are regional - in the pancreatic space itself, in its surroundings, or in the residual pancreas in case of a partial pancreatectomy. Metastases first invade the liver and the lungs. Three of 81 patients whom we followed up died from secondary brain localizations.

Clinical, biological, and morphological examinations play a role in follow-up. A clinical follow-up looks for functional or systemic symptoms such as pains, recent onset of digestive disorders, jaundice, neurological deficiency, anorexia, and weight loss. One must also look for hepatomegalia, epigastric palpable mass, suspicious adenopathies (Troisier), and ascites. A biological follow-up, in addition to a check of the sedimentation rate, includes tumor marker assays, for an elevation after pancreatectomy would reveal a recurrence of the disease. This has been suggested by Shintoku et al. in a study on the variations of CA-19-9 and POA in 14 patients with pancreatectomies [18]. Glycemia must also be surveyed, as changes in the regulation of diabetes can indicate a recurrence of the disease. A morphological follow-up takes into account the upper abdomen. A CT scan of the liver and pancreatic area appears to give the best evaluation. As for the lungs, an X-ray film is sufficient. Faced with a neurological deficiency or simple disorientation, a CT scan of the brain is required.

These controls must be very frequent during the first 3 years, when recurrence is most likely; one examination every 4 months is congruent with the costs, the demands on the patient and the screening for recurrences or metastases at an early stage. After this, they can be done twice a year.

Treatment of metastases or recurrences is related to their onset, diffuse or localized. When diffuse, it is better to avoid radiation therapy and chemotherapy. But when localized, there does not exist any hope for cure, but a palliative effect can be awaited with treatments being in process.

References

1. Baker JP, Detsky AS, Wesson DE (1982) Nutritional assessment, a comparison of clinical judgment and objective measurements. N Engl J Med 306: 969–972
2. Barkin JS, Kalser MH, Redlhammer D, Heal A (1978) Initial levels of CEA and their rate of change in pancreatic carcinoma following surgery, chemotherapy and radiation therapy. Cancer 42: 1472–1476
3. Belghiti J (1983) Que doit-on attendre des indices nutritionnels prédictifs du risque opératoire en chirurgie digestive? Gastroenterol Clin Biol 7: 841–842
4. Buzby GP, Mullen JL, Mattens DC (1980) Prognostic nutritional index in gastrointestinal surgery. Am J Surg 139: 160–167

5. Cubilla AL, Fitzgerald PH, Fortner JG (1978) Pancreas cancer. Duct cell adenocarcinoma: survival in relation to site, size, stage and type of therapy. J Surg Oncol 10: 465-482
6. Di Constanzo J, Martin J, Cano N, et al (1983) Indice nutritionnel pronostique et chirurgie digestive. Gastroenterol Clin Biol 7: 851-856
7. Edis AJ, Kiernan PD, Taylor WF (1980) Attempted curative resection of ductal carcinoma of the pancreas. Mayo Clin Proc 55: 531-536
8. Faivre J, Milan C, Hilton P, Klepping C, et al (1982) Les cancers digestifs dans le département de la Côte d'Or. Incidence, traitement, survie. Presses Universitaires, Dijon
9. Ford GT, Whitelaw WA, Roselal TW, Cruse PJ, Guenter CA (1983) Diaphragm function after upper abdominal surgery in humans. Am Rev Respir Dis 127: 431-436
10. Gilsdorf RB, Spanos P (1973) Factors influencing morbidity and mortality in pancreatoduodenectomy. Ann Surg 177 (3): 332-337
11. Goldmann L, Caldera DL, Nusbaum SR, et al (1977) Multifactorial index of cardiac risk in noncardiac surgical procedures. N Engl J Med 297: 845-850
12. Hastings PR, Beazley RM, Cohn I (1982) Progress with pancreatic cancer. Prog Clin Cancer 8: 319-332
13. Hodgkinson DJ, Remine WH, Weiland LH (1978) A clinico-pathologic study of 21 cases of pancreatic cystadenocarcinoma. Ann Surg 188: 679-684
14. Malt RA (1983) Treatment of pancreatic cancer. JAMA 250 (11): 1433-1437
15. Moossa AR, Lewis MH, Mackie CR (1979) Surgical treatment of pancreatic cancer. Mayo Clin Proc 54: 468-474
16. Mullen JL, Buzby GP, Mattews DC, Smale BF, Rosato EF (1980) Reduction of operative morbidity by combined pre-operative and post-operative nutritional support. Ann Surg 192: 604-613
17. Mullen JL (1981) Consequences of malnutrition in surgical patients. Surg Clin North Am 61: 465-487
18. Shintoku J, Takami S, Uematsu T, et al (1985) Evaluation of carbohydrate antigen 19-9 (CA-19-9) and pancreatic oncofetal antigen (POA) in follow-up of pancreatic cancer patients. In: American Society of Clinical Oncology Proceedings, vol 4, C 36
19. Trede M (1985) The surgical treatment of pancreatic carcinoma. Surgery 97 (1): 28-35

12 Conclusion

H. Baumel and B. Deixonne

Cancer of the pancreas has not yet given up all of its secrets. Far from it! A great deal remains to be done to improve our knowledge of its epidemiology, diagnosis, and treatment.

It is a peculiar cancer, requiring a unique approach which justifies a large investment of time and effort. This has been done in the United States (Pancreatic Cancer Task Force, National Pancreatic Cancer Project) and in Japan (Japan Pancreas Society), where research into a cancer screening program has been started. This impetus should be taken up worldwide.

Modern diagnostic and treatment techniques have progressed so much that we can be disappointed not to have more rapidly improving results. However, even if the slight gain in the length of survival during the past 10 years is not spectacular, it is a factor of hope for three reasons:

1. Our methods today are very effective and should modify, little by little, the proportion of operations performed using the therapeutic options, either curative or palliative, that have been employed up until now.
2. Our knowledge of the natural history of pancreatic cancer has also increased. This is particularly true in the case of intraglandular localizations (multifocal tumors) and extraglandular invasion, especially lymphatic.
3. All this favors the more aggressive and radical surgery now being done by many surgeons, an attitude even more justified in the case of small tumors and young patients.

It appears that the three periods of Porter and the fourth of Longmire (see Preface) will soon be succeeded by a fifth, one of improvement in therapeutic results.

We must therefore pursue our efforts to establish earlier diagnoses and to compile more homogeneous patient groups with respect to staging, so that they may undergo controlled therapeutic trials. Different teams around the world are now undertaking this work but their results will not be available for several years.

It would be of tremendous interest if international and national research groups could be formed and if a large number of cases could be used for a prospective study. Only specialized centers which understand the problems posed by this cancer should undertake such a task.

Many authors have written about this subject before us, and we concur with the following advice: all surgeons who intervene in a case of obstructive jaundice originating in the pancreas must be able to histologically confirm this diagnosis during the operation and to perform an extensive and precise workup of the lesion. The surgeon's experience and time, and the environment at hand may make a regional total resection possible. If these conditions are not fulfilled the surgeon must refuse to operate on the patient. If he does operate, having done a locoregional workup as completely as possible, he should be content to perform the vital bypasses and then refer his patient to a specialized center. As severe as this point of view appears, it is justified by the extreme difficulty and the poor overall results in the treatment of this cancer.

We hope, therefore, that the progress achieved for other forms of cancer after similar work will also follow from the efforts being made now regarding cancer of the pancreas, which remains today as it was in the past, the most serious of all the digestive cancers.

Note in proof: Since the time we wrote this work, an issue of the World Journal of Surgery (Vol. 8, Nr. 6, 1984) particularly dedicated to "The Cancer of the Pancreas" came to our knowledge as well as an important work from Andreani T et al. on "Non Surgical Palliative Treatments of Neoplastic Jaundices" in Gastroentérologie Clinique et Biologique (Vol. 10, Nr. 4, 1986) and from Chigot JP, Spay G, Bory M, de Calan L on "Le Cancer du Pancréas" in Actualités Chirurgicales 1, Chirurgie Générale et Digestive, Masson Ed., Paris 1986.

13 Subject Index